Kazmeister

Dyslexia
A Neuroscientific Approach
to Clinical Evaluation

Dyslexia
A Neuroscientific Approach to Clinical Evaluation

Edited by
Frank H. Duffy, M.D.
Associate Professor of Neurology, Harvard Medical School; Director of Developmental Neurophysiology, The Children's Hospital, Boston

Norman Geschwind, M.D.
Late James Jackson Putnam Professor of Neurology, Harvard Medical School; Professor of Psychology and Health Sciences and Technology, Massachusetts Institute of Technology; Director, Neurological Unit, Beth Israel Hospital, Boston

Little, Brown and Company
Boston/Toronto

Copyright © 1985 by Little, Brown and Company (Inc.)

First Edition

All rights reserved. No part of this book may be reproduced in any form or by any electronic or mechanical means, including information storage and retrieval systems, without permission in writing from the publisher, except by a reviewer who may quote brief passages in a review.

Library of Congress Catalog Card No. 85-50041

ISBN 0-316-19454-9

Printed in the United States of America

HAL

The cover image, a BEAM statistical probability map, illustrates the region activated by reading in a 10-year-old learning disabled boy with a left hemisphere cystic lesion. The image shows change (reduction) in alpha while reading as compared to resting. Note the unusual reversed hemispheric activation.

Dedication

During the course of 1984, two of our primary authors passed away unexpectedly. In May, Dr. Rita G. Rudel died of cancer and in November, Dr. Norman Geschwind, the co-editor of this volume, died suddenly at his home in Brookline, Massachusetts. This volume is dedicated to these two exceptional people. The following are offered as memoria to them:

The loss of Norman Geschwind has been very deeply felt within the international scientific community. At the funeral ceremony Jerome Lettvin of MIT eloquently expressed our shared view of Dr. Geschwind as an intellectual leader in the common search to understand the human brain. It was my privilege to know Dr. Geschwind throughout my medical career as a student, resident, colleague, collaborator, and always mentor. At each stage his lectures and discussions were critical stimulants to my own thought. For me, Norman Geschwind was always there and he shall always be.

Frank H. Duffy, M.D.

Rita Rudel was a leader in the nascent field of developmental neuropsychology, bringing to its complex issues her classical training by two great pioneers, Kurt Goldstein and Hans-Lukas Teuber. To this background Rita added her own special creativity in experimental design, her incisive analytic reasoning, and her deep feeling for people. To her colleagues and students, she will always represent the model of the clinical investigator, both scientist and artist. And her loss will be deeply felt by everyone who knew her.

Martha B. Denckla, M.D.

Contents

Preface ix
Contributing Authors xi

1. Dyslexia in Neurological Perspective 1
   Norman Geschwind

2. Written Language Underachievement: An Overview of the Theoretical and Practical Issues 3
   Drake Duane

3. The Definition of Dyslexia: Language and Motor Deficits 33
   Rita G. Rudel

4. On Some Relationships Between Acquired and Developmental Dyslexias 55
   John C. Marshall

5. Patterns of Infant Behavior: Analogues of Later Organizational Difficulties? 67
   Heidelise Als

6. Should So-Called Modality Preferences Determine the Nature of Instruction for Children with Reading Disabilities? 93
   Isabelle Y. Liberman

7. Brain Electrical Activity Mapping (BEAM): The Search for a Physiological Signature of Dyslexia 105
   Frank H. Duffy and Gloria B. McAnulty

8. Sound-Film Microanalysis: A Means for Correlating Brain and Behavior 123
   William S. Condon

9. Neurometric Evaluation of Brain Electrical Activity in Children with Learning Disabilities 157
   E. Roy John, Leslie Prichep, Jacob Fridman, Hansook Ahn, Herbert Kaye, and Henry Baird

10. Motor Coordination in Dyslexic Children: Theoretical and Clinical Implications 187
    Martha Bridge Denckla

11. Biological Foundations of Reading 197
    Norman Geschwind

Index 213

Preface

In the last decade, there has been considerable advancement in the understanding of the learning disabilities in general, particularly of the reading/language disorder dyslexia. There has not been a general consensus, however, among the medical, psychological, and educational professionals in the field on numerous dyslexia-related issues, ranging from the primary issue of defining the term *dyslexia* to the delineation of appropriate remedial methods. The only point of agreement is that there is a continuing need for research and dissemination of research findings and theoretical constructs in this area.

The relevance of this topic is unquestionable. Community surveys conservatively estimate that dyslexia affects 3 to 6 percent of school-age children. Between 800 and 1,000 children are referred each year to The Children's Hospital in Boston alone for school achievement and learning difficulties. Some 50 percent of these children prove to have specific reading disability. An informal survey indicates that 20 to 30 percent of the children seen by pediatric neurologists at this institution present with the chief complaint of learning, attention, or other school-related problems.

The intent of this book is to present a discussion of recent developments and to suggest future directions of dyslexia research based on the differing viewpoints and findings of an interdisciplinary group of researchers, educators, and medical professionals involved in this area. As a context for other professionals and the lay reader, the initial chapters provide a historical review and some current views on the definition of what is, and what is not, dyslexia. Subsequent chapters are directed to questions of early prediction, diagnostic methods, and theoretical considerations. More detailed discussions of the conceptual framework of the book are provided in the first two chapters.

In May 1981, the Institute for Child Development Research (ICDR) sponsored a symposium on dyslexia in Philadelphia. The symposium was designed as a forum to allow the easy communication of ideas by a diverse group of professionals who are approaching the same problem from varied perspectives. The various presentations at that symposium constitute the germinal sources of the chapters in this volume. In addition to acknowledging an indebtedness to our colleagues who were the contributors to the symposium and this book, we wish to strongly express our gratitude to Mr. and Mrs. Peter Pattison, the founders and directors of ICDR, whose unstinting commitment to the amelioration of childhood neurological diseases has been the basis for their generous efforts in disseminating knowledge in this area. We further wish to acknowledge the many people who served as research subjects, giving of their time to further our endeavors. It is through the selfless giving of these many individuals as professionals, as patients, and as concerned parents that this book is possible. We also wish to acknowledge the organizational and editorial efforts of David McAnulty in bringing the manuscript together.

F. H. D.
N. G.

Contributing Authors

Hansook Ahn, Ph.D.
Professor of Liberal Arts and Sciences, Ajou University, Suweon, Korea; Research Associate Professor of Psychiatry, Brain Research Laboratories, New York University Medical Center, New York, New York

Heidelise Als, Ph.D.
Assistant Professor of Pediatrics (Psychology), Harvard Medical School; Associate in Psychiatry and Director of Neurobehavioral Infant and Child Studies, The Children's Hospital, Boston, Massachusetts

Henry Baird, M.D.
Professor of Pediatrics, Temple University School of Medicine; Attending Physician (Neurology), St. Christopher's Hospital for Children, Philadelphia, Pennsylvania

William S. Condon, Ph.D.
Associate Professor of Psychiatry, Boston University Medical School; Consultant, Schizophrenia Research, Solomon Carter Fuller Community Mental Health Center, Boston, Massachusetts

Martha Bridge Denckla, M.D.
Chief, Section on Autism and Related Disorders, National Institute of Neurological and Communicative Disorders and Stroke; Clinical Associate Professor of Neurology (part-time), Johns Hopkins University School of Medicine; Clinical Associate Professor of Neurology, Uniformed Services of the Medical Sciences, Bethesda, Maryland

Drake D. Duane, M.D.
Associate Professor of Neurology, Mayo Medical School; Consultant in Neurology, Mayo Clinic and Mayo Foundation, Rochester, Minnesota

Frank H. Duffy, M.D.
Associate Professor of Neurology, Harvard Medical School; Director of Developmental Neurophysiology, The Children's Hospital, Boston, Massachusetts

Jacob Fridman, Ph.D.
Vice President/Engineering, Neurometrics, Inc., New York, New York

†Norman Geschwind, M.D.
James Jackson Putnam Professor of Neurology, Harvard Medical School; Professor of Psychology and Health Sciences and Technology, Massachusetts Institute of Technology; Director, Neurological Unit, Beth Israel Hospital, Boston, Massachusetts

E. Roy John, Ph.D.
Professor of Psychiatry, Brain Research Laboratories, New York University Medical Center, New York, New York

Herbert Kaye, Ph.D.
Associate Professor of Psychology, State University of New York, Stony Brook, Stony Brook, New York

Isabelle Y. Liberman, Ph.D.
*Professor, Department of Educational Psychology, University of Connecticut, Storrs;
Research Associate, Haskins Laboratories, New Haven, Connecticut*

John C. Marshall, Ph.D.
*External Scientific Staff of the Medical Research Council, Neuropsychology Unit,
University Department of Clinical Neurology, The Radcliffe Infirmary, Oxford, England*

Gloria B. McAnulty, Ph.D.
*Research Associate in Neurology, Harvard Medical School and The Children's Hospital,
Boston, Massachusetts*

Leslie S. Prichep, Ph.D.
*Associate Professor of Psychiatry, Brain Research Laboratories, New York University
Medical Center, New York, New York*

†Rita G. Rudel, Ph.D.
*Clinical Professor of Medical Psychology, Columbia College of Physicians and Surgeons;
Head of Neuropsychology, Department of Psychiatry, Columbia Presbyterian Medical
Center, New York, New York*

†Deceased

1 Dyslexia in Neurological Perspective
Norman Geschwind

The history of the concept of dyslexia has been curious, its very existence having been repeatedly questioned not only in the past, but even today. Throughout the history of medicine and the sciences of behavior, arguments as to the existence of particular syndromes have been common, and the pendulum has often swung repeatedly until some consensus was reached. Dyslexia has, however, been subjected to more vicissitudes than many other conditions that have aroused controversy. The reasons are not difficult to specify, as we shall see.

Firstly, as a behavioral syndrome, dyslexia has been the victim of upheavals in attitudes about behavior. Thus, in the 1920s and 1930s, there was a widespread tendency to reject neurologically based explanations of behavior and a tendency to stress purely environmental explanations. Since each individual's behavior was thought to be uniquely determined by his own experience, the attempt to designate syndromes was looked on with disfavor.

It was also widely assumed that accepting neurological causation would imply adopting a stance of therapeutic nihilism. Yet a review of the history of dyslexia in the United States should have made clear that belief in neurological causation implied neither therapeutic negativism nor a lack of interest in the individual. The investigator who put dyslexia on the map, so to speak, in the United States was Samuel Torrey Orton, a neurologist and neuropathologist, who recognized a distinctive syndrome that closely resembled the classical condition of acquired alexia with agraphia. Orton immediately mobilized his energies to develop all aspects of work on dyslexia, that is, clinical description, diagnostic methods, educational remediation, and neurological research.

In retrospect, it is perhaps the oddest part of the story that Orton succeeded with some professional groups while failing with others in his attempts to have this common and disabling disorder recognized and treated. His greatest impact was undoubtedly on the educational profession. While not everyone recognized the importance of his work, at least a devoted handful of individuals saw the importance of his findings and began to develop the methods of remediation so well known today. Where he succeeded least was with his own colleagues in medicine and indeed in his own areas of specialization—neurology, psychiatry, and neuropathology. One might have expected an enthusiastic response in the medical world for Orton's remarkable demonstration that millions of people were suffering from a neurologically based disorder, a disorder that had previously been known to only a few, who had thought it extremely rare, while it was totally unknown to the great majority.

The educators, or at least a sufficiently large group of them, faced the reality of what Orton had demonstrated, that is, the existence of enormous numbers of otherwise bright children who had excessive difficulty in acquiring the language skills that most children, even the dull ones, acquired with only a reasonable expenditure of effort. It was, one must recognize in retrospect, the educators and the parents, faced with daily contact with this mystifying and frustrating condition, who refused to ignore the problem. The widespread neglect of this disorder was reinforced by a common belief at that period that the so-called general factor in intelligence ensured that bright children would be good at everything. The obvious counterexamples such as the existence of individuals with remarkable and sometimes isolated talents in music, art, mathematics, and athletics somehow did not lead to the realization that no simple division into the bright and the dull could explain the array of disabilities and talents to be found in the population.

This book and the conference that was its source document the fact that this long period of relative neglect of dyslexia outside the educational world has begun to end and that neurological clinicians and laboratory investigators, pediatricians, psychologists, and linguists have come to be aware of both the practical and theoretical importance of dyslexia.

The clues had indeed been available from the very start. Orton in his very first paper made enough remarkable observations to stimulate research in a wide variety of disciplines. Dyslexics were predominantly male and were most likely to be left-handed and have left-handedness in the family. They were more likely to stutter. Although not present in every dyslexic, the tendency of some to reverse letters was a mark of some remarkable phenomena in the brain. Indeed, Orton called attention in that first paper to the fact that some dyslexics read better when the text was reversed by a mirror, a phenomenon that remained an oddity, occasionally revived and often denied, and which has only very recently begun to receive proper attention. The fact that reversals, when present, tended to occur only in verbal material refuted any simple "visual" interpretation as accounting for all dyslexia, but this finding did not receive the attention it deserved. The existence of many dyslexics with well-developed talents in mechanical and spatial activities had long ago impressed itself on many therapists, but the profound implications of this fact did not attract the attention of those in other disciplines until much later. The fact that dyslexics commonly had problems with other aspects of language, such as delayed speech development and a special difficulty with foreign languages, suggested that many of the clues to their problems might be deciphered by those with competence in linguistics. Every one of these areas has now come to be recognized as deserving of study. But major mysteries remain. How are we to account for those who recover spontaneously? And how are we to explain the mechanism by which certain forms of remediation are successful in so many cases? Perhaps more important, how are we to explain those who fail to improve even in the best of hands?

Some may argue that concern for mechanism must be secondary to concern for treatment. It is, however, an error to attempt to create such an opposition. Unless treatment is perfect, which it is not, knowledge of mechanism is likely to advance diagnosis, prevention, and therapy. Furthermore, as long as we do not understand clearly what leads to success and what leads to failure, we leave many dyslexics and their families prey to the popular fads that inevitably arise when adequately founded scientific knowledge is not available.

We hope that the following chapters will provide useful indications of some of the directions in which research is presently moving in this field, a field that is now beginning to assume its rightful place in the world of science.

2 Written Language Underachievement: An Overview of the Theoretical and Practical Issues

Drake D. Duane

A contemporary challenge to those in the sciences is the translation of theoretical constructs and research data into their practical implications. This is particularly true for a pragmatic American society, which expects a palpable product of its investigators. As a clinical neurologist, sensitive both to the neurosciences and to the needs of educationally handicapped patients, I will attempt to perform that explanatory function regarding written language underachievement and dyslexia.

Physicians and Dyslexia

In the later nineteenth and early twentieth centuries, the initial descriptions of children who encountered unusual difficulty in learning to read came from the field of medicine [7, 17, 51, 57, 70, 96]. From these physicians' perspective came the view that the observed behavior might be comparable to that noted in adults who had lost the ability to read as a result of focal brain lesions. These observations were the earliest basis of the postulation of a neurological basis for reading underachievement in children. The initial term chosen was that of *congenital word blindness,* suggesting that the condition was present from birth.

Between the mid-1920s and late 1940s, the neuropsychiatrist and neuropathologist Samuel T. Orton evaluated some 3,000 children and adults with reading, writing, and speech problems [75]. Orton rejected the previous hypothesis by Hinshelwood [51] of a causal unilateral cerebral lesion. He was struck by the laterospatial errors in writing that were observed in his patient population, and he coined the term *strephosymbolia.* However, inspection of his records and book suggests that he quite commonly used the terms *specific reading disability* and *specific writing disability.* Orton was apparently the first to suggest that the genesis of the observed underachievement was faulty language lateralization. In part, this perception was related to his clinical observation of an apparently high frequency of mixed eye, hand, and foot preference and also relative ambidexterity in his patients. Although others have subsequently questioned the importance of mixed eye, hand, and foot preference as representing a significant associated feature or causal factor in reading disability [6, 84], the frequency of occurrence of such cross laterality in my own clinical patients and those observed by Denckla (see Chap. 10) appears to be higher than that encountered in the general population. Furthermore, in contrast to those negative studies [6, 84], many others have found elevated rates of non-right-handedness among dyslexics. Although not predictive of reading failure, it may be one of the corollaries of that condition and may constitute a relative risk factor. Additionally, Orton emphasized the language learning handicap of dyslexia. Further, despite his speculations on potential variation among individuals in cerebral organization for language, he suggested that the disability was potentially treatable through special educational techniques.

The British neurologist Macdonald Critchley [15, 16] focused on the term *developmental dyslexia*. He took the position that the condition represented a specific and "pure" neurological syndrome innate to the neurobiology of the affected individual. His speculations as to the nature of the disorder were relatively consonant with those of Orton.

This line of reasoning emanating from the medical profession, focusing as it did on reading but recognizing a variety of so-called epiphenomena (e.g., right-left disorientation, relative clumsiness), eventuated in the definition of a condition referred to as specific developmental dyslexia by the World Federation of Neurology. The condition was defined as follows: "A disorder manifested by difficulty in learning to read despite conventional instruction, adequate intelligence, and socio-cultural opportunity. It is dependent upon fundamental cognitive disabilities which are frequently of constitutional origin" [16].

Perhaps because of its origins in medicine and the physicians' perception that dyslexia represented a disease state, the concept of specific developmental dyslexia has often not been accepted by those in education. Indeed, the notion that innate biological variation might intrude on the usual development of scholastic aptitude has been actively or passively rejected by the majority of workers in the teaching profession.

Even in the medical profession, the exclusionary and unquantified language of the World Federation of Neurology definition was criticized [37, 82, 83, 86]. The thoughtful extension of this criticism was the epidemiological study on the Isle of Wight by Rutter and associates [85]. This British study attempted to clarify whether there did indeed exist a higher number of underachieving readers than would be predicted by statistical means. For this purpose, a longitudinal study was carried out, employing a regression equation in which achievement was predicted on the basis of observed correlations among educational attainment, age, and IQ in the general population. Individual rather than group tests were employed, and comparisons were made between age-matched groups. The investigators were able to define, in terms of underachievement of at least 2 standard deviations below prediction, that a group of intelligent students experiencing underachievement in reading did exist. The occurrence level on the Isle of Wight among 10-year-olds was 4 percent. Such students were designated as possessing *specific reading retardation* and were contrasted with students who underattained in reading but who demonstrated general low intellectual capacity. The latter group was referred to as "backward readers" [84, 85, 87, 108, 109].

With the statistical criterion of 26 months or more of retardation on standardized reading tests, the characteristics of the specific reading retardation group included a higher ratio of boys than girls (3.5:1), no evidence of overt neurological disorder, often a history of delay in speech, often a family history of reading disability, a universally concomitant underachievement in spelling ability, and importantly, with regard to natural history, less progress in reading over time with the result that the frequency increased in older children.

Although a prominent socioeconomic factor could not be found operating on the Isle of Wight, a comparable study in inner London suggested a 10-percent incidence among 10-year-olds, this contrasting with the 4-percent rate among 10-year-olds on the Isle of Wight. This higher incidence in a metropolitan area [9] suggested that geographical and social factors affect the frequency of reading retardation. These data reinforce the earlier observations of Eisenberg [36] that the incidence of reading underachievement was much higher within a given United States metropolitan area when contrasted with that city's surrounding suburbs.

The Isle of Wight studies, although avoiding the use of the term *dyslexia*, reaffirmed many of the characteristics that had been attributed to that condition. Surprisingly, despite the fact that these more dispassionate studies have verified the existence of a population of intelligent students who were selectively underachieving in at least two aspects of written language (reading and spelling), they appear to have made a negligible impact on educational attitudes, policies, and practices.

Brain Damage and Special Education

In contrast to the negativism expressed toward the medically generated terms of *dyslexia* and *specific reading retardation*, the field of education was more receptive to research by workers from education and psychology. During the period from the late 1930s through the 1960s, Strauss and others [91, 92, 93, 94] studied the characteristics of children thought to be suffering from an unequivocal central nervous system insult. Their observations on the "brain injured" suggested variability in the degree of backwardness in one scholastic aptitude as opposed to another. In addition, within this population, many children had social-behavioral aberrations, apparent difficulty in attending to specific tasks, obvious motor incoordination, and presumptive perceptual deficits. Whether the greater acceptance by educationalists of the notion of this brain-damaged population of students was engendered by the fact that there was something visibly different about these students, as had been the case with the physically handicapped who were previously allocated special educational services, or because the hypothesis was generated by those closer to the field of education is not clear. Also, potentially appealing to those charged with serving students in the classroom was the direct educational interventional measures that were proposed to address the needs of these brain-injured students.

However, just as the danger of overgeneralization was a reasonable criticism of the term *developmental dyslexia*, there evolved the erroneous concept that the diverse behaviors of the brain-injured and slow learners were phenomena of a similar mechanism. By extrapolation, the group was then considered somewhat uniform. This resulted in recommendations of certain educational strategies, such as those subsumed under the term *perceptual motor training*, that were thought to compensate for or remediate many or all of the backward behaviors, including that of reading retardation.

This concept led to the undocumented assumption that many students with reading disabilities had sustained some putative central nervous system insult that was causal to their symptoms. The corollary was that if perceptual motor techniques were of assistance to those poor-reading students who demonstrated clinical motor incoordination, such techniques could be applied in the presence or absence of incoordination alike with the equal expectation of improving reading skills. However, an increasing body of knowledge now suggests that many persons with selective reading disability appear to possess a linguistic rather than a perceptual deficit [62, 63, 68, 71, 100]. As a consequence, language-pertinent remediation rather than perceptual-motor–pertinent remediation appears more rational and effective in most instances [56, 61, 68]. I am aware of no evidence suggesting the contrary concept that therapy directed specifically to deficits in written language has any effect on gross motor impairment.

Minimal Brain Dysfunction

Questions have been raised about perinatal and other acquired physical factors that might result in the selective underachievement in reading [55]. However, it became apparent that a distinction could not readily be made between putative innate biological predisposition, perhaps under genetic influence, as had been suggested by the term *specific developmental dyslexia,* and those instances of academic underachievement in which a potentially encephalopathic event had occurred. For this latter group, the term *minimal brain damage* (MBD) had been applied.

In an attempt to resolve this difficulty, Clements [12] emphasized dysfunction rather than damage, while preserving the term *MBD*. Dencka [20, 21] has nicely reviewed the evolution of the concept, pointing out that Clements and Peters [13] had been careful to use the plural in referring to minimal brain dysfunction*s* and that they were primarily attempting to preserve the implication of a brain-behavior relationship.

Although I commend Dencka's appropriate usage of the term *minimal brain dysfunction,* my personal concern is that the term has, in general, been misused by our colleagues in the medical profession. Rather than as had been intended, it is often employed as a solitary diagnostic entity without the appropriate refinement as to which of the minimal brain dysfunctions the diagnostician finds in evidence. Unfortunately, the term has, until recently, been employed as almost synonymous with the hyperkinetic syndrome, particularly by those in psychiatry. When used by neurologists, it has often had the connotation of the earlier damage hypothesis. Whether justifiable or not, the damage postulate has carried a negative prognostic connotation to those in education, to the parents of the affected children, and to the identified patient. Indeed there is a need to clarify with greater precision whether an encephalopathic event is in itself causal or is additive to other potential risk factors in the production of underachievement in written language. Furthermore, the issue of whether such insult to the nervous system truly carries any differential prognosis requires further clarification.

Specific Learning Disability

Despite the fact that there was disagreement concerning terminology among the various disciplines of student assessment, parents of students who were educational underachievers were being advised that, for whatever reason, their underachieving child had the potential for higher achievement. Furthermore, it was suggested that the means of reaching educational potential was through modification of educational procedures. It was in the context of the civil rights movement in this country in the 1960s that consumer advocates, agitating for the rights of a variety of minority groups, including the handicapped, moved Congress to recognize the existence of underachieving students. The question was, which term would be used to designate the educationally handicapped and who would serve those designated?

The term selected was one, it was hoped, that would not be tainted by the controversy surrounding each of the previous terms discussed, but would be new, neutral, and educationally pertinent. That term was *specific learning disability*. As to the question of who would provide the services, it would be those who were serving other handicapped students in the field of special education. By federal law in 1969, special educational services could be provided for no more than 12 percent of the public school enrollment, and no more than one-sixth of that group—that is, 2 percent of the school-age population—could be considered learning disabled. This percentage contrasts with the 4 percent incidence of specific reading retardation on the Isle of Wight.

Initially associated with the amendments of the Elementary and Secondary Education Act of 1969, Title VI, the Education of the Handicapped Act of 1970, Public Law 91-230, and then with the more recently enacted Public Law 94-142, *learning disability* was defined as "a disorder in one or more of the basic psychological processes involved in understanding or using spoken or written language." This implied that the emphasis was on language skill. The congressional enactment defined the manifestations as "disorders of listening, thinking, speaking, reading, writing, spelling or arithmetic." Subsequent revision has deleted the word *thinking*, and spelling became subsumed under "written expression." Manifestations of reading disability were in the area of decoding or comprehension. Deficit in arithmetic skills could be either in computational skills or arithmetic reasoning. In contrast to the other manifestations that bear a relationship to language function, it is not apparent that the dyscalculic student has a language disorder or that language remediation has any pertinence to improvement in deficits in calculation or mathematical reasoning. Furthermore, if the analogy to adult-acquired disorders is appropriate to the developmental disorders, the brain mechanisms related to dyscalculia are likely to be different from those associated with reading disability. Although dyscalculia may be seen in isolation in children, a confounding observation is that underachievement in arithmetic ability may coexist with one or more of the language-related disabilities.

The law, for purposes of encompassment, indicated that specific learning disability had previously been referred to as "perceptual handicap, minimal brain dysfunction, dyslexia, and developmental aphasia." Finally, a so-called exclusionary clause was provided, indicating that a specific learning disability is "not a learning problem due primarily to visual, hearing or motor handicap, mental retardation, emotional disturbance or environmental disadvantage."

This last clause is subject to the same criticisms as the World Federation of Neurology definition of specific developmental dyslexia. Potentially, it could mean that environmental factors or coexistent health problems could exclude a student from receiving appropriate special educational services. A practical problem then confronted the educational establishment: who was to become the learning disability specialist when none had existed previously? Ultimately, three kinds of "specialists" were brought into the programs: (1) those previously in general education, most commonly from programs referred to as remedial reading (in which the pace rather than the strategy of teaching had been emphasized); (2) those from other preexisting special educational programs working with other types of handicapped students; and (3) new instructors at institutions of higher education to be trained for the new field of learning disabilities. The result was that the services provided to these newly defined students came from educators of diverse ages, experience, backgrounds, and training. Consequently, a nonuniform mode of remedial services came into existence.

In spite of the fact that the term *specific learning disability* was generated by educationalists, considerable resistance remains even to this day in accepting the existence of this population, whether designated as learning disabled or any of the other antecedent terms used in an attempt to describe underachieving students [25, 59]. (For a brief review of the history of terminology, see Duane [31].)

Because of these attitudes, the concern expressed by Hinshelwood [50] remains a pragmatic challenge to those in current practice. He stated, "It is a matter of the highest importance to recognise the cause and the true nature of this difficulty in learning to read which is experienced by these children, otherwise they may be harshly treated as imbeciles or incorrigibles and either neglected or flogged for a defect for which they are in no wise responsible."

Because of these concerns regarding terminology and resistance to much of the theoretical conceptualization that is considered pertinent by investigators, workers in the research areas must choose their terminology carefully and translate the implications of their efforts in terms that are persuasive to those in the educational field. On the other hand, the appropriately strong emotions felt by parents and individuals affected by selective academic underachievement should caution investigators against arriving at premature conclusions or drawing inferences broader than the data would reasonably permit. For those in clinical practice who are engaged in the assessment of these students, care with regard to precision of diagnosis must be exercised. Up-to-date information should be maintained as it evolves in the field. Clinician and researcher alike should note that if the figure of 5 percent of selective underachievers in written language within a school-age population is accurate, that rate exceeds the combined occurrence of the seizure disorders, cerebral palsy, and mental retardation. Such an incidence rate constitutes an important public health problem for which both clinical services and research funding are warranted.

National Joint Committee on Learning Disabilities

One positive outcome of the deliberations pertaining to the regulations for provision of services to the learning-disabled population was the bringing together of six organizations representing the consumers and clinical professionals in the field of learning disability. In 1975, a National Joint Committee on Learning Disabilities was formed, made up of three representatives from each of the following organizations: Association for Children and Adults With Learning Disabilities; American Speech, Language, and Hearing Association; Division of Children With Communication Disorders; Council for Learning Disabilities (the last two are members of the Council for Exceptional Children); International Reading Association; and Orton Society. The combined membership of these six organizations is approximately 180,000 consumers and professionals with a potential for considerable influence. The agreed purposes for the committee are as follows:

1. To facilitate communication and cooperation of the member organizations.
2. To provide an interdisciplinary forum for the review of issues for governmental agencies and act as a resource committee for those agencies and other interested groups.
3. To provide a unified response to national issues in the area of learning disabilities when and as the need arises.
4. To seek agreement on major issues and problems pertinent to the area of learning disabilities.
5. To prepare and disseminate statements to various publics in order to clarify issues in the area of learning disabilities.
6. To identify research and to service delivery needs in learning disabilities.

This committee (of which I was selected the chairman for 1981) has recently completed its initial position paper, which is devoted to issues of definition [72]. The thrust of that position paper was to reemphasize the heterogeneity of the term *learning disability* and the fact that among the manifestations one may observe in the learning disabled are difficulties in self-regulatory behaviors, with altered patterns of social perception and social interaction. The implication here is that the term cannot be generically used and that due recognition must be paid to the subgroups within that designation. Furthermore, individuals with what are now referred to as attention deficit disorders are also to be regarded as being handicapped in the educational environment. This suggests that the social behavior of such individuals within the learning-disabled population (dyslexia being one of the learning disabilities) warrants research and intervention.

The National Joint Committee also pointed out that the use of the word *children* in the current federal definition focuses on academic performance and fails to give appropriate attention to the developmental nature of these conditions, which are, in all likelihood, in evidence before school entry and in many instances appear to persist beyond conventional school age. For those involved in clinical services and research regarding the disability of dyslexia, this affirmation of the broader problem encourages investigation of preschool and adult age groups. Indeed, the present federal definition and associated regulations (Public Law 94-142) mandate a "child find" for preschool identification, which, for lack of an appropriate research base and implementation teams, has foundered in most school districts.

The National Joint Committee reemphasized that learning disabilities such as dyslexia are intrinsic to the individual and that the basis of the disorder is presumed to be central nervous system dysfunction. In contrast to traditional educational thought, the committee went on to encourage an understanding of etiological mechanism to (1) facilitate the determination of prognosis, (2) clarify the nature of the condition for those affected and their families, and (3) give direction for research that will influence educational practice.

The committee also reacted to the so-called exclusionary clause of the federal definition, which might lend itself to the misinterpretation that individuals with any of the learning disabilities could not be multiply handicapped or come from diverse cultural and linguistic backgrounds. This need for sensitivity to the existence of reading retardation in diverse geographical, socioeconomic, and bilingual populations has also been asserted by Benton [8], Eisenberg [37], and Rutter [83]. As a consequence of their expressed concerns, the members of the committee proposed the following definition of learning disabilities:

Learning disabilities is a generic term that refers to a heterogeneous group of disorders manifested by significant difficulties in the acquisition and use of listening, speaking, reading, writing, reasoning, or mathematical abilities. These disorders are intrinsic to the individual and presumed to be due to central nervous system dysfunction.

Even though a learning disability may occur concomitantly with other handicapping conditions (e.g., sensory impairment, mental retardation, social and emotional disturbances) or environmental influences (e.g., cultural differences, insufficient/inappropriate instruction, psychogenic factors), it is not the direct result of those conditions or influences.

I can foresee the possibility that contributions such as those made in this volume might well be more widely distributed to investigators in the field and increase the likelihood of a change in clinical diagnostic and therapeutic practice through the efforts of the National Joint Committee on Learning

Disabilities and its component members, especially the Orton Society (which has altered its name to the Orton Dyslexia Society).

DSM-III Diagnostic Classification for Developmental Disorders

For those of us in the field of medicine, the situation in diagnosis with regard to developmental disorders, although improved, still does not correspond directly with that in education as expressed by the third edition of the *Diagnostic and Statistical Manual of Mental Disorders* (abbreviated DSM-III) [3]. The following are the diagnostic options:

1. Attention deficit disorder
   a. With hyperactivity
   b. Without hyperactivity
   c. Residual type
2. Developmental reading disorder
3. Developmental arithmetic disorder
4. Developmental language disorder
   a. Expressive type
   b. Receptive type
5. Developmental articulation disorder
6. Mixed specific developmental disorder
7. Atypical specific developmental disorder

The above classification equates developmental reading disorder with dyslexia. The diagnostician is advised that there is a significant impairment of reading when a 1- to 2-year discrepancy in reading skill, in contrast to chronological age, mental age, and school experience for ages 8 to 13 years, is encountered. No specific guidance for those below or beyond ages 8 to 13 is provided. The descriptive characteristics are those of faulty oral reading, including omissions, additions, and distortions of words. The rate of reading is described as slow, often with reduced reading comprehension and sparing of the ability to copy written words. Associated features in this syndrome are said to be errors in spelling to dictation, which are described as numerous and bizarre and are not explained by phonetics or by simple reversal of letters. Other common associated features are said to include subtle language difficulties, such as impaired sound discrimination and difficulties with sequencing words properly, in addition to behavioral problems, such as those associated with attention deficit disorder and conduct disorder. Thus, the *DSM-III* classification encompasses Denckla's [20, 21] dyslexia-plus and dyslexia-pure. Unfortunately, use of the term "soft" neurological signs is employed, citing as an example finger agnosia, which is alleged to be more common among younger children. As to prevalence, the manual states that "the disorder is apparently common." As a consequence, developmental reading disorder as defined by the *DSM-III* would appear to be a middle ground between specific developmental dyslexia and specific reading retardation.

A Definition of Dyslexia

For my own purposes, I frequently make use of the term *developmental dyslexia*. The denotation of developmental can be construed as equivalent to that of primary, as contrasted to secondary or acquired dyslexia. However, in dealing with children, adolescents, and young adults, I have not readily been able to discern clinically when the individual has experienced an acquired event that was causal to his or her symptoms. This is not an uncommon conundrum in clinical practice, and it poses a question about a potential dual role of genetic risk and brain insult.

A working definition for developmental dyslexia that I currently favor is somewhat modified from the one I offered previously [26, 29]. For me, developmental dyslexia connotes the constitutional and often familial disparate reduction in the rate and quality of the acquisition and use of written language skills. The disorder is frequently associated with antecedent or coexistent disparate underperformance in oral language. There may or may not be associated other problems of symbolic manipulation, along with disordered development of the concepts of time and space.

Although such a definition can be criticized as subjective and descriptive, the term *disparate reduction* refers to measured intelligence and age in contrast to age-, IQ-, and environmentally matched peers. The extent to which a disparate reduction must be present before the diagnosis can be applied will depend on whether the definition is to be used for research or for clinical practice. In research, more stringent and extreme variation will be required, as was utilized in the Isle of Wight studies. This is to maximize the probability that the selected population for investigation will be truly dyslexic. However, as Rutter [83] has admitted, such rigid statistical treatment provides a minimum estimate of the prevalence of dyslexia. In clinical practice, greater liberality would appear appropriate for the provision of remedial services.

Some [20] have suggested that the intellectually gifted child who is performing at grade level in reading requires no special concern. However, many of these bright but relatively retarded readers, when confronted with demands involving expressive written language, especially at secondary or postsecondary levels of education, may underperform and have difficulty in course work in which essay writing is required. Further, some of these students demonstrate unusual difficulty in the mastery of a second language in the classroom [24].

The use of the words *written language* in my definition is done advisedly. My concern is not only with decoding written language but also with comprehending it, possessing the ability to oralize it, and being able to produce it with regard to both lexical orthography (grapheme-phoneme rules for words) and the semantic, grammatic, and metalinguistic elements of receptive and expressive written language. By such a statement I reveal my bias for a language construct for the dyslexias. The use of the plural will soon be apparent. Thus, I find no fault with the concept of specific reading retardation, except for the fact that that term does not immediately communicate the invariable association of spelling underachievement and that it implies statistical treatment, which does not have equivalent application to children below the age of 7 years or to young adults at secondary levels of education. I would offer similar support and reservation for the Symmes and Rapoport [95] proposition of "unexpected reading failure."

The Utility of Subtyping Dyslexia

Over the last 15 years, research attempts at the clarification of the behaviors crucial to the manifestation of underachievement in written language have met with frustration. The result has been the increasing awareness that the manifest underachievement is not uniform in its clinical presentation. As a result, attempts have been made to recognize subgroups within the dyslexic population. There are a number of reasons why this may be a profitable undertaking. As Denckla [20] has suggested, the diagnosis of dyslexia by subtype reinforces the definitive attributes of the condition rather than leaving one to make a diagnosis by exclusion. If there are subtypes of dyslexia, investigation may reveal that there are differential prognoses based on the types identified. Furthermore, the characteristics of the subtypes may offer directions for improved therapeutic strategies. As a consequence, a retrospective or, better still, prospective analysis of subgroupings may permit earlier, more appropriate intervention.

In a more theoretical vein, more rigorous study of subgroupings within dyslexia may clarify other aspects of brain-behavior relationships. As examples, the following questions might be addressed: Are there subtypes of dyslexia in which the alleged positive attributes of the dyslexic person, such as unusual spatial skills, are more apt to be observed? Do subtype characteristics remain constant within a given individual over time, or do they change over time, including shifts to another of the subgroups, and does that hold implications for change in the remedial plan? Do any of the subtypes suggested correlate with brain anatomy, physiology, or chemistry?

In view of the evidence suggesting that in many cases of reading retardation a familial or perhaps genetic factor is observed [38, 39, 47, 111], it is reasonable to inquire whether any of the subtypes is heritable. Further, because of the observed differential occurrence in males, a condition that has not been explained by genetic mechanisms, one may investigate whether certain subtypes of dyslexia are more likely to be observed in females. If that should be the case, it may have implications regarding the nature of cerebral organization in females as compared with males. It is another aspect of this point that has thus far captured attention, that is, the greater occurrence of dyslexia among males has suggested that there are risk factors associated with male cerebral organization. For a detailed discussion of differential sex occurrence of dyslexia, see Ansara and associates [4].

Dyslexic Subtypes

Attempts at classification of dyslexics into subtypes began with Kinsbourne and Warrington [58], who in 1963 contrasted two groups of disabled readers on the basis of Wechsler's Intelligence Scale for Children (WISC) verbal-performance IQ discrepancies of 20 points or more in either direction. Children with the lower verbal IQs demonstrated signs of impaired language expression and reception, whereas those with lower performance IQs appeared intact linguistically but demonstrated impaired finger differentiation, greater disability in mathematics, visuoconstructive defects, and left-right disorientation.

Other attempts at subtype differentiation that bear at least superficial resemblances are those of Johnson and Myklebust [54], Ingram, Mason, and Blackburn [52], and Boder [11]. Using somewhat different techniques, each was able to distinguish between an audiophonological and a visuospatial type of disability, as reflected in the types of errors made by dyslexic children in their reading and spelling. From her experience, Boder [10] has suggested a much higher frequency of occurrence of dysphonetic dyslexia in English-speaking and English-reading children. This auditory versus visual type of classification would tentatively suggest modes of educational intervention [54].

A novel approach to the classification of dyslexics was provided by Mattis, French, and Rapin [66]. Their study of 113 subjects aged 8 to 18 years included a control group of "brain-damaged" readers and "brain-damaged" dyslexics, who were contrasted with "developmental" dyslexics. The frequency of positive family history in the developmental dyslexic group was 79 percent. When a neuropsychological battery that was designed to measure language, articulation, graphomotor skills, and visuospatial perceptual skills was employed, three syndromes emerged that accounted for 90 percent of subjects in both the brain-damaged dyslexic and the developmental dyslexic populations. One was primary language disorder, a second was articulatory and graphomotor discoordination, and a third suggested visuospatial perceptual disorder. In the brain-damaged dyslexic category, 43 percent of subjects were in the language disorder subtype, 30 percent in the articulation and graphomotor disorder subtype, and 17 percent in the visuospatial perceptual disorder subtype. By contrast, the developmental dyslexic group showed percentages of 28 percent, 48 percent, and 14 percent, respectively. When the two groups were combined, the relative frequency of the language disorder was 39 percent, the articulation and graphomotor category 37 percent, and the visuospatial perceptual disorder 16 percent.

The following difficulties are encountered with the report of Mattis, French, and Rapin [66]: (1) data on breakdown by sex were not provided for any of the categories; (2) no information was provided on whether there was a family history of reading disability in the brain-damaged dyslexic population, a point that would be of particular interest because it may be that potentially latent genetic dyslexic tendencies are more apt to express themselves clinically as a result of encephalopathic insult; (3) the designation of "brain damage," regardless of the attempts at uniformity of designation, is often subjective and nonuniform; (4) one cannot determine from the report whether, in either dyslexic population, the authors are referring to what Denckla has called dyslexia-pure or dyslexia-plus or both; and (5) the age range was broad, and the study was nonlongitudinal, so that if individuals had shifted classification over time, this point would have been obscured.

However, Mattis [65] defended the validity of this classification on the basis of a follow-up study in another patient population, suggesting similar subgroupings but a higher frequency of occurrence of individual students overlapping between categories.

A related but smaller and more carefully conducted retrospective study of dyslexic subtype was that of Denckla [20]. There were 52 dyslexia-pure subjects, ages 7 to 14 years, with a male-female ratio of 4:1. Positive family history was found in 40 of the 52 subjects. History of an encephalopathic event was present in 7, and a suspicious event or a risk factor was present in 17. Interestingly, 15 of the subjects had both a positive family history and a history of encephalopathic event or risk factor. This again raises the issue of potential combined effects of familial and acquired physical risk factors. Behavioral complaints were noted in 7 subjects. Historical evidence of delay in speech was present in 26 subjects.

On the basis of the behavioral measures utilized, 4 of the 52 subjects could not be classified within one of the five major categories defined by the author [20]. Although two were classified as having a visuospatial disorder, both were also anomic. Six were classified as having an articulatory-graphomotor disorder, 31 a language disorder, 5 deficient verbal memorization, and 3 a right hemisyndrome with mixed language disorder. Thus, a large proportion, 34 of 52 subjects, or 65 percent, had evidence of language disorder according to the definition used by the author, and 12 percent had an articulatory-graphomotor syndrome, indicating freedom from oral language difficulty aside from speech sound production. The verbal memorization syndrome occurred in 5 of the population, or 10 percent, all teenagers. Three of them had no abnormalities on neurological examination, including those findings construed as developmental. In this study, perhaps because of the sample size, there were no cases of the non-language-impaired visuospatial syndrome described by Mattis, French, and Rapin [66].

The validity of Denckla's research measures had been reinforced by prior studies, many in collaboration with Rudel, which utilized not only normal controls but also nondyslexic controls with minimal brain dysfunction [18, 19, 22, 23]. On the basis of the mixed pattern of syndromes observed, Denckla could not conclude that there was one syndrome with one cause. She correctly pointed out that the absence of longitudinal follow-up at the time of the report limited the ability to comment on the issue of prognosis in relation to etiology. This study confirms the suspicion of many, myself included, that there is a strong speech and language correlate of dyslexia.

An important clinical and research point made by Denckla [20, 21] is that the reading underachievement that is characteristic of dyslexia may not occur in isolation. Rather, her observations suggest that dyslexic syndromes may coexist with hyperkinesis. Thus, a clinically useful distinction, with research implications, was her separation of "dyslexia-pure" and "dyslexia-plus." Both subgroups warrant further investigation as to their similarities and differences in respect to cause, manifestation, prognosis, and treatment. I would submit that within each category an additional potentially meaningful distinction is that distinguishing persons with and without evident speech disorder. By speech disorder I am implying a similar hierarchical approach to oral language as was suggested in the previous discussion of written language.

Pirozzolo [78] combined the previous efforts of Kinsbourne and Warrington [58], Boder [10], and Mattis, French, and Rapin [66] with his own work and suggested that dyslexia could be dichotomized into an auditory-linguistic and a visuospatial type. His auditory-linguistic group was characterized by deficits in verbal learning ability similar to those of the dysphonetic dyslexics described by Boder [10] and the language disorder dyslexics described by Kinsbourne and Warrington [58] and Mattis, French, and Rapin [66]. Pirozzolo's visuospatial group was characterized by deficits in visuospatial perceptual ability and was considered roughly similar to the dyseidetic group described by Boder, the developmental Gerstmann group of Kinsbourne and Warrington, and the visuospatial perceptual group described by Mattis, French, and Rapin. Pirozzolo went on to contrast his two groups on the basis of lateralized visuoperceptual tasks, eye movement latency tasks, and eye movement patterns during reading.

Hemispheric Specialization and Dyslexic Subtypes

From those subclassifications of dyslexia emphasizing a bimodal separation, an extrapolation to left- and right-hemispheric specialization of function might be made; that is, subgroups that are suggested to be verbally deficient might be characterized by a reduction in quality of function in the left hemisphere, and conversely, those with relative dysfunction in visuospatial skills might be correlated with right-hemispheric dysfunction. There is, however, an alternative view that suggests that some of the differences may reflect unusual capability and a lack of occlusion of contralateral hemispheric function. Either interpretation should also take into account callosal function, along with those attributes usually ascribed to the right or left hemisphere.

Indeed, on the basis of observations in patients who had commissurotomy or hemispherectomy, Zaidel [110] suggested that the dysphonetic dyslexia of Boder [10] corresponds to a left-hemispheric deficit, whereas the dyseidetic dyslexia represents either a right-hemispheric or a bilateral hemispheric deficit. In contrast, Witelson [104], on the basis of dihaptic studies in dyslexic boys, offered a more uniform interpretation of their reading errors as reflecting the use of right-hemispheric strategies in reading, which are presumably less efficient than those performed by the left hemisphere. The characteristics of right-hemispheric language, based on studies of split-brain patients may be summarized as: (1) comprehension of spoken nouns, verbs, short sentences, and phrases, (2) comprehension of written nouns and verbs, (3) written naming by use of block letters by the left hand to name objects presented only to the right hemisphere, (4) difficulties with speech phonology and production, (5) difficulties with syntactic analysis and production, (6) poor understanding of function words, (7) poor performance on phonetic analysis and recognition of consonant-vowel syllables, and (8) restrictions in short-term memory [64].

It is not my intent to proceed into a detailed discussion of the described differential language capacities of the two hemispheres but rather to offer the observation that at this juncture it would appear premature to suggest that the data provide a clear delineation of the causes of reading underachievement. However, further work in the area of hemispheric specialization for language and its potential correlation to dyslexia is to be encouraged.

Using a neurophysiological basis, Fried [41] suggested that the dysphonetic dyslexic group could be differentiated from dyseidetic dyslexics and normal readers. Normal readers demonstrated greater waveform differences between verbal and nonverbal auditory event–related potentials over the left hemisphere as contrasted to the right; no such asymmetry was found in the dysphonetic dyslexics.

I have elsewhere reviewed the potential relationship of central auditory dysfunction and reading disabilities, especially as assessed by dichotic listening tests [27]. The nonhomogeneity of the populations studied and the variability in the research paradigm make it difficult to draw a meaningful conclusion from dichotic listening studies as to their association, causal or otherwise, with reading underachievement. Language pathologists have often reacted negatively to such studies as representing prelinguistic challenges that are not pertinent to the language process [80]. For the most part, the usual pattern of right-ear advantage on dichotic listening tests has been confirmed in the dyslexic population. In one dichotic listening study, a small sample of boys averaging 9 years of age with presumed auditory processing disorders was contrasted to an age-matched normal-achieving control group. The results indicated a right-ear advantage in both groups. However, differential accuracy of performance related to stimulus onset–time separation was demonstrated. It appeared for this small population that increasing onset–time separation improved the performance of the students with an auditory processing disorder to nearly equal that of the nonunderachieving students [97]. However, from the data presented, one cannot ascertain whether this differential performance represents differences in perceptual function or auditory linguistic underperformance. With the assistance of my associate in audiology, Dr. Wayne Olsen, I have observed similar types of performance on dichotic consonant-vowel nonsense syllables in some dyslexic students. On clinical grounds, however, not all of these students had apparent "auditory processing" deficits, and some would fit into the Denckla category of dyslexia-plus.

Neuroanatomical Studies

Stimulated by the inquiry of Norman Geschwind, the last 15 years have witnessed a remarkable series of observations relating to gross and microscopic hemispheric asymmetries of the human brain and their potential relationship to normal and disordered language development. In 1968, Geschwind and Levitsky [44] demonstrated, in a study of 100 adult brains, asymmetries in the surface area of the planum temporale, a language-pertinent site. The planum was larger on the left side in 65 percent of brains, approximately equal on the two sides in 24 percent, and larger on the right in 11 percent. Subsequent studies confirmed that a similar frequency and type of asymmetry were present at birth and indeed could be detected as early as 31 weeks of gestation [11, 101, 105]. The last findings suggest an innate biological characteristic that is not secondary to environmental factors. For an excellent review of the subject of asymmetries of the central nervous system and their significance, see Galaburda and colleagues [43].

The next tantalizing observation pertinent to the question of developmental dyslexia was the report by Hier and associates [49] in which computed tomography (CT scans) of the brain was performed in 24 patients with developmental dyslexia. Ten of these patients showed a reversal of the pattern of asymmetry observed in normal right-handed individuals, such that the right parieto-occipital region was wider than the left. The 10 dyslexic patients with this reversal of cerebral asymmetry had a lower mean verbal IQ than the 14 other dyslexic patients in the study. The authors suggested that the apparent reduction in volume in the left hemisphere may have posed a relative risk factor for the development of linguistic capability in the left hemisphere or, conversely, that greater language demands may have been placed on the right hemisphere of these subjects. Whether this dyslexic subgroup bears any relation to those discussed previously, such as the Kinsbourne and Warrington [58], Johnson and Myklebust [54], or Boder [10] dysphonetic subgroups, is not clear. Similarly, whether they correspond to the linguistically less competent subgroups described by Mattis, French, and Rapin [66] or to those individuals with language deficits in the classification of Denckla [20] is not apparent. However, the possible correlation of gross brain anatomy with subtype classification warrants investigation.

Similar reversal of asymmetry has been described in childhood autism [48] as well as in children and young adults with learning disability [81]. In the latter study, reversed asymmetry correlated best with a history of delay in speech. These in vivo, noninvasive studies raise questions as to the extent to which brain anatomy may contribute to behavior, specifically the acquisition of language. However, in no instance can reversed asymmetry be construed as diagnostic of coexistent academic underachievement, for such asymmetry is also found in the asymptomatic, normal-achieving population.

The culmination of these neuroanatomical studies was that of the pathological description of a dyslexic patient's central nervous system by Galaburda and Kemper [42]. This study was the first careful microscopic examination of the central nervous system of a dyslexic person. The patient was left-handed, possessed a positive family history of reading underachievement, and historically was delayed in speech and had documented difficulties with reading and spelling. Dichotic digits showed right-ear superiority, which suggested left-hemispheric lateralization of language. With no known complication of gestation, delivery, or neonatal health, the patient experienced nocturnal seizures at the age of 16 years. Routine electroencephalograms (EEGs) were normal except for one sleep recording, which suggested borderline slowing over the right hemisphere. An isotope brain scan was normal. The subject died at the age of 20 from a fall in which no insult to the central nervous system occurred. At autopsy, the left cerebral hemisphere was found to be consistently wider than the right. The planum temporale on the left was approximately equal in size to that on the right, a finding observed in 24 percent of the general population. However, polymicrogyria in the left temporal speech region was detected. Cortical dysplasias were observed in the limbic, primary, and association cortices of the left hemisphere. The extent to which the physical alterations were causal to the educational underachievement cannot be stated. However, the observations clearly raise the possibility of such a causal relationship and suggest that continuing studies of a similar nature should be carried out.

The membership of the Orton Society, in the belief that such work must be carried on, has directed funds received from the Underwood Company to Dr. Galaburda and his laboratory at the Beth Israel Hospital in Boston so that this work may continue. Additionally, the Society is actively engaged in the accumulation of in-life descriptive data of dyslexic individuals who have pledged their central nervous systems for anatomical study after death. As a consequence of such continued research, it is hoped that a clearer relationship will be established between brain morphology and dyslexic behavior. However, it would seem prudent that such individuals be studied for their positive attributes; dyslexic subtype; eye, hand, and foot preference; sex; CT scan findings; and refined EEG studies to maximize the breadth of the inferences that may be drawn.

These anatomical studies should also include careful examination of the corpus callosum in view of the potential for differential hemispheric functioning on the basis of dysgenesis of that major means of physical communication between the two hemispheres. Given the recent report by Sidtis and associates [89] on the importance of the anterior commissure in semantic access between the hemispheres, both the anterior and posterior portions of the corpus callosum and their connections warrant careful inspection. Additional support for a potential role of the corpus callosum in dyslexia has been suggested by the report of Yingling [106], which notes the occurrence of prolonged latencies and reduced amplitudes in the contralateral hemisphere after tactile stimulation to the hand in dyslexic subjects. These studies were thought to represent a potential maturational lag of the corpus callosum in the childhood-age population studied.

Aside from examination of cortical structures in the corpus callosum, future anatomical descriptions of the central nervous system of dyslexic persons should include descriptive comment of the basal ganglia, which have important motor functions. Similarly, the thalamic nuclei would be worthy of description because of the role of the thalamus in speech [98], memory [99], general activation of the cortex, and somatosensory function.

Although one rarely encounters evidence of true cerebellar dysfunction in the neurological examination of the dyslexic person, some authors have proposed the notion (without good clinical or research support) of a cerebellovestibular dysfunction correlate to dyslexia [40, 60]. Because of the simplicity of such a hypothesis, it has recently gained some measure of popularity. Similarly, occupational therapy strategies for intervention in this population have been proposed, based on the notion of some failure of "sensory integration" presumed to lie within the brainstem [5]. The last two speculations, although suffering from imprecise use of terminology and poor research technique, could be given objective support or rejected by neurophysiological, pathological-anatomical, and neurochemical study. Certainly in those persons who come to postmortem study with a life history suggesting hyperkinesis coexistent with dyslexia, study of the brainstem reticular activating pathways to the central thalamic nuclei would be worthwhile [90].

Neurochemical Studies

Despite the recent explosion of information in the field of neurochemistry, little direct information is available regarding neurochemical relationships to language in general or to dyslexia in particular. In 1971, Wender [102] speculated on a number of potential neurochemical correlates to minimal brain dysfunction. However, because of his generalization in the use of the term, it is impossible to determine whether any of his hypothesized neurochemical mechanisms are applicable to any of the MBD subgroups. As the central nervous systems of dyslexic persons become available for anatomical study, neurochemical analysis of the material will be an important adjunctive study. Although there will be some constraints pertaining to time and handling of the tissue, this potential use of the specimens made available through the Orton Society dyslexia neuroanatomy study has not escaped the attention of the advisory board to that investigation.

I have previously summarized the major research in asymmetries of brain structure in dyslexics. There is also evidence of asymmetry of neurotransmitter distribution in lower animals and humans. Glick, Jerussi, and Zimmerberg [46] have described asymmetric distribution of dopamine in lower mammals. Human studies have suggested higher levels of norepinephrine in the left pulvinar as contrasted with the right [74]. This is potentially important, since this region of the thalamus is known to have implications for language function [73, 98]. Conversely, these same investigators demonstrated a higher concentration of norepinephrine in the right somatosensory regions of the thalamus as compared with the left [74]. Most recently, choline acetyltransferase, the enzyme important in the production of the neurotransmitter acetylcholine, has been shown to be more highly concentrated in the left first temporal gyrus than in the right in human subjects. The enzyme activity was specifically highest in cortical layers II and IV [2]. It is not yet clear whether these observations provide a direct neurochemical analogue of the anatomical and functional asymmetries of the human nervous system. Further basic information of the neurochemistry of the "normal" population will be required against which comparisons can be made in the dyslexic population. Within the dyslexic population, these neurochemical studies should take into account the issue of subtype and associated gross and microscopic anatomical variations.

In the near future, positron computed tomography (PCT) may permit studies of brain chemistry in the intact subject. This is somewhat analogous to the structural analysis permitted by CT scanning in vivo. That is, CT scans provide morphological information that can be correlated with, but is not identical to, direct anatomical inspection. Similarly, it is likely that PCT will offer some insights into dynamic brain chemistry in vivo, which will not be identical to the data available from postmortem studies. At present, PCT is primarily a measure of cerebral glucose metabolism. Preliminary work suggests no cerebral asymmetry of glucose metabolism during the *resting state* [67]. Also recent research [77] has documented increases in metabolism at the level of the visual cortex in a manner that would be predicted in association with visual tasks.

Another new technique of assessing tissue metabolism, including brain tissue metabolism, is the use of nuclear magnetic resonance (NMR). By this technique, the magnetic properties of atomic nuclei are observed in a uniform magnetic field. Such nuclei are polarized, and their behavior is observed by low-energy radio waves. As with PCT, correlation with brain structure may be possible by visual imaging. Also as with PCT, NMR provides in vivo information of brain chemistry that differs from that obtained in studies performed at postmortem examinations [76].

The clinical side of basic neurochemistry is applied neuropharmacology. The potential contribution of neuropharmacology to the treatment of dyslexia is not clear. Interpreting the results of such therapy is difficult because of the often empirical nature of the reports and the use of diagnostic terminology that is too broad to allow inferences to be made with regard to specific behaviors. On the other hand, the behavior of hyperkinesis (now referred to as attention deficit disorder) seems most likely to benefit from drug treatment. For such behavior, the central nervous system stimulants methylphenidate and dextroamphetamine are most commonly employed and may have a favorable effect on attention span and social behavior [69]. The reason why these compounds are effective is as yet unknown. Further, prediction as to which children with hyperkinetic syndromes will experience favorable effects and at what dosages of the alerting compounds is, at this point, totally empirical. It is a reasonable concern that drugs may be injudiciously prescribed, poorly monitored, and inappropriately construed as "healing" the child, with the result that the necessary concomitant home- and school-based therapies are not undertaken. Evidence suggests that treatment with methylphenidate has no positive effect on the nonhyperkinetic dyslexic child [45]. Thus, there is no evidence to indicate the use of alerting agents in the treatment of dyslexia-pure.

Another pharmacological agent that has recently received attention is the compound piracetam. Wilsher, Atkins, and Manfield [103] suggested that dyslexic boys treated with this compound showed improvement in verbal learning. The compound appears to be safe, but its active mechanism is unknown. A multicenter study within the United States is presently comparing the efficacy and safety of piracetam with placebo in children who have specific written language difficulties (dyslexia). However, on the basis of the information currently available, it is not possible to differentiate whether piracetam has an independent favorable effect on reading performance or enhances the effects of concomitant remedial instruction.

Electroencephalography

With the exception of the rare instances of reading-, writing-, or calculation-induced seizures, routine EEG neither assists in making the diagnosis of specific educational underachievement nor offers reliable clues as to why the underachievement is present (for reviews, see Connors [14] and Duane [32]). However, increasingly sophisticated analysis of EEG outputs by computers, along with more novel studies of EEG correlates with specific behaviors, have recently emerged [1, 34, 35].

Particularly intriguing are the results obtained by Duffy and associates [34] in utilizing the brain electrical activity mapping (BEAM) technique in dyslexic students. The subject selection is clean, the tasks selected for recording are appropriate, the EEG technique is sound, and the visual display is both informative and aesthetically pleasing. In their small patient population, differences were observed predominantly in the left hemisphere, but also in the frontal speech regions. These results raise the question of whether the students investigated would have fallen into the anomic classification of Denckla [20]. The described bilateral midline changes may or may not have some correlation with the reduction in heel-toe alternation described by Denckla (see Chap. 10). As stimulating as this work is, sample sizes should be increased for both the control and the original dyslexia-pure category; also, subtype variation and a comparison between results obtained in the dyslexia-pure versus the dyslexia-plus categories should be investigated. It would also be useful to have the findings replicated at other reputable centers. Chapter 7 provides further discussion of BEAM analysis of dyslexia.

The BEAM technique clearly has potential relevance to the investigation of physiological concomitants of dyslexia. However, from the material published so far, one cannot yet regard this as a clinical diagnostic tool. This statement applies particularly to the neurometrics technique of John (see Chap. 9), which is less readily interpretable because of the lack of specificity of the population studied by that device.

Those of us in medicine have learned by experience with other health problems that diagnostic tests assist in reinforcing clinical impressions that are based on the history and physical examination. However, they never replace anamnesis and hands-on evaluation. For example, when we are presented with the clinical question of the presence or absence of a seizure disorder, we cannot rely on the EEG to reveal specific epileptiform discharges. Depending on the frequency of the episodes and their character, the clinician may elect to recommend anticonvulsant pharmacological management on the basis of the history. Conversely, on occasion the patient with an apparently valid history of no known seizurelike episodes may demonstrate an EEG pattern suggesting a latent seizure diathesis. In this case, many clinicians would withhold medicinal treatment until a clinical event compatible with a seizure has occurred. This process is referred to as clinical judgment. There is no reason to believe that in questions of educational underachievement testing results should replace the judgment of a trained and experienced clinician. However, I sincerely trust that the elegant research work that has begun will continue to further clarify the neurophysiological concomitants of dyslexia and result in the appropriate clinical use of these EEG derivatives in the assessment of dyslexic persons. At this time, direct tests of reading, writing, and academic potential are the only absolute measures of the presence or absence of dyslexia. All of the other measures discussed previously are, as yet, imperfect correlates. I have more recently provided a comprehensive review of the use of CT and EEG in dyslexia and pointed out how deficiencies of prior studies might be averted [33].

Future Studies

In many of the previous sections, suggestions regarding further studies have more commonly been of a retrospective than a prospective nature. In this final section, I wish to make some additional incidental clinical observations, offer suggestions for future research, and finally, propose means by which many of the questions raised can perhaps be better answered.

Because it is frequently speculated that hemispheric organization for language is a cause or correlate of dyslexia and/or a means by which compensation is achieved, the study of dyslexic individuals who have in later life acquired focal cerebral disease may be of value. Put simplistically, if the compensatory mechanism or underlying strategy for reading in the dyslexic person, or *some* dyslexic persons, is in the right hemisphere, it will be desirable to learn what effects right cerebral lesions, such as stroke, may have on the dyslexic's written language competence. Eye, hand, and foot preference should be noted, and if available, antecedent information as to language lateralization, as might be assessed by dichotic listening tests, would be desirable. If there are instances of dyslexic individuals with acquired right brain lesions who decline further in their written language competence after suffering such lesions, this would at least suggest that the intactness of that portion of the right hemisphere was important to the level of competence the individual had previously been able to achieve.

The only example of an adult with probable constitutional dyslexia and subsequent cerebral disease with which I am acquainted is that of a 47-year-old man with a left parieto-occipital infarct who was seen by my colleagues at the Mayo Clinic [30]. The patient was right-handed, was diabetic, had a history of transient ischemic attacks, and then acquired more profound reading and spelling dysfunction, along with dyscalculia, right homonymous hemianopsia, signs of diabetic peripheral neuropathy, and retinopathy, without hemiparesis or expressive speech deficit. A CT scan of the head demonstrated a well-demarcated zone of decreased attenuation in the left parieto-occipital region compatible with infarction. Unfortunately, the specific characteristics of the written language disability present previous to cerebral infarct that might have permitted a classification as to subtype were not available; nor could a definitive definition of subtype be made after infarction. However, the described qualities of the reading and spelling errors were compatible with Boder's dyseidetic type of dyslexia. Differential response in such patients to rehabilitative efforts would be of interest, as it would in previously nondyslexic individuals with acquired alexias (as described by Marshall in Chap. 4).

At this point, it would appear that the risk factors associated with childhood dyslexia are (1) male sex, (2) other family members affected with dyslexia, and (3) to some extent, gestational or perinatal cerebral insult. However, it may be fruitful to investigate family histories for other identifiable medical conditions. Based on my own clinical experience, there may be a higher than expected familial occurrence or coexistent disorder of narcolepsy. Adult manifestations of narcolepsy consist of inordinate nocturnal sleep requirements, difficulty in maintaining alertness during the day, and to a variable extent, cataplexy, sleep paralysis, and hypnagogic hallucinations. The treatment of choice is that of an alerting agent such as methylphenidate. Narcolepsy appears to be a dominantly inherited trait without sex predilection [107]. I have observed families in which some members are affected with narcolepsy, others with dyslexia, and some with both. At this point, such observations must remain anecdotal until they are systematically reviewed. However, the potential association of dyslexia-plus with narcolepsy would be of particular interest because of the similarity of treatment of hyperkinesis and narcolepsy.

The Need for More Precise Early Identification

Professionals such as myself who predominantly evaluate students at or beyond the age of 14 years find it particularly dismaying how often inaccurate predictions are made with respect to later characteristics of a student who was evaluated as a child. How is it that at the age of 5 or 6 years a child can be described as restless and awkward with the use of pencil and paper and yet as an adolescent that person can be captain of the football team or be preparing for a career in architecture and design? Denckla, in Chapter 10, suggests that these instances are the results of observations in which overgeneralization is made regarding incoordination observed in early childhood that may have no application in adolescence or with other behaviors. It would be useful, however, to improve the prognostic accuracy with respect to childhood assessments. This goes beyond predicting decoding reading failure [53] to higher-order receptive written language competence, expressive written language ability, calculation skill, arithmetic reasoning skill, impulsivity, artistic ability, musical ability, and the like.

Although such information is not solely dependent on the school environment, it may help in the construction of both general and special school strategies in maximizing innate skills and minimizing innate ineptitudes. Even with early diagnosis of decoding behavior in reading, longer-term follow-up has proved disappointing. The study of Satz and associates [88] revealed that only 6.1 percent of students classified as having severe reading retardation in grade two had improved by the end of grade five. Thirty percent of the average readers in grade three had become problem readers by the end of grade five. Thus, there was virtually no improvement in the performance of problem readers between grades two and five, and delayed reading problems occurred in grade five for many students who had been average readers in grade two. These data suggest that predictive batteries contain flaws in predicting subsequent reading failure or that the quality of instruction was inappropriate for the students in this study (or both). When we also observe the natural history of specific reading retardation from the Isle of Wight studies [85], we must be concerned about the quality of instruction at the elementary school level and about the logic of the nationwide practice of reducing the intensity of educational intervention in the postelementary school years.

Although it has been suggested that brain-based mechanisms have been underlying causes of significant reading underachievement, this, if correct, does not necessarily imply refractoriness to educational intervention. Rawson [79] has demonstrated that, at least for some dyslexic boys, a favorable outcome can nonetheless be achieved.

Pertinent to the subject of intervention is the observation of antecedent oral language underperformance in those who later demonstrate reading underachievement. If such a subgroup does exist, a reasonable question is whether effective intervention of the oral language disability lessens the risk or improves the prognosis for written language underperformance.

Longitudinal Prospective Population Study

Salient questions that have been raised include the following: What are the antecedents (familial and physical) to the types of dyslexia? How do any of these affect prognosis? What is the relationship of the dyslexic patterns to brain anatomy and physiology? How may we positively affect educational practice?

My suggestion for clarification of these questions is likely to be costly, time-consuming, and physically and mentally taxing to the investigators and subjects alike. In part, these suggestions are articulated in an April, 1978 letter to Arthur Prensky in response to an inquiry by the National Institute of Neurologic and Communicative Disorders and Stroke (NINCDS) of the Orton Society [28]. The following points present only the broad outlines for such an investigation:

1. The study must either be a population study, as was conducted on the Isle of Wight, or provide a representative sample within a given geographical area.
2. The study should be prospective.

3. The study should be longitudinal.
4. Entry of subjects would be at the time pregnancy is identified.

Parents and first-degree relatives would have been screened for dyslexic traits and, as best as possible, classified as to dyslexic subtype for those meeting the criteria as dyslexic. Detailed analysis of coexistent health problems among family members of all persons in the study would be carried out. Computed tomography scans of the brain and advanced EEG studies such as BEAM and perhaps PCT and NMR would be required for all parents and first-degree relatives selected for and agreeing to participation in the study.

On the basis of the presence or absence of dyslexia in the family, offspring would be categorized as being either at genetic risk or not. Pregnancy and delivery would also be carefully monitored for both genetic risk or no genetic risk. Then, offspring would be classified as being either at no gestational/perinatal risk or at gestational/perinatal risk.

Early infancy studies, such as those described by Als (see Chap. 5), would be carried out. At appropriate age intervals, developmental motor skills, speech and language, and attentional and cognitive ability would be assessed throughout the preschool years. Of necessity, these studies would require a multidisciplinary collaborative effort at least involving professionals in the areas of medicine, psychology, speech, and language. If an impact is to be made on the delivery of educational services, those from the teaching profession must also be actively involved. At points deemed to be appropriate, CT scans and EEG studies such as BEAM would be performed. Tentative predictions of later school failure might be made during the preschool years on the basis of analysis of the aforementioned skills. My suspicion is that more careful analysis of speech development would carry greater predictive weight. At the time of entry into school, a prediction of potential reading underachievement would be made.

Depending on the criteria established for the earliest age appropriate to the use of the term *dyslexia,* frequency of occurrence within each of the four dyslexic subcategories previously discussed would be established (the four categories might be expanded if a definite encephalopathic event occurred in any of the four groups). Furthermore, attempts at classification of type of dyslexia would be made, including the designation of dyslexia-pure or dyslexia-plus.

Once dyslexia is diagnosed, a retrospective analysis of the characteristics antecedent of the diagnosis would be undertaken. These characteristics would be contrasted with those in persons in whom dyslexia is not present.

Ideally, the study would progress throughout the school years, taking note of the frequency of arithmetic underachievement, motor development, and attentional ability. Serial BEAM studies would be carried out on the population, and improvement or decline in the basic skills would be noted.

As the subjects enter postelementary schooling, the quality level of higher-order written and oral language demands would be assessed. Exceptional skills in such areas as the graphic arts, music, and athletics would be noted. Similarly, performance in the acquisition of a second language would be assessed.

At a point deemed safe for those being investigated, PCT or NMR studies would be carried out. Higher education and vocational attainments would subsequently be recorded. At perhaps more than one point in the study, dichotic listening tests would be performed.

The final terminus would be at the end of the subject's life span, at which time there would be a postmortem investigation of gross and microscopic anatomical detail and neurochemical analysis.

Only under the above conditions can there be a reasonable expectation of clarifying the multiple questions previously raised. However, there is no guarantee that definitive answers would be provided. As technology improves, additional or alternative means of assessing central nervous system function could be introduced. One would hope that within such a paradigm educators would be stimulated to stretch their skills and transmit to their colleagues their observations concerning those educational rationales and techniques that appear to provide better outcomes.

For reasons of cost and potential influence on governmental funding patterns in education, financial assistance would be sought from governmental agencies, including those in education. In light of the present attitude toward economics, it would appear appropriate to solicit collaborative (matching) financial support from the private sector. Such groups as the Orton Society, the Foundation for Children With Learning Disabilities (New York City), and perhaps the sponsors of the symposium on which this book is based, the Institute for Child Development Research, would be able to direct private philanthropy in this direction.

Short of the prospective longitudinal community study just suggested, the duration of which is likely to be beyond the life span of many of us studying dyslexia today, we must be content with shorter-term longitudinal prospective and retrospective studies that address more restricted questions. In any case, these investigations should probe into the biological and social development of human behavior with sensitive, informed innocence.

References

1. Ahn, H., et al. Developmental equations reflect brain dysfunctions. *Science* 210:1259, 1980.
2. Amaducci, L., et al. Choline acetyltransferase (ChAT) activity differs in right and left human temporal lobes. *Neurology* 31:799, 1981.
3. American Psychiatric Association. *Diagnostic and Statistical Manual of Mental Disorders (DSM-III)* (3rd ed.). Washington, D.C.: American Psychiatric Association, 1980.
4. Ansara, A., et al. (Eds.). *Sex Differences in Dyslexia*. Towson, Md.: Orton Dyslexia Society, 1981.
5. Ayres, A. J. Deficits in sensory integration in educationally handicapped children. *J. Learn. Disabil.* 2:160, 1969.
6. Belmont, L., and Birch, H. G. Lateral dominance, lateral awareness, and reading disability. *Child Dev.* 36:57, 1965.

7. Benton, A. L. Developmental dyslexia: Neurological aspects. *Adv. Neurol.* 7:1, 1975.
8. Benton, A. L. Some Conclusions About Dyslexia. In A. L. Benton and D. Pearl (Eds.), *Dyslexia: An Appraisal of Current Knowledge.* New York: Oxford University Press, 1978. P. 451.
9. Berger, M., Yule, W., and Rutter, M. Attainment and adjustment in two geographic areas: II. The prevalence of specific reading retardation. *Br. J. Psychiatry* 126:510, 1975.
10. Boder, E. Developmental Dyslexia: A Diagnostic Screening Procedure Based on Three Characteristic Patterns of Reading and Spelling. In B. Batemant (Ed.), *Learning Disorders.* Seattle: Special Child Publications, 1971. Vol. 4, p. 297.
11. Chi, J. G., Dooling, E. C., and Gilles, F. H. Left-right asymmetries of the temporal speech areas of the human fetus. *Arch. Neurol.* 34:346, 1977.
12. Clements, S. D. *Minimal Brain Dysfunction in Children: Terminology and Identification.* NINDB, Monograph No. 3, Public Health Service Publication No. 1415. Washington, D.C.: U.S. Department of Health, Education, and Welfare, 1966.
13. Clements, S. D., and Peters, J. E. Minimal brain dysfunctions in the school-age child: Diagnosis and treatment. *Arch. Gen. Psychiatry* 6:185, 1962.
14. Connors, C. K. Critical Review of "Electroencephalographic and Neurophysiological Studies in Dyslexia." In A. L. Benton and D. Pearl (Eds.), *Dyslexia: An Appraisal of Current Knowledge.* New York: Oxford University Press, 1978. P. 251.
15. Critchley, M. *Developmental Dyslexia.* Springfield, Il.: Thomas, 1964.
16. Critchley, M. *The Dyslexic Child* (2nd ed.). London: Heinemann, 1970.
17. Critchley, M. Developmental Dyslexia: Its History, Nature and Prospects. In D. D. Duane and M. B. Rawson (Eds.), *Reading, Perception and Language.* Baltimore: York, 1975. P. 9.
18. Denckla, M. B. Development of speed in repetitive and successive finger-movements in normal children. *Dev. Med. Child Neurol.* 15:635, 1973.
19. Denckla, M. B. Development of motor co-ordination in normal children. *Dev. Med. Child Neurol.* 16:729, 1974.
20. Denckla, M. B. Minimal Brain Dysfunction and Dyslexia: Beyond Diagnosis by Exclusion. In M. E. Blaw, I. Rapin, and M. Kinsbourne (Eds.), *Topics in Child Neurology.* New York: Spectrum, 1977. P. 243.
21. Denckla, M. B. Minimal Brain Dysfunction. In J. S. Chall and A. F. Mirsky (Eds.), *Education and the Brain* (National Society for the Study of Education, 77th Yearbook, Pt. 2). Chicago: University of Chicago Press, 1978. P. 223.
22. Denckla, M. B., and Rudel, R. G. Naming of object-drawings by dyslexic and other learning disabled children. *Brain Lang.* 3:1, 1976.
23. Denckla, M. B., and Rudel, R. G. Rapid 'automatized' naming (R.A.N.): Dyslexia differentiated from other learning disabilities. *Neuropsychologia* 14:471, 1976.
24. Dinklage, K. T. Inability to Learn a Foreign Language. In G. B. Blaine, Jr. and C. C. McArthur (Eds.), *Emotional Problems of the Student* (2nd ed.). New York: Appleton-Century-Crofts, 1971. P. 185.
25. Divoky, D. Education's latest victim: The "LD" kid. *Learn. Mag. Creative Teach.* 3:20, 1974.
26. Duane, D. D. Developmental dyslexia: Etiologic theories and therapeutic implications. *Psychiatr. Ann.* 7:448, 1977.

27. Duane, D. D. A Neurologic Perspective of Central Auditory Dysfunction. In R. W. Keith (Ed.), *Central Auditory Dysfunction*. New York: Grune & Stratton, 1977. P. 1.
28. Duane, D. D. Letter to Arthur Prensky on behalf of the Orton Society in response to NINCDS Inquiry, April 14, 1978.
29. Duane, D. D. The dyslexic child: Diagnostic implications. *Pediatr. Ann.* 8:632, 1979.
30. Duane, D. D. Theories about the causes of dyslexia and their implications. *Pediatr. Ann.* 8:641, 1979.
31. Duane, D. D. Toward a definition of dyslexia: A summary of views. *Bull. Orton Soc.* 29:56, 1979.
32. Duane, D. D. Toward the Demystification of the Clinical Electroencephalogram. In W. M. Cruickshank and A. A. Silver (Eds.), *Bridges to Tomorrow: Selected Papers from the 17th International Conference of the Association for Children with Learning Disabilities*. Syracuse, N.Y.: Syracuse University Press, 1981. P. 151.
33. Duane, D. D. Neurodiagnostic Tools in Dyslexic Syndromes in Children: Pitfalls and Proposed Comparative Study of Computed Tomography, Nuclear Magnetic Resonance, and Brain Electrical Activity Mapping. In G. T. Pavlides and F. D. Fisher (Eds.), *Dyslexia: Neuropsychology and Treatment*. New York: Wiley, in press.
34. Duffy, F. H., et al. Dyslexia: Regional differences in brain electrical activity by topographic mapping. *Ann. Neurol.* 7:412, 1980.
35. Duffy, F. H., et al. Dyslexia: Automated diagnosis by computerized classification of brain electrical activity. *Ann. Neurol.* 7:421, 1980.
36. Eisenberg, L. The Epidemiology of Reading Retardation and a Program for Preventive Intervention. In J. Money (Ed.), *The Disabled Reader: Education of the Dyslexic Child*. Baltimore: Johns Hopkins Press, 1966. P. 3.
37. Eisenberg, L. Definitions of Dyslexia: Their Consequences for Research and Policy. In A. L. Benton and D. Pearl (Eds.), *Dyslexia: An Appraisal of Current Knowledge*. New York: Oxford University Press, 1978. P. 29.
38. Finucci, J. M. Genetic considerations in dyslexia. *Prog. Learn. Disabil.* 4:41, 1978.
39. Finucci, J. M., et al. The genetics of specific reading disability. *Ann. Hum. Genet.* 40:1, 1976.
40. Frank, J., and Levinson, H. Dysmetric dyslexia and dyspraxia: Hypothesis and study. *J. Am. Acad. Child Psychiatry* 12:690, 1973.
41. Fried, I. Cerebral dominance and subtypes of developmental dyslexia. *Bull. Orton Soc.* 29:101, 1979.
42. Galaburda, A. M., and Kemper, T. L. Cytoarchitectonic abnormalities in developmental dyslexia: A case study. *Ann. Neurol.* 6:94, 1979.
43. Galaburda, A. M., et al. Right-left asymmetries in the brain: Structural differences between the hemispheres may underlie cerebral dominance. *Science* 199:852, 1978.
44. Geschwind, N., and Levitsky, W. Human brain: Left-right asymmetries in temporal speech region. *Science* 161:186, 1968.
45. Gittelman-Klein, R. Short- and long-term effects of methylphenidate on cognitive performance in learning disability children. In *Proceedings of the 20th International Congress of Psychology*. Tokyo: University of Tokyo Press, 1974.
46. Glick, S. D., Jerussi, T. P., and Zimmerberg, B. Behavioral and neuropharmacological correlates of nigrostriatal asymmetry in rats. In S. Harnad, et al. (Eds.), *Lateralization in the Nervous System*. New York: Academic, 1977. P. 213.

47. Hallgren, B. Specific dyslexia ("congenital word-blindness"): A clinical and genetic study. *Acta Psychiatr. Neurol. Scand.* [Suppl.] 65:1, 1950.
48. Hier, D. B., LeMay, M., and Rosenberger, P. B. Autism and unfavorable left-right asymmetries of the brain. *J. Autism Dev. Disord.* 9:153, 1979.
49. Hier, D. B., et al. Developmental dyslexia: Evidence for a subgroup with a reversal of cerebral asymmetry. *Arch. Neurol.* 35:90, 1978.
50. Hinshelwood, J. Congenital word-blindness. *Lancet* 1:1506, 1900.
51. Hinshelwood, J. *Congenital Word-Blindness.* London: Lewis, 1917.
52. Ingram, T. T. S., Mason, A. W., and Blackburn, I. A retrospective study of 82 children with reading disability. *Dev. Med. Child Neurol.* (Minneap.) 12:271, 1970.
53. Jansky, J. J., and de Hirsch, K. *Preventing Reading Failure: Prediction, Diagnosis, Intervention.* New York: Harper & Row, 1972.
54. Johnson, D. J., and Myklebust, H. R. *Learning Disabilities: Educational Principles and Practices.* New York: Grune & Stratton, 1967.
55. Kawi, A. A., and Pasamanick, B. Association of factors of pregnancy with reading disorders in childhood. *J.A.M.A.* 166:1420, 1958.
56. Keogh, B. K. Non-cognitive aspects of learning disabilities: Another look at perceptual-motor approaches to assessment and remediation. Presented at the Psychologist, the School and the Child with MBD/LD, Asilomar, Calif., October 1976.
57. Kerr, J. School hygiene, in its mental, moral, and physical aspects. *J. R. Statist. Soc.* 60:613, 1897.
58. Kinsbourne, M., and Warrington, E. K. Developmental factors in reading and writing backwardness. *Br. J. Psychol.* 54:145, 1963.
59. The LD movement: Brilliant star or glaring copout? (letter to the editor). *Learning* 3:26, 1975.
60. Levinson, H. N. *A Solution to the Riddle Dyslexia.* New York: Springer, 1980.
61. Liberman, I., and Shankweiler, D. Speech, the Alphabet, and Teaching to Read. In L. Resnick and P. Weaver (Eds.), *Theory and Practice of Early Reading.* Hillsdale, N.J.: Erlbaum, 1979.
62. Liberman, I. Y., Mark, L. S., and Shankweiler, D. Reading disability: Methodological problems in information-processing analysis. *Science* 200:801, 1978.
63. Liberman, I. Y., et al. Letter confusions and reversals of sequence in the beginning reader: Implications for Orton's theory of developmental dyslexia. *Cortex* 7:127, 1971.
64. Ludlow, C. L. Research Directions and Needs Concerning the Neurological Bases of Language Disorders in Children. In C. L. Ludlow and M. E. Doran-Quine (Eds.), *The Neurological Bases of Language Disorders in Children: Methods and Directions for Research.* NINCDS Monograph No. 22, National Institute of Health Publication No. 79-440. Bethesda, Md.: U.S. Department of Health, Education, and Welfare, 1980. P. 183.
65. Mattis, S. Dyslexia Syndromes: A Working Hypothesis that Works. In A. L. Benton and D. Pearl (Eds.), *Dyslexia: An Appraisal of Current Knowledge.* New York: Oxford University Press, 1978. P. 43.
66. Mattis, S., French, J. H., and Rapin, I. Dyslexia in children and young adults: Three independent neuropsychological syndromes. *Dev. Med. Child Neurol.* (Minneap.) 17:150, 1975.
67. Mazziotta, J. C., et al. Tomographic mapping of human cerebral metabolism: Normal unstimulated state. *Neurology* (N.Y.) 31:503, 1981.

68. Menyuk, P. Relations Between Acquisition of Phonology and Reading. In J. T. Guthrie (Ed.), *Aspects of Reading Acquisition*. Baltimore: Johns Hopkins University Press, 1976. P. 89.
69. Millichap, J. G. Drugs in management of minimal brain dysfunction. *Ann. N. Y. Acad. Sci.* 205:321, 1973.
70. Morgan, W. P. A case of congenital word blindness. *Br. Med. J.* 2:1378, 1896.
71. Morrison, F. J., Giordani, B., and Nagy, J. Reading disability: An information-processing analysis. *Science* 196:77, 1977.
72. National Joint Committee for Learning Disabilities. Learning disabilities: Issues on definition. *Perspect. Dyslexia Orton Soc.* 6:1:4, 1981.
73. Ojemann, G. A., Fedio, P., and Van Buren, J. M. Anomia from pulvinar and subcortical parietal stimulation. *Brain* 91:99, 1968.
74. Oke, A., et al. Lateralization of norepinephrine in human thalamus. *Science* 200:1411, 1978.
75. Orton, S. T. *Reading, Writing and Speech Problems in Children: A Presentation of Certain Types of Disorders in the Development of the Language Faculty*. New York: Norton, 1937.
76. Partain, C. L., et al. Nuclear Magnetic Resonance Imaging. In C. M. Coulam et al. (Eds.), *The Physical Basis of Medical Imaging*. New York: Appleton-Century-Crofts, 1981. P. 243.
77. Phelps, M. E., et al. Tomographic mapping of human cerebral metabolism: Visual stimulation and deprivation. *Neurology* (N.Y.) 31:517, 1981.
78. Pirozzolo, F. J. *The Neuropsychology of Developmental Reading Disorders*. New York: Praeger, 1979.
79. Rawson, M. B. *Developmental Language Disability: Adult Accomplishments of Dyslexic Boys*. Baltimore: Johns Hopkins University Press, 1968.
80. Rees, N. S. The speech pathologist and the reading process. *A.S.H.A.* 16:255, 1974.
81. Rosenberger, P. B., and Hier, D. B. Cerebral asymmetry and verbal intellectual deficits. *Ann. Neurol.* 8:300, 1980.
82. Rutter, M. The concept of dyslexia. *Clin. Dev. Med.* 33:129, 1969.
83. Rutter, M. Prevalence and Types of Dyslexia. In A. L. Benton and D. Pearl (Eds.), *Dyslexia: An Appraisal of Current Knowledge*. New York: Oxford University Press, 1978. P. 3.
84. Rutter, M., Tizard, J., and Whitmore, K. (Eds.), *Education, Health and Behaviour*. London: Longmans, Green, 1970.
85. Rutter, M., et al. Research report: Isle of Wight Studies, 1964–1974. *Psycholog. Med.* 6:313, 1976.
86. Rutter, M., and Yule, W. Specific Reading Retardation. In L. Mann and D. A. Sabatino (Eds.), *The First Review of Special Education*, Vol. 2. Philadelphia: J.S.E., 1973.
87. Rutter, M., and Yule, W. The concept of specific reading retardation. *J. Child Psychol. Psychiatry* 16:181, 1975.
88. Satz, P., et al. Some developmental and predictive precursors of reading disabilities: A six-year follow-up. In A. L. Benton and D. Pearl (Eds.), *Dyslexia: An Appraisal of Current Knowledge*. New York: Oxford University Press, 1978. P. 313.
89. Sidtis, J. J., et al. Cognitive interaction after staged callosal section: Evidence for transfer of semantic activation. *Science* 212:344, 1981.
90. Silver, L. B. A proposed view on the etiology of the neurological learning disability syndrome. *J. Learn. Disabil.* 4:123, 1971.

91. Strauss, A. A. Typology in mental deficiency: Its clinical, psychological and educational implications. *Proc. Am. Assoc. Ment. Defic.* 63:85, 1939.
92. Strauss, A. A., and Kephart, N. C. *Psychopathology and Education of the Brain-Injured Child,* Vol. 2. New York: Grune & Stratton, 1955.
93. Strauss, A. A., and Lehtinen, L. E. *Psychopathology and Education of the Brain-Injured Child,* Vol. 1. New York: Grune & Stratton, 1947.
94. Strauss, A. A., and Werner, H. Disorders of conceptual thinking in the brain-injured child. *J. Nerv. Ment. Dis.* 96:153, 1942.
95. Symmes, J. S., and Rapoport, J. L. Unexpected reading failure. *Am. J. Orthopsychiatry* 42:82, 1972.
96. Thomas, C. J. Congenital "word-blindness" and its treatment. *Ophthalmoscope* 3:380, 1905.
97. Tobey, E. A., et al. Effects of stimulus-onset asynchrony on the dichotic performance of children with auditory-processing disorders. *J. Speech Hear. Res.* 22:197, 1979.
98. Van Buren, J. M., and Borke, R. C. Alterations in speech and the pulvinar: A serial section study of cerebrothalamic relationships in cases of acquired speech disorders. *Brain* 92:255, 1969.
99. Van Buren, J. M., and Borke, R. C. The mesial temporal substratum of memory: Anatomical studies in three individuals. *Brain* 95:599, 1972.
100. Vellutino, F. R. Alternative conceptualizations of dyslexia: Evidence in support of a verbal-deficit hypothesis. *Harvard Educ. Rev.* 47:334, 1977.
101. Wada, J. A., Clarke, R., and Hamm, A. Cerebral hemispheric asymmetry in humans: Cortical speech zones in 100 adult and 100 infant brains. *Arch. Neurol.* 32:239, 1975.
102. Wender, P. H. *Minimal Brain Dysfunction in Children.* New York: Wiley-Interscience, 1971.
103. Wilsher, C., Atkins, G., and Manfield, P. Piracetam as an aid to learning in dyslexia: Preliminary report. *Psychopharmacology* (Berlin) 65:107, 1979.
104. Witelson, S. F. Developmental dyslexia: Two right hemispheres and none left. *Science* 195:309, 1977.
105. Witelson, S. F., and Pallie, W. Left hemisphere specialization for language in the newborn: Neuroanatomical evidence of asymmetry. *Brain* 96:641, 1973.
106. Yingling, C. D. EEG research and learning disabilities. Read at the International Conference of the Association for Children With Learning Disabilities, San Francisco, February 28–March 3, 1979.
107. Yoss, R. E., and Daly, D. D. Hereditary aspects of narcolepsy. *Trans. Am. Neurol. Assoc.* 85:239, 1960.
108. Yule, W. Predicting reading ages on Neale's Analysis of Reading Ability. *Br. J. Educ. Psychol.* 37:252, 1967.
109. Yule, W. Differential prognosis of reading backwardness and specific reading retardation. *Br. J. Educ. Psychol.* 43:244, 1973.
110. Zaidel, A. The Split and Half Brains as Models of Congenital Language Disability. In C. L. Ludlow and M. E. Doran-Quine (Eds.), *The Neurological Bases of Language Disorders in Children: Methods and Directions for Research.* NINCDS Monograph No. 22, National Institute of Health Publication No. 79-440. Bethesda, Md.: U.S. Department of Health, Education, and Welfare, 1980. P. 55.
111. Zerbin-Rüdin, E. Kongenitale wortblindheit oder spezifische dyslexie (congenital word-blindness) (translated by S. G. Vandenberg.) *Bull. Orton Soc.* 17:47, 1967.

3
The Definition of Dyslexia: Language and Motor Deficits

Rita G. Rudel

There is by now substantial evidence supporting the view that delayed or impaired reading is consistently seen in the context of delayed or impaired language acquisition [48, 51]. Research on language performance has distinguished reading-disabled children not only from normal controls, but also from children with other learning disabilities [9, 14, 15, 17, 41, 42] and has also differentiated dyslexic children with different types of reading disability [12, 19, 34, 43, 46].

Difficulties with fine motor coordination [6], including poor copying ability, have also been reported [38]. That dyslexic children might have problems with hand-eye coordination is an implicit deduction of Orton's [36] hypothesis that "mixed dominance" is in some way involved in the etiology of reading disability. Levels of language development and motor proficiency appear, in fact, to be interrelated. In studies of preschool children (ages 3–6 years), we have found a robust correlation between speed of finger, hand, and foot movements and verbal fluency measures [7], and Annett [2] has reported vocabulary to be positively correlated with speed of foot movements.

There have also been electrophysiological [20, 21, 30, 39] and neuroanatomical [23] data reporting differences between children who readily learn to read and those who do not. Despite what thus appears to be considerable progress in defining dyslexia in terms of language, motor, electroencephalographic, and structural differences, dyslexia continues to be ill-defined in the public and even the medical mind. We are sometimes asked for clinical diagnoses of patients as young as 4 or as old as 40 years, with problems ranging from poor performance in nursery school to failures at school, at work, or at climbing the ladder of social success, all referred to us as "possibly dyslexic."

To some extent, an exclusionary consensus has emerged that defines dyslexia as reading impairment in the absence of certain negative factors [11, 22, 40] but does not define the *presence* of symptoms that have been found to be consistently correlated with the disorder. Thus, and quite reasonably, dyslexia is considered as a plausible diagnosis or as a category for research when limiting factors such as neurological, psychiatric, sensory, and intellectual impairment, as well as an inadequate environment for learning, have been ruled out. But the definition has no provision for the inclusion of a specific set of deficits except for the deficit in reading, which is expressed as some degree of discrepancy between mental age, chronological age, or grade level and measures of reading ability. These are, however, numerical values, which may not have the validity they are presumed to possess. How the discrepancy is to be determined has never been satisfactorily resolved.

This work was in part supported by a grant from the U.S. Department of Health, Education and Welfare, Public Health Service, USPHS HD 12278-02.

Rutter [43] has, in fact, insisted that discrepancy scores or ratios can be misleading inasmuch as they assume a parallel between IQ and reading that does not exist and they fail to take into account a "regression effect" that leads to an overestimate of reading retardation in very intelligent children and an underestimate in the less intelligent populations. A regression value [52] predicts achievement from correlations between reading, chronological age, and IQ in the social and educational population appropriate for each child. A discrepancy between the reading grade level (RGL) of the child and the expected reading grade level (ERGL) of that population then defines the degree of impairment. The amount of discrepancy between RGL and ERGL that defines reading impairment still has to be arbitrarily set, however, and the question persists: how much difference is sufficient to create a problem, and does that discrepancy differ for various groups of children?

There are almost as many questions raised by the discrepancy approach as there are questions answered. Is one justified in classifying as dyslexic an upper-middle-class child with a reading age equal to his chronological age when most of the others in his school are reading considerably above level? Or, in contrast, do we judge as perfectly adequate the poor performance of an economically disadvantaged child with a low RGL that is nonetheless on a par with, or even above the ERGL of others in his school district? What if both these hypothetical children can sustain the tested level of reading only with constant, intensive reading remediation? This may be somewhat akin to questioning whether a diabetic is still a diabetic if he responds favorably to insulin but cannot live without it. In fact, we do not know whether children with reading scores at or close to grade level, but with histories of difficulty in learning to read, have the same or different correlated deficits from those demonstrated in children with clearly deficient reading scores. In other words, do the correlated symptoms go away when remediation has brought reading level up to grade level?

There are other problems with the definition of dyslexia by discrepancy score. One problem is the reliance on test scores that do not necessarily measure the same thing. Even the two sets of scores (verbal and performance) on the Wechsler's Intelligence Scale for Children–Revised (WISC-R) test are often very different. Belmont and Birch [3] reviewed 12 studies in which the mean verbal scale was lower than the performance scale in retarded readers. They confirmed this in their own study, and similar discrepancies have been subsequently reported by Warrington [50] and Ackerman, Peters, and Dykman [1]. Kaufman [28] has noted, however, that the *average* WISC-R discrepancy, regardless of direction, was 9.7 IQ points for all children ages 6 to 16 years, and a discrepancy of 12 points or more occurred in 33 percent of the standardization sample. He notes that additional research is needed to determine whether verbal-performance IQ discrepancies really do characterize learning-disabled children. Many studies of dyslexic children use the verbal *or* performance IQ to "rule out" retardation in their reading-disabled groups. Obviously, very different biases are "ruled in" by such a procedure.

Methods of the Present Study

Similarly, reading tests, even when they measure only decoding skills and not comprehension, may yield very discrepant scores because they are standardized on different populations. There is also the issue regarding content and reading rate. Some tests require the reading of single words, others of passages; some are timed, others untimed. The selection of children as reading impaired, and therefore the definition of dyslexia, may depend on which type of test is used. To determine whether such test variables made any difference in who is, and who is not, diagnosed as dyslexic by discrepancy score and to evaluate once again the relationship of reading disorder to language and motor proficiency, we undertook a retrospective study based on our patient files.

The test results of 50 children, ages 6 years and 11 months to 14 years, who had been seen for diagnostic evaluation during a period of 18 months were recorded. Rather than establish a priori discrepancy criteria for selection, only the following constraints were established:

1. The intake information had to include some reference to a specific problem with reading, and at upper age levels, to unusually slow reading.
2. On the WISC-R, the subject had to have scored a full scale IQ score of over 80, but either a verbal or performance score of at least 90.
3. There could be no hard neurological signs or sensory or psychiatric disorders.
4. There had to have been adequate educational opportunity.

Assuming, as does the third edition of the *Diagnostic and Statistical Manual of Mental Disorders* (*DSM-III*), that dyslexia and emotional problems may coexist without their necessarily being causally related, children with emotional problems were not excluded. Referrals were from neurologists, psychiatrists, school guidance counsellors, and parents themselves. Children referred by personnel at pediatric and pediatric neurology clinics were also included, and therefore, the population selected did *not* have socioeconomic homogeneity.

The original assessment, which included a WISC-R as well as other standardized tests (e.g., Peabody Picture Vocabulary Test [PPVT], Ravens), generally took an entire day to complete. Most of the children were also given two reading tests: the Wide Range Achievement Test (WRAT), which is untimed and consists of individual words graded for difficulty, and the Gray Oral Reading Test (GORT), a timed passage reading test also graded for difficulty.

Tests developed in research studies of learning-disabled children were also administered. For this retrospective study, however, the scores on two expressive language tests, the Oldfield-Wingfield Test [35] and the Rapid Automatized Naming [14], and time scores on six motor tests, these being the speed of repetitive and alternating movements of fingers, hand, and feet [9, 10], were tabulated. Each child had been characterized as left- or right-handed, -footed, or -eyed prior to administration of the timed motor tests, and we examined these data to determine the prevalence of mixed dominance (right hand–left eye preference) among them. In sum, we selectively utilized data obtained by at least five different testers for diagnosis of reading impairment: (1) intelligence quotient, (2) two sets of reading scores, (3) lateral preference, (4) scores on two expressive language tests, and (5) six timed tests of fine motor coordination. We sought to determine the extent to which the data from this clinical group with reading problems would differ from data on more homogeneous reading-disabled research groups selected by accepted discrepancy criteria. The goal was to take a step beyond the diagnosis of dyslexia by exclusion and discrepancy [11] to a more substantive definition in terms of associated deficits.

Subjects

The children in the present analysis were randomly selected from a group meeting the IQ criteria discussed above and lacking hard neurological signs or sensory or psychiatric disorders. There turned out to be 40 boys and 10 girls, a sex ratio not representative of our overall referrals. During the same 18-month period, we saw for complaints other than reading difficulty 62 children, of whom 35 were boys and 27 girls, a male-female proportion of 56:44 percent, compared with 80:20 percent for children with reading problems. The predominance of males in dyslexic populations has been noted in many previous studies [5, 8, 45].

Table 3-1 provides average WISC-R IQ scores according to age groupings, sex, and source of referral (clinical versus private) for the children analyzed

Table 3-1. **WISC-R IQ scores of of 50 children with reading problems according to age, sex, and source of referral**

Characteristic	n	Sex		Verbal		Performance		Full scale	
		M	F	Mean	SD	Mean	SD	Mean	SD
Age									
6–8 years	19	15	4	97.4	14.5	103.1	14.1	100.0	14.2
9–11 years	22	18	4	94.2	12.5	98.3	13.9	95.2	10.0
12–14 years	9	7	2	105.1	7.1	106.0	9.1	105.6	4.8
Sex									
Male	40			97.0	12.1	99.8	12.8	97.7	9.8
Female	10			98.8	16.5	108.2	14.0	103.6	17.0
Referral source									
Clinical	20	14	6	89.0	12.6	103.4	12.2	94.8	11.6
Private	30	26	4	103.0	9.8	100.3	14.1	101.6	10.9
Total	50	40	10	97.4	12.9	101.5	13.4	98.9	11.6

WISC-R = Wechsler's Intelligence Scale for Children–Revised; n = number in sample; SD = standard deviation.

in the present study. The group as a whole is clearly of normal intelligence. Thirty of the 50 children were private referrals, implying higher socioeconomic status, and 20 were from pediatric and pediatric neurology clinics. The preponderance of males was much less marked among the clinical referrals; in fact, 6 of the 10 girls were clinical patients. The IQ data were analyzed using three-way analysis of variance (ANOVA) (age × sex × referral source [clinical or private]). As compared to clinical patients, private patients had significantly higher full scale ($p < .05$) and verbal ($p < .001$) IQ scores. A significant ($p < .05$) sex × referral source interaction was found for the full scale IQ and performance IQ scores in that female private patients scored higher than female clinical patients, while there were not significant differences for male patients. More than half of the subjects had relatively equal verbal and performance IQ scores, exhibiting less than the 10-point discrepancy on the two scales that were given as the mean difference reported for a normal population [28]. Of the patients whose test scores showed discrepancies greater than 10 points, twice as many had higher performance than verbal IQ scores, but none of those referred by the clinics had higher verbal than performance scores, and in this respect, they were significantly different than the private patients ($p < .004$).

The children of this sample had received and were receiving extra educational help through remedial reading, private tutoring, or resource-room time, but the range of ages and variety of school districts from which they were referred make it impossible to characterize the quality or amount of remediation they received.

The Classification of Dyslexia

Reading Tests

Table 3-2 provides the mean RGL scores on the WRAT and the GORT for the group as a whole, as well as for the subgroups by age, sex, and referral source. Analyses of variance applied to the RGL scores of the children yielded a significant test effect ($p < .002$); virtually every child scored higher on the WRAT than on the GORT. As would be expected, there was also a significant ($p < .001$) age effect on the RGL scores, but there were no significant differences between sex or referral source groups. There was a significant test versus referral source interaction, indicating that the difference between the test scores was greater among the private patients ($p < .01$). This may be attributable in part to the fact that a high percentage of the clinical referrals were girls, whose mean RGL did not differ on the two tests. What appeared to be an increasing disparity with age between the tests was not statistically significant according to the analysis of test versus age interaction. However, when corrected for age (either chronological age or mental age), there is a significant age effect ($p < .001$), indicating that younger children exhibit less reading retardation. The severity of reading disorder appears to be greater in older children. It is impossible to tell whether this result reflects a slow

Table 3-2. **Reading grade level scores on the WRAT (single words) and GORT (passages)**

Characteristic	WRAT (n = 46)		GORT (n = 50)	
	Mean	SD	Mean	SD
Age (years)				
6–8	2.72	1.1	1.92	0.8
9–11	3.67	1.2	2.67	1.6
12–14	7.08	2.8	4.72	2.0
Sex				
Male	3.96	2.2	2.58	1.4
Female	3.37	1.8	3.45	2.5
Referral source				
Clinical 20	3.03	1.4	2.12	1.0
Private 30	4.46	2.4	3.18	2.0
Total	3.87	2.2	2.75	1.7

WRAT = Wide Range Achievement Test; GORT = Gray Oral Reading Test; n = number in sample; SD = standard deviation.

rate of improvement (and therefore an increase in degree of reading disability with age) or a selection bias, given that the most severely impaired children are still reading disabled at older ages.

It may be reasonably concluded that this group, referred on the basis of reading problems, read single words better than passages and, therefore, that determination of dyslexia based on their scores would differ depending on which test was used. The group as a whole could be characterized as reading disabled (23.9-month discrepancy between mental age and reading age) if one used the passage reading scores as tested by the GORT. However, the group could not be readily diagnosed as reading disabled using the WRAT, which tests the reading of single words and for which the mean discrepancy was only 8.6 months (for 46 of the 50 children).

If one calculates a reading quotient $\left(RQ = \dfrac{\text{reading age}}{\text{mental age}}\right)$ for each child, using an RQ of 0.85 as a cutoff to divide the group for severity of impairment, 13 out of 46, or 28 percent, would be classified as dyslexic from their single-word (WRAT) reading, whereas 31 of 50, or 62 percent, would be so classified based on passage reading (GORT) (χ^2 = 10.99, p < .001). As shown in Table 3-3, the mean RQs calculated with GORT scores are significantly lower than comparable RQs using WRAT scores (p < .001). Still, RQs determined by using the scores on the two tests are highly correlated (r = .74). Although their absolute reading scores were lower, the clinical group had the same proportion of deficient readers by discrepancy criteria as did the private patients.

The amount or direction of difference between verbal and performance IQ in the screening did *not* predict reading scores on either test and did not predict the discrepancy between single-word and passage reading. There was

Table 3-3. Number and percent of children impaired in reading on the WRAT and GORT

Characteristic	RQ[a] < 0.85 on WRAT		RQ[a] < 0.85 on GORT		Not reading impaired by either test	
	Frequency[b]	Percent	Frequency[b]	Percent	Frequency[b]	Percent
Age (years)						
6–8	2 (19)	11	7 (19)	37	12 (19)	63
9–11	6 (19)	32	16 (22)	73	6 (22)	27
12–14	5 (8)	63	8 (9)	89	1 (9)	11
Sex						
Male	10 (39)	26	25 (40)	62	15 (40)	38
Female	3 (7)	43	6 (10)	60	4 (10)	40
Referral source						
Clinical	5 (19)	26	12 (20)	60	8 (20)	40
Private	8 (27)	30	19 (30)	63	11 (30)	37
Total	13 (46)	28	31 (50)	62	10 (50)	38

[a] $RQ = \dfrac{\text{reading age}}{\text{mental age}}$

[b] The values shown in parentheses provide the total number of children in each subgroup. WRAT = Wide Range Achievement Test; GORT = Gray Oral Reading Test; RQ = reading quotient.

only one instance of a nonsignificant trend involving those pupils with lower verbal than performance IQ scores. These pupils appeared to exhibit lower RQs on single-word (WRAT) reading, possibly a reflection of inadequate vocabulary affecting both tests.

How can one explain the difference between scores on two reading tests? In addition to the fact that they were standardized on different sample populations, there are other differences. The GORT is a timed test and therefore penalizes slowness, which the WRAT does not. Many of the children, particularly those who require tutoring in phonetic decoding, read with painful slowness, one word at a time. Intuitively one would expect the reading of prose, given the effect of context and the syntactic and semantic constraints, to be simpler than reading unrelated words. This may not be true for children with reading problems [18]. Using an auditory test of object naming in which incomplete sentences or definitions are read aloud, we have found that the semantic and syntactic cues provided by simple, declarative sentences are not utilized as well by dyslexic children as by nondyslexic controls [42]. Vogel [49] reported that dyslexics also do not use syntax as well as controls in speaking.

Analysis of reading errors on the GORT revealed that most often the dyslexics misread function words, short auxiliary verbs, pronouns, prepositions, and articles, thereby rendering their reading much like the speech of certain adult asphasic patients [4]. The fact that the difference between the WRAT and GORT scores in Table 3-2 tended to *increase* with age, although not significantly, suggests that with schooling, age, and reading remediation, single-word decoding may approach normative levels more rapidly than the reading of prose.

To ascertain whether reading single words and prose would yield different scores in other populations and with other tests, the Woodcock (single word) and Gilmore (prose) reading tests were administered to 57 students without learning problems and to 19 with learning problems in a local parochial school. The Gilmore reading test was chosen because reading speed does not affect the accuracy score. There was a statistically insignificant trend among those in regular classes to read prose passages *better* than single words. The reverse was true for children in classes for the learning disabled. However, the latter result, that single-word reading was better than prose reading among the 19 learning disabled, only approached statistical significance ($p < .05$).

Whether or not greater difficulty with prose reading is symptomatic of dyslexia, this unexpected finding makes it imperative that any definition of dyslexia that is dependent on a reading score specify which test was used, that is, whether it involves reading single words or prose and whether latency measures affected the scores.

Tests of Language

Naming of Pictured Objects

The Oldfield-Wingfield Picture Naming Test [35] was employed on the study group to characterize the nature of naming errors, as had been done in previous dyslexia studies [14, 17]. In this test, there are 36 drawings of objects to be named, 10 practice items and 26 to be scored, the names of which range in Lorge-Thorndike word-frequency groups from *bed* (Group 1) through *gyroscope* (Group 7). Errors were recorded and categorized as circumlocutory, substitutions (paraphasic-in-kind), phonological, or sequential, all of which we have classified as "dysphasic" (linquistic) errors. Misidentifications of the objects were classified as perceptual errors. There were also "don't know" responses and unclassified errors.

Earlier studies [15, 52] have demonstrated that children defined as dyslexic [15] in terms of an RQ of 0.80 or below (median = 0.69) or, as in Yule's study [52], in terms of a multiple regression equation [17] made significantly more dysphasic errors on the Oldfield-Wingfield test of naming pictured objects than did matched groups of learning-disabled children who were not dyslexic. In both of these previous studies [15, 52], the nondyslexic made significantly more perceptual errors, that is, misidentification of the objects. The Yule study yielded a reversal of relative frequency of dysphasic and perceptual errors in the two learning-disabled groups. The dyslexic group made 0 to 50 percent dysphasic errors (mean = 41%) and 0 to 33 percent perceptual errors (mean = 15%), while the nondyslexic learning-disabled group made 0 to 55 percent perceptual errors (mean = 38%) and 0 to 29 percent dysphasic

Table 3-4. Percent dysphasic (language) and perceptual (mistaken identity) errors to total errors on a test (Oldfield-Wingfield) of naming pictured objects

Characteristic	Percent of dysphasic errors			Percent of perceptual errors	
	n (48)*	Mean	SD	Mean	SD
Age (years)					
6–8	17	41.2	14.0	17.5	15.1
9–11	22	53.0	15.8	24.9	17.7
12–14	9	64.3	22.0	18.6	15.8
Sex					
Male	38	51.3	16.6	22.0	16.7
Female	10	49.6	24.4	17.5	16.3
Referral source					
Clinical	19	43.4	17.8	17.9	15.0
Private	29	55.9	17.0	23.1	17.4
Degree of impairment					
RQ <0.85	30	53.27	20.26	20.8	15.8
RQ >0.85	19	47.06	13.85	21.5	18.1
Total	48*	50.9	18.2	21.1	16.5

*Two subjects were not given this test; both were male and in the age range 6–8 years; 1 was a clinical patient and 1 private.
n = number in sample; SD = standard deviation; RQ = reading quotient.

errors (mean = 20%). A linear discriminant function analysis revealed that the proportion of dysphasic errors was the best single indicator of dyslexia in the two learning-disabled groups.

As can be seen from Table 3-4, among the subjects of this retrospective study, selected only on the basis of referral for evaluation of reading problems, a mean of 50.9 percent of total errors were dysphasic and only 21.1 percent of total errors were perceptual ($p < .001$). A four-way analysis of variance (ANOVA) performed on the data revealed a significant age effect ($p < .01$). While the proportion of dysphasic errors increased with age, the proportion of perceptual errors did not. However, the age by error type interaction was not statistically significant. There were not differences attributable to sex, source, referral (clinical or private), or severity of impairment as determined by an RQ above or below 0.85.

Latencies on Rapid Automatized Naming

The stimulus categories on the Rapid Automatized Naming (RAN) test are colors, numbers, lower case letters, and pictured objects (from the 4-year-old level of the Stanford-Binet Vocabulary Test) with five items per category, thereby generating 20 of each stimulus. Children were instructed to name each item on each card as rapidly as possible; time and errors were recorded

Table 3-5. Number and percent of children slow on Rapid Automatized Naming (RAN) and proportion of tests on which they were slow

Characteristic	n[a]	Children slow on two or more tests		Mean proportion (%) of tests children were slow on
		Frequency	Percent	
Age (years)				
6–8	17	10	59	34
9–11	20	18	90	64
12–14	3	3[b]	100	72
Sex				
Male	31	23	74	53
Female	9	8	89	44
Referral source				
Clinical	17	15	88	57
Private	23	16	70	48
Degree of impairment				
RQ <0.85	23	19	83	64
RQ >0.85	17	12	70	35
Total	40	31	78	52

[a]Only 40 of the 50 subjects were given this test.
[b]Based on norms for children 10–11 years of age.
n = number in sample; RQ = reading quotient.

[14]. Scores were compared with data obtained from a previous study [13] on children without learning problems. This control group consisted of 180 children, 90 boys and 90 girls, distributed in six age groups from age 5 years and 11 months to 10 years and 11 months. Only children from the middle range of school achievement were included. The school population from which they were chosen had a mean IQ of 106 ($\pm$9). For this study, we measured only response latencies.

Table 3-5 provides RAN test results for the study group. The test was not administered to 6 of the 9 children in the oldest group (12–14 years) or to 4 of the youngest children (6–8 years). Therefore, data on only 40 subjects were available. A child was characterized as "slow" on any one of the four parts of the test if his score was more than 1 standard deviation above the mean latency for his age. Of the total study group, 78 percent were slow on two or more of the subtests, whereas 16 percent of the control group were slow on one of each by the same criteria. An ANOVA was used to compare time scores on the RAN of the 40 study group children against controls, matched for age and sex, selected from the previous study [13]. Time scores of the 12- to 14-year-olds in the study group were compared to those of the 10- to 11-year-old controls, the oldest group tested in the normative sample. These comparisons are provided in Table 3-6.

Table 3-6. Analysis of variance of Rapid Automatized Naming (RAN) time scores of 40 children with reading problems compared with controls*

Factors	Colors		Objects		Letters		Numbers	
	F value	Significance	F value	Significance	F value	Significance	F value	Significance
Group	13.96	*.0003*	14.49	*.0002*	40.04	*.0001*	24.56	*.0001*
Age	5.48	*.0051*	10.77	*.0001*	15.22	*.0001*	7.84	*.0006*
Sex	2.47	.1182	0.22	.6367	0.23	.6305	1.16	.2843
Group × age	0.57	.5664	0.42	.6575	0.77	.4630	0.70	.5001
Group × sex	0.01	.9094	0.71	.4007	0.04	.8517	1.19	.2777
Age × sex	4.07	*.0190*	1.63	.1996	0.79	.4537	1.35	.2612
Group × age × sex	2.96	.0548	4.92	*.0085*	1.99	.1410	2.01	.1378

*Control data were available only to ages 10–11 years; time scores of the older experimental children, ages 12–14 years, were compared to those of younger controls. Significant results are in italics.

There were highly significant age and group differences, implying that rate improved with age for both groups, and children with reading problems were significantly slower than controls. There were no age or sex differences nor any interactions except within the reading-impaired group, where 9- to 11-year-old girls were significantly faster than boys of the same age.

In sum, children with reading problems are slow at word, letter, or number retrieval even when the stimuli constitute as small a universe as five. Without time constraints they also have difficulty retrieving the exact names of objects. They tend to circumlocute, use the wrong word in the same class ("nail" for "screw"), mispronounce the word ("deathoscope"), or missequence syllables. They do not, however, make a higher proportion of errors in perception than do control subjects of the same age.

Tests of Lateral Preference and Motor Skill

Lateral hand preference of the study subjects was determined on the basis of handwriting and nine mimed actions (e.g., cutting with a scissors, throwing a ball). Designation was based on 7 out of 10 of these actions. For the study group as a whole, there was the same proportion of left-handers as in non-dyslexic populations, 10 percent, but 20 percent of the girls were left-handed. Eye preference was determined in three trials of sighting dominance by having the child look through holes of different size cut into large sheets of paper held in both hands. Of the 49 children for whom data were collected, mixed dominance occurred in 47 percent (all male). Forty-three percent were right-handed and left-eyed, another 4 percent left-handed and right-eyed, and 2 percent (all male) had no consistent eye preference. This proportion of mixed dominance lies midway between the 30 percent generally reported for normal populations and the 60 percent that Denckla has recorded in her clinical practice with learning-disabled children.

The tests of motor coordination used in our diagnostic service were developed by Denckla [9, 10], who also ascertained the norms. They consist of three repetitive and three alternative movements of the feet, hands, and fingers, left and right: toe taps, hand pats, and finger taps, heel-toe alternation, hand pronation-supination, and finger-thumb opposition. The time required to carry out 20 of each of the repetitive movements, 10 complete alternations, or five finger successions on each side is recorded.

The subjects constituting Denckla's standardization sample were average-achieving children from middle-class suburban communities attending schools where the mean IQ range was 106 to 112. They ranged in age from 5 years to 10 years, and 11 months, and therefore, comparisons of our oldest group (ages 12–14 years) were made with Denckla's 10-year-olds. Table 3-7 presents the statistical results comparing the study group to the control group in motor skills. There was the expected increase in speed with age on all measures, and except for heel-toe alternation, the study groups were significantly slower than the controls. The 10 girls in our population were faster than the boys on four of the six tests, but not on hand and finger repetitive movements.

As seen in Table 3-7, group by age interactions were significant. However, the children with reading problems were slower than controls only up to age 11 years. This may reflect the fact that 12- to 14-year-olds were compared with younger children, the 10- to 11-year-olds in the standardization sample. Norms on older children are needed before it can be concluded that slowness on these tests is not symptomatic of reading-impaired children after age 10.

In Table 3-7, group by sex interactions on toe taps, heel-toe alternation, and finger succession movements reflect the more rapid performance of the study group girls, who on these measures were not slower than the controls. Boys were slower than girls in the two younger age groups only, accounting for the age group by sex interactions.

Wherever an effect of laterality (side) was noted in Table 3-7, the left side was significantly slower than the right for both groups, but there was a greater difference between the rate of left and right movements among the reading impairment than among the controls. This was true for toe taps, heel-toe alternations, hand pronation-supination, and finger tapping. For hand pats only, the reading impaired were slower than the controls only with the right hand.

One may note from the size of the F values in the table that children with reading problems are better discriminated from a control population by repetitive rather than alternative movements. Stated another way, the number of unaffected movements, or those within normal limits, were twice as great among alternating than among repetitive movements.

The motor data were also analyzed for a difference between those with RQs greater than 0.85 and those whose RQs fell below that level. For foot movements, toe taps, and heel-toe alternation, the group with higher RQs was paradoxically slower. On finger repetition, only the youngest children with

Table 3-7. Analysis of variance of motor coordination time scores of 49 children with reading problems compared with controls*

Factors	Toe taps		Heel-toe alternations		Hand pats		Hand pronation-supination		Finger taps	
	F value	Significance	F value	Significance	F value	Significance	F value	Significance	F value	Significance
Group	27.899	*.001*	1.562	.213	21.535	*.001*	6.902	*.010*	33.86	*.001*
Age	10.523	*.001*	21.939	*.001*	9.346	*.001*	13.676	*.001*	7.264	*.001*
Sex	8.492	*.004*	15.601	*.001*	1.137	.283	4.923	*.028*	1.929	.167
Group × age	5.6	*.005*	1.687	.188	3.302	*.039*	3.513	*.032*	2.412	.093
Group × sex	12.92	*.001*	4.239	*.041*	0.473	.493	2.891	.091	1.869	.174
Age × sex	4.914	*.009*	0.074	.5	0.125	.5	0.148	.5	7.032	*.002*
Group × age × sex	5.127	*.007*	0.407	.5	0.98	.377	0.026	.5	8.166	*.001*
Side (left or right)	4.799	*.03*	24.074	*.001*	N.S.	N.S.	14.201	*.001*	32.256	*.001*
Group × side	All laterality interactions were not significant		N.S.	N.S.	7.072	*.009*	All laterality interactions were not significant		All laterality interactions were not significant	

*Control data were available only on children ages 7–11 years; time scores of the older experimental children, ages 12–14 years, were compared to those of younger controls. Significant results are in italics.
N.S. = not significant.

higher RQs were slower than the others. The left side (finger, hand, or foot) in our reading-impaired population was slower than the right, regardless of severity of impairment indicated by RQ.

Mixed dominance, difficulties with fine motor coordination, and the slower left side in reading-disabled children are further explored in Chapter 10, and I shall therefore restrict myself here to evaluating their significance in formulating a definition of dyslexia.

Conclusions

Difficulties in Defining Dyslexia

However one sets the extent and limits of reading disability, there are difficulties of definition, and while these may differ somewhat in their application to diagnosis and research, both demand consensus. Consensus has been achieved to some degree in a priori fashion in relation to the exclusion of conditions that are presumed to inhibit learning to read at a normal pace and at acceptable levels, but not in relation to discrepancy measures. The question of *how much* difference between reading quotient and reading expectancy is necessary or sufficient to create a problem for the child can only be answered arbitrarily, even within well-defined social contexts. A discrepancy definition of dyslexia, even with exclusionary clauses, cannot account for different degrees of remediation effects on the achievement of grade or near grade level reading scores. Reading at grade level cannot mean the same thing for children who attain it without special help as for those whose grade level standing depends on continued infusions of special training.

To continue the analogy made earlier, assessments of blood sugar level do not distinguish the insulin-injected diabetic from the nondiabetic who produces his own insulin. As has been demonstrated, assessment of reading levels, or of discrepancies between them and expectancy based on age and intelligence, is fraught with arbitrariness. Which test should one use? Should such tests be timed or untimed? Reading, except for the reading of road signs, rarely involves single words, and although one usually may read at one's own pace, it is not a very useful skill if it is too slow for keeping up with others, for timed examinations, or for comprehension or recall. Besides, slow reading is laborious and even boring, as those of us who have plowed through foreign language texts can attest. One can reduce the statistical size of dyslexic populations by requiring only the untimed reading of single words or, conversely, increase their size by the use of timed prose reading tests. This dilemma furthermore involves only decoding and not comprehension.

Under the most ideal conditions, with the most statistically sophisticated selection methods, definition by reading quotient can only confirm that a problem exists and that the child does not read as well as he should, given his level of intelligence. It does not tell us whether the child's problem is one of motivation, lack of effort, or the expression of an inadequately functioning biological system. The reading discrepancy approach has had heuristic value in establishing correlates of dyslexia, but ultimately the disorder will have to be defined in terms of these related deficits. Language impairment appears to be a critical place to start, since it can be demonstrated in both acquired alexia as well as developmental dyslexia [26]. Luria [33] speculated that naming difficulties adversely affected the entire speech system and that reading and writing were simply other aspects of speech activity. Liberman and Shankweiler [31] restated this concept as "reading is somehow parasitic on speech."

Naming Impairment as a Deficit Correlate

The children seen in our diagnostic service for "reading problems" were as impaired on both naming tests as groups of children selected by the usual statistical procedure for research. They made more errors naming 26 pictured objects [35] than did control groups of adequate readers, and the proportion of these errors classified as "dysphasic" was as great as had been establishd in research studies with dyslexic children [15, 17]. In contrast, the number of "perceptual" errors they made did not differ from controls. Children with reading problems, whatever their discrepancy scores, appear to be dysnomic, tending to describe rather than name objects, to substitute the name of another object in the same class, to mispronounce, or to missequence the syllables. Their lexicons do not have adequate semantic or phonological organization, a characteristic also of dysphasic adult patients [35]. Like most adult patients with alexia [25], they have word retrieval problems. Also like dysphasic adults, however, they have at least average intelligence.

That the speed of naming is a critical variable in the reading process is indicated by the study group results on the RAN test. Compared to the expected 16-percent level of the control group, 78 percent of this study group were slow on two or more of the four tests. The RAN protocols provide one possible explanation for the study group's slowness in naming repeated stimuli. Although each subtest included only five items (five numbers, five letters, five colors, five objects), these children would often, after first naming them correctly, provide one or more incorrect names in the same class, but not from among the five subtest items' names (e.g., calling the clock a "watch," red "orange," *a* "e"). Almost as often, they would immediately correct the error, but it was as if they had difficulty maintaining a set for the very limited universe of names from which their responses had to be rapidly retrieved. Possibly this reflects poor establishment or maintenance of language expectancy or "set," which is also critical in passage reading, where semantic and syntactic cues provide another, even more complex, form of language expectancy. These results and those of other word-finding tests [42] suggest that poor readers may not adequately employ either type of cue.

Wolf [51] has also reported a strong relationship between reading and speed of word retrieval. A battery of naming tests (including parts of the RAN) yielded a correlation coefficient of .74 ($p < .001$) between naming and reading tests, replicating Goodglass and Kaplan's [24] correlation of .74 between naming and reading scores in an aphasic population. Wolf [51] also reported that "the older the child the more latency differences increased between reading groups," supporting the data provided here of an increasing proportion of paraphasic errors and longer naming latencies with age. Concomitantly, there was a trend for the difference between single-word and passage decoding skill to increase with age. Consistent with the evidence that our oldest group was the most impaired, Wolf [51] reported a plateau on naming tests between 8 and 10 years of age among reading-disabled children, suggesting to her a "qualitatively distinct pattern of lexical retrieval . . . not simply a maturational lag." As noted before, there is a possible selection bias in cross-sectional studies (like this one and Wolf's), which attempt to assess age differences as if they were longitudinal changes. Possibly those children of 12 years or older who are still having trouble reading are the most impaired and may have always had greater deficits. There is as yet no evidence from longitudinal studies that the deficits increase as dyslexic children grow older.

The degree of reading impairment, measured as an RQ of more than or less than 0.85, did *not* significantly distinguish the degree of language impairment as measured on the two tests used in the study, although the trend was in that direction. With ongoing remediation, children may improve to normal or near normal reading levels while their underlying deficits remain the same, accounting, possibly, for the lack of correlation between speed of naming (RAN) and reading scores. Wolf [51] reports to have found, using naming tests, previously undetected language problems in average readers who were described as never having worked to their potential. She says, "In reality, these children were working very hard to achieve their on-grade-level status." As we have noted, all the children in our sample needed and were receiving remediation to achieve or sustain their reading performance, but whether or not they had "caught up" to grade level in reading, their language impairment had not caught up and remained untreated.

Motor Deficit Correlates

The relevance of mixed hand-eye dominance to reading disability is discussed in Chapter 10. We found it in almost half of this population with reading problems, and while not as striking a difference from the normative 30 percent as other differences we found, it continues to be a "where there is smoke there may be fire" sign.

Our motor data are consistent with a great many other findings of slowing in learning-disabled children, including excess slow-wave activity on the electroencephalogram [27, 44]; (see also Chap. 9). The most robust deviations from normal were found on the simpler, repetitive tasks, especially foot tapping. This is of particular interest in view of Annett's [2] finding that speed of foot movements correlated with size of vocabulary. In another study (see Chap. 10), in which Denckla compares the motor skill of 40 carefully selected reading-disabled children with these same norms, the dyslexics were distinguished from controls only on repetitive toe taps and only at ages 7 and 8 years. Duffy (see Chap. 7) reports differences between dyslexic boys and controls near the foot area (supplementary motor strip) in his brain electrical activity mapping (BEAM) studies, and Denckla speculates on the relationship between finely tuned foot movements and reading, a skill heavily dependent on language. It may, as she suggests, have something to do with the cephalocaudal axis of development, the most distant relay from the cortical control (the foot) being the most vulnerable. Disturbances of motor control, after all, are almost always present with acquired aphasia and/or alexia.

While the motor data thus appear to fit nicely with other evidence in suggesting a link between speed of fine coordinated movements and language (or reading), there is a curious difference between these data and Denckla's that demands close scrutiny. The children with reading problems in this study were clearly more deviant and were impaired on more of the motor tests than were the dyslexic children reported by Denckla. Yet both groups were selected to meet the same exclusionary criteria. Denckla, however, aiming at a "pure" dyslexic group, also screened her patients for any evidence of attention deficit disorder. In the generally accepted practice, I did not apply this screening. This difference in the extent, if not the direction, of results may reflect the relative "purity" of the two groups.

We demonstrated earlier [16] that hyperactive boys (now defined as attention deficit disorder [ADD] in the *DSM-III*) were significantly slower than controls in these same motor tests. Apparently, children with reading problems *plus* attention disorders are slower on motor tests than are children with reading problems but without attention disorders. Attention deficit disorder in some of these children may also explain the inverse relationship, noted before, between severity of reading impairment (as determined by an RQ < 0.85) and motor speed. Slowing on motor tasks appears to reflect a relatively greater degree of attention disorder. Those with lower RQs (< 0.85) were probably more "purely" reading disabled and thus more directly comparable to Denckla's group. Attention disorder may play a large role in determining what is investigated as "dyslexia" and therefore in the outcome of studies. Yet, attention disorder is rarely recognized as the confounding factor that it is in the selection of dyslexia children for research. It is *not* one of the items in the consensus for exclusion, nor do studies usually indicate whether or not experimental groups were screened for attentional problems.

In this study, the direction of change with age of the language data appears to be different than that of the motor data. Although the reading-disabled population was distinguished from controls on both, changes with age were in opposite directions, with increasing differences on tests of language (confirming Wolf [51]) and diminishing differences on the motor tests (confirming the report by Denckla, Chap. 10). In view of the fact that on the motor tests, as well as on the RAN, children older than 11 years were being compared with younger controls, it is not likely that the difference in direction is due to opposite floor and ceiling effects. It would seem, rather, that the plateau in naming speed and naming accuracy reached by normal readers on our tests at about age 11 is not achieved by older poor readers, who may, in fact, plateau at lower levels [51]. In contrast, the motor slowness, at least on these tests, appears to be outgrown by age 9 to 10 years, a possible indicator of "maturational lag" [29]. It may, in fact, be a stronger predictor than a correlate of reading disability.

Defining Dyslexia

It has long been acknowledged that developmental dyslexia cannot be defined without the inclusion of those variables that make the acquisition of reading skills difficult or impossible, that is, neurological, psychiatric, or sensory pathology; intellectual retardation; and, of course, lack of opportunity to learn. In addition to these commonly accepted exclusionary factors, the presence or absence of attention deficits must at least be specified. Dyslexia ought to be defined as "with or without attention deficit disorder," much as the *DSM-III* definition of attention deficit disorder is "with or without hyperactivity."

Measures of reading are essential, of course, but these must specify whether they are based on timed or untimed tests of single-word or prose passage reading. One could also characterize the dyslexic child in terms of level of phonetic decoding ability with the use of standardized tests consisting of nonsense syllables. If one uses a variety of reading tests, the discrepancies among them may, in themselves, help to define the pattern of dyslexia in the individual instance and may aid in the derivation of subtypes of dyslexia.

Discrepancy scores, however determined or expressed, are irrelevant as long as it can be established that (1) the child cannot achieve or sustain the level demanded of him at school *and* (2) the child has other correlated symptoms of dyslexia. What these correlated symptoms are has been the subject of considerable research and can by now be fairly approximated.

Clearly, deficits of language are critical and can be demonstrated in slowed automatized naming, dysphasic errors of naming (as demonstrated here and elsewhere), poor learning of verbal associations [48], inadequate use of phonic structure and word segmentation [32], slow word and sound processing [47], inadequate temporal processing in the production and perception of speech [53], and impaired word finding [51]. Tallal [47] suggests, as had Orton [37], that were language tests regularly administered to children with reading disorders, they would be "found to have subtle, or even not so subtle, receptive and/or expressive language delay." Just as the the exclusionary factors tell us what dyslexia is not, these correlated deficits tell us what dyslexia is and may also eventually distinguish among *types* of dyslexia.

Deficits on motor tests, as described here, may be symptomatic of dyslexia only before age 9 to 10 years or may characterize those dyslexic children who also have attentional disorders. A study is now well underway to determine whether tests such as these are predictors of reading disability.

Undoubtedly, other replicable correlated deficits will emerge from the great variety of electroencephalographic, evoked potential, computed tomographic, visual processing, and eye movement studies that continue to preoccupy the field. Until then, one can employ the tests of the language and auditory processing correlates that have been established and are relatively simple to administer. The presence of such deficits, rather than discrepancy scores, actually defines dyslexia.

Acknowledgment

I want to thank Dr. Jeffrey Halperin for his valuable assistance in the statistical analysis of these data.

References

1. Ackerman, P. T., Peters, J. E., and Dykman, R. A. Children with specific learning disabilities. *J. Learn. Disabil.* 4:150, 1971.
2. Annett, M. Laterality of childhood hemiplegia and the growth of speech and intelligence. *Cortex* 9:4, 1973.
3. Belmont, L., and Birch, H. G. The intellectual profile of retarded readers. *Percept. Mot. Skills* 22:787, 1966.
4. Benson, D. F. Aphasia. In K. M. Heilman and E. Valenstein (Eds.), *Clinical Neuropsychology*. New York: Oxford University Press, 1979.
5. Benton, A. L. Developmental Dyslexia: Neurological Aspects. In W. J. Friedlander (Ed.), *Advances in Neurology*. New York: Raven, 1975.
6. Benton, A. L. Summary. In A. L. Benton and D. Pearl (Eds.), *Dyslexia: An Appraisal of Current Knowledge*. New York: Oxford University Press, 1978.
7. Berger-Gross, P. N., Haggerty, R., Rudel, R. G., and Kreiger, J. Ontogenesis of Associated Movements: Is it a Cognitive Calendar? American Psychological Association 1984 Annual Conference, Toronto, Ontario.
8. Bettman, J. W., et al. Cerebral dominance in developmental dyslexia. *Arch. Ophthalmol.* 78:722, 1967.
9. Denckla, M. B. Development of speed in repetitive and successive finger movements in normal children. *Dev. Med. Child Neurol.* 15:635, 1973.
10. Denckla, M. B. Development of motor coordination in normal children. *Dev. Med. Child Neurol.* 16:729, 1974.
11. Denckla, M. B. Minimal Brain Dysfunction and Dyslexia: Beyond Diagnosis by Exclusion. In M. E. Blaw, I. Rapin, and M. Kinsbourne (Eds.), *Topics in Child Neurology*. New York: Spectrum, 1977.
12. Denckla, M. B. Childhood Learning Disabilities. In K. Heilman and E. Valenstein (Eds.), *Clinical Neuropsychology*. New York: Oxford University Press, 1979.
13. Denckla, M. B., and Rudel, R. G. Rapid "automatized" naming of pictures, objects, colors, letters, and numbers by normal children. *Cortex* 10:186, 1974.
14. Denckla, M. B., and Rudel, R. G. Naming of object drawings by dyslexic and other learning-disabled children. *Brain Lang.* 3:1, 1976.
15. Denckla, M. B., and Rudel, R. G. Rapid "automatized" naming (R.A.N.): Dyslexia differentiated from other learning disabilities. *Neuropsychologia* 14:471, 1976.

16. Denckla, M. B., and Rudel, R. G. Anomalies of motor development in hyperactive boys. *Ann. Neurol.* 3:231, 1978.
17. Denckla, M. B., Rudel, R. G., and Broman, M. Tests that discriminate between dyslexic and other learning-disabled boys. *Brain Lang.* 13:118, 1981.
18. Doehring, D. G. Acquisition of rapid reading responses, Serial 165. *Monogr. Soc. Res. Child Dev.* 41(2):1, 1976.
19. Doehring, D. G., and Hoshko, I. M. Classification of reading problems by the Q technique of factor analysis. *Cortex* 13:281, 1976.
20. Duffy, F. H., et al. Dyslexia: Regional differences in brain electrical activity by topographic mapping. *Ann. Neurol.* 7:412, 1980.
21. Duffy, F. H., et al. Dyslexia: Automated diagnosis by computerized classification of brain electrical activity. *Ann. Neurol.* 7:421, 1980.
22. *Federal Register* 41:230, 1976.
23. Galaburda, A., and Kemper, T. Cytoarchitechtonic abnormalities in development dyslexia. *Ann. Neurol.* 6:94, 1979.
24. Goodglass, H., and Kaplan, E. *The Assessment of Aphasia and Related Disorders*. Philadelphia: Lea & Febiger, 1972.
25. Hécaen, H. Aspects des troubles de la lecture (alexies) au cours des lésions cérébrales en foyer. *Hommage à André Martinet*, numéro spécial de Word. 23:265, 1967.
26. Holtzman, R. N. N., Rudel, R. G., and Goldensohn, E. S. Paroxysmal alexia. *Cortex* 14:592, 1977.
27. Hughes, J. R. Electroencephalography and Learning Disabilities. In H. R. Myklebust (Ed.), *Progress in Learning Disabilities*, Vol. 2. New York: Grune & Stratton, 1971.
28. Kaufman, A. S. Intelligent Testing with the Weschler Scale for Children–Revised. In I. B. Weiner (Ed.), *The Wiley Series on Personality Processes*. New York: Wiley, 1979.
29. Kinsbourne, M. Minimal brain dysfunction as a neurodevelopmental lag. *Ann. N.Y. Acad. Sci.* 205:268, 1973.
30. Leisman, G., and Ashkenazi, M. Aetiological factors in dyslexia: IV. Cerebral hemispheres are functionally equivalent. *Neuroscience* 11:157, 1980.
31. Liberman, I. Y., and Shankweiler, D. Speech, the Alphabet, and Teaching to Read. In L. Resnick and P. Weaver (Eds.), *Theory and Practice of Early Reading*. Hillsdale, N.J.: Erlbaum, 1979.
32. Liberman, I. Y., et al. Phonetic Segmentation and Recoding in Beginning Readers. In A. S. Reber and D. Scarborough (Eds.), *Reading: Theory and Practice*. Hillsdale, N.J.: Erlbaum, 1976.
33. Luria, A. R. Towards the mechanisms of naming disturbance. *Neuropsychologia* 11:417, 1973.
34. Mattis, S., French, J.H., and Rapin, I. Dyslexia in children and young adults: Three independent neuropsychological syndromes. *Dev. Med. Child Neurol.* 17:150, 1975.
35. Newcombe, F., et al. Recognition and naming of object drawings by men with focal brain wounds. *J. Neurol. Neurosurg. Psychiatry* 34:392, 1971.
36. Orton, S. T. Word-blindness in school children. *Arch Neurol. Psychiatry* 14:581, 1925.
37. Orton, S. T. *Reading, Writing and Speech Problems in Children*. New York: Norton, 1937.
38. Owen, F. W., et al. Learning disorders in children: Sibling studies, Serial 144. *Monogr. Soc. Res. Child Dev.* 1971.
39. Rebert, C., Wexler, B., and Sproul, A. EEG asymmetry in educationally handicapped children. *Electroencephalogr. Clin. Neurophysiol.* 45:436, 1978.

40. Rudel, R. G. Learning disability: Diagnosis by exclusion and discrepancy. *J. Am. Acad. Child Psychiatry* 19:547, 1980.
41. Rudel, R. G., Denckla, M. B., and Broman, M. Rapid silent responses to repeated target symbols by dyslexic and nondyslexic children. *Brain Lang.* 6:52, 1978.
42. Rudel, R. G., Denckla, M. B., and Broman, M. The effect of varying stimulus context on word-finding ability in normal, dyslexic and other learning-disabled children. *Brain Lang.* 13:130, 1981.
43. Rutter, M. Prevalance and Types of Dyslexia. In A. L. Benton and D. Pearl (Eds.), *Dyslexia: An Appraisal of Current Knowledge.* New York: Oxford University Press, 1978.
44. Satterfield, J. H. EEG issues in children with minimal brain dysfunction. *Semin. Psychiatry* 5(1):35, 1973.
45. Stephenson, S. Congenital word-blindness. *Lancet* 2:827, 1904.
46. Symmes, J. S., and Rapoport, J. Unexpected reading failure. *Am. J. Orthopsychiatry* 42:82, 1972.
47. Tallal, P. Auditory temporal perception, phonics, and reading disabilities in children. *Brain Lang.* 9:182, 1980.
48. Vellutino, F. R. Toward an Understanding of Dyslexia: Psychological Factors in Specific Reading Disability. In A. L. Benton and D. Pearl (Eds.), *Dyslexia, an Appraisal of Current Knowledge.* New York: Oxford University Press, 1978.
49. Vogel, S. Syntactic abilities in normal and dyslexic children. *J. Learn. Disabil.* 7:103, 1974.
50. Warrington, E. The incidence of verbal disability associated with reading retardation. *Neuropsychologia* 5:175, 1967.
51. Wolf, M. The Word Retrieval Process and Reading in Children and Aphasics. In K. Nelson (Ed.), *Children's Language* (Vol. 3). New York: Gardner, 1980.
52. Yule, W. Predicting reading ages on Neale's analysis of reading ability. *Br. J. Educ. Psychol.* 37:252, 1967.
53. Zurif, E. B., and Carson, G. Dyslexia in relation to central dominance and temporal analysis. *Neuropsychologia* 8:351, 1970.

4

On Some Relationships Between Acquired and Developmental Dyslexias

John C. Marshall

Although the history of writing systems can be traced back to about 3500 B.C.E. and perhaps some 5,000 years earlier yet [38], the history of *mass* literacy is considerably briefer. In western Europe, the leaders of the Protestant Reformation translated the Latin Bible into the vernacular and encouraged their followers to learn to read the Scriptures for themselves. In England, the first "Sunday school" was founded by Robert Raikes in 1780, with the primary objective of teaching children (and adults) to read the English (or perhaps one should say Scottish) Bible; by the end of the nineteenth century very substantial numbers of children were, more or less, in full-time education in Europe and North America. Thus it is that by the turn of the century, a sufficiently large population of beginning readers was available for teachers, doctors, and ophthalmologists to notice that a sizable minority of this population experienced great difficulty in learning to read. Developmental dyslexia, under the rubrics "congenital word blindness," "congenital symbol amblyopia," "congenital dysorthographia," and dozens more, was discovered, or at least named [9, 18, 21, 27, 37]. Once dyslexia was discovered, the first question that arose was, Within what overall framework shall the condition (or better, conditions) be described?

Somewhat earlier, neurologists had begun to outline the varieties of acquired dyslexia [14, 28, 46] and the lesion sites that were responsible for impairment of reading, writing, and spelling. It was therefore reasonable to conjecture that there might be both behavioral and neurological similarities between the acquired and developmental dyslexias. In both conditions, word blindness without letter blindness was described [14, 27]; that is, patients were reported who could name on confrontation both individual letters and sequence of letters in words but could not "recognize" words. The crucial role of the left angular gyrus and its ipsilateral and contralateral inputs was discovered by Dejerine in careful autopsy studies of patients with acquired dyslexia [13, 14]. Hinshelwood [22] and Fisher [17] then speculated that a congenital or perinatal aplasia of the angular gyrus (either bilateral or unilateral left) might be the proximate cause of severe problems in learning to read. Hinshelwood [22] thus interpreted the developmental dyslexias as consequent on the child's attempting to read with "a part of the brain which does not usually discharge that function."

Classification by Association

The promise of these early studies was, in my opinion, squandered as the field came to be determined by what I shall call the "correlational" approach to the dyslexias. Relatively "pure" cases of dyslexia, that is, cases without other signs of major cognitive impairment, had been sporadically observed since Schmidt [39] first described in 1676 a man who, after an attack of apoplexy, could neither read words nor name individual letters, yet who could write faultlessly words that were dictated to him. Indeed the patient could not read back, after a short interval, words that he himself had written. Hence when cases were reported in which reading impairment was *not* an isolated symptom, it seemed very natural to construct a taxonomy of the acquired dyslexias in terms of the symptomatology *associated with* reading disorder. Thus a popular classification of the acquired dyslexias distinguishes between "pure" dyslexia [19], dyslexia with agraphia [13], dyslexia in the context of Wernicke's aphasia [42], and dyslexia in the context of Broca's aphasia [3]. Other taxonomies (e.g., De Massary [12], 1932) have incorporated yet further associated signs, distinguishing between dyslexia with spatial disorder, with agnosia, with apraxia, with acalculia, and so on.

The primary justification for these classifications by associated symptoms was that the different varieties of acquired dyslexia so defined could be mapped with fair accuracy onto a set of distinct lesion sites [4]. Before the advent of modern radiological techniques, to predict in vivo the locus of damage to the brain on behavioral grounds was clearly an achievement of some magnitude. Yet the detail and sophistication of anatomical description within this tradition often served to conceal a paucity of information about the behavioral characteristics of the patients. With rare exceptions [29], little or no attention was paid to the actual phenomena that could be observed when the patient was asked to read (or write). Little account was taken of which word clauses were impaired or preserved; little consideration was given to the strikingly different types of error made by different patients. No serious effort was made to relate pathologies of reading to normative models of the underlying processes involved in fluent performance. The theory of reading became locked into Dejerine's [13, 14] distinction between a central "store" of visual language representations (damage to which caused dyslexia with dysgraphia) and the various pathways to this store from left and right occipital areas (damage to which caused dyslexia without dysgraphia).

A similar concentration on correlational classifications can be seen in many current studies of the development dyslexias. Thus, Mattis, French, and Rapin [32] distinguish between dyslexia in association with language disorder, with articulatory and graphomotor dyscoordination, and with visuospatial perceptual disorder. Similar groups have been isolated by Denckla [15], and two further groups added: dyslexia in association with "dysphonemic sequencing difficulty" and with "verbal memorization disorder." The most striking characteristic of many of the developmental taxonomies reviewed in Benton and Pearl [5] is that they are *not* systematic analyses and classifications of reading impairment per se. Rather, they are groupings of *children with a reading disorder*, where the grouping is determined by the associated symptomatology. As with comparable studies of the acquired dyslexias, work within this tradition has typically failed to specify what actually happens when the dyslexic child tries to read. Although some investigators have distinguished different error types, such as audiophonic confusions versus visuospatial confusions [25] or phonic versus semantic paralexias [6], there have been few if any systematic attempts to build models of developmental reading disorder on such qualitative variation in the data base.

More seriously, the correlational approach, with its essential commitment to group studies, has failed to establish whether the deficits that are often associated with dyslexia constitute necessary and/or sufficient conditions for the emergence of reading impairment. The mere existence of a "cognitive profile" in which, for example, verbal repetition deficits are associated with a reading deficit does not suffice to show either that the disorder of repetition is the cause of the reading disorder or that some more general underlying problem is the cause of both disorders.

Our own approach [31, 34] has temporarily laid many of these issues to one side in favor of describing the qualitative and quantitative characteristics of acquired and developmental reading disorder per se. But this enterprise demands, of course, some general framework within which observations can be systematically compared and interpreted. That framework is provided by information-processing models of *normal* reading performance.

Routes to Reading

The core of the reading process can be seen as the assignment of linguistic structure to the written word. An orthographic form must be associated with a phonological, a morphological, and a semantic representation. Current models of reading suggest that the system whereby such structure is computed has a highly modular organization in which multiple routes operate in parallel to assign sound, form, and meaning with speed and accuracy. A simple model of normal reading, expressed as a flow diagram, is shown in Figure 4-1. The boxes indicate processing stages where distinct linguistic representations are assigned to their input; the arrows show the flow of information between processing stages [28].

Early visual analysis (EVA) is the component that extracts local and global visual features from the stimulus array. Early visual analysis feeds three distinct routes employed in the assignment of linguistic form: the "phonic" route, the "direct" route, and the "lexical" route.

The Phonic Route

Local features, that is, features that support individual letter recognition, derived from EVA are fed to letter representations (LR). Here explicit but abstract (e.g., indiscriminate with respect to case) letter identities are assigned. Multiletter strings are assumed to be formally segmented into their component letters (e.g., $d + o + g$). This representation is then input to the graphemic parser (P). The function of P is to resegment, as necessary, the letter sequence into regular graphemic "chunks." A graphemic chunk in this sense is a letter or multiletter sequence that maps onto a *single* phoneme in words (or regularly spelled neologisms) that contain the relevant segment [10, 45]. The repre-

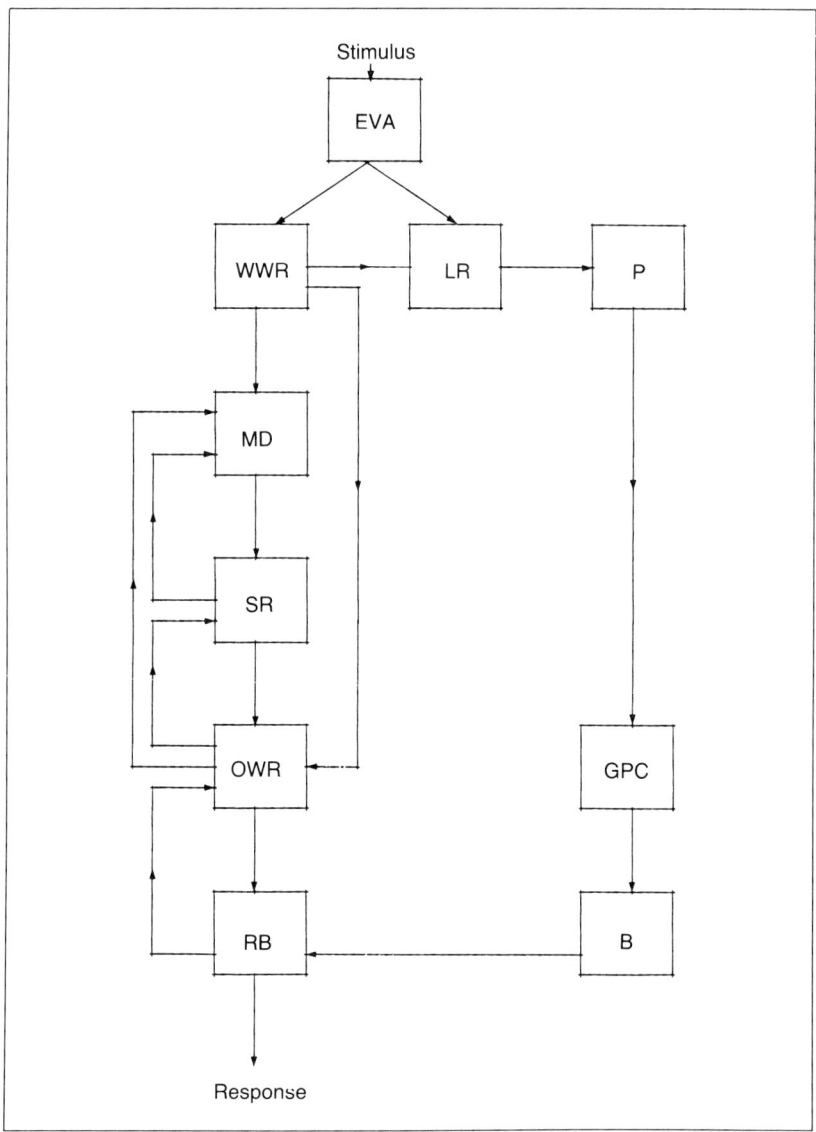

Fig. 4-1. Mechanisms implicated in normal reading. (*EVA* = early visual analysis; *WWR* = whole word representations (visual); *LR* = (abstract) letter representations; *P* = (graphemic) parser; *MD* = morphological decomposition; *SR* = semantic representations; *OWR* = output word representations (oral); *GPC* = grapheme-phoneme conversion; *B* = blender (phonological); *RB* = response buffer.)

sentation of *dog* (i.e., $d + o + g$) will not require further resegmentation, but sequences such as $f + o + e$ must be reanalyzed as $f + oe$. That is, *oe* is normally a vowel digraph with the regular pronunciation [ou]. It is, of course, not a digraph in such words as *poet* or *coerce*. Such graphemic "exception" words will be misparsed by P.

The output of P is input to the grapheme phoneme correspondence rules (GPC). There, each single or multicharacter grapheme is associated with the (single) phoneme that is its most frequent phonological realization (e.g., *j* → [dz]; *ea* → [i:]; *oa* → [ou]). It follows from the definition of this route that written words whose phonological realization is "irregular" will be associated with an incorrect phonological code. Thus, in *canoe* and *shoe*, for example, the digraph *oe* will, incorrectly, be given the value [ou] when the exceptional pronunciation [u:] is required.

The output of GPC, a regular segmented phonological code, is then input to the blender (B). The function of this mechanism is to assign an articulatory code with specified phonetic values for coarticulation phenomena that will serve to instruct the vocal tract's smooth pronunciation of the word. This representation is in turn input to the response buffer (RB) from where the final triggering of the articulatory system for overt output takes place.

The Direct Route

Early visual analysis also feeds a "global" mechanism, whole word representations (WWR), that can be characterized as the visual recognition device that underlies the notion of "sight vocabulary." Parallel processing of visual stimulus information, including word length and overall configuration, especially important in lowercase script, serves to locate the representations of attested words of the language. This "holistic" recognition device outputs an arbitrary code that serves to locate the phonological realization of the whole word in the component oral word representations (OWR). The route from WWR to OWR can be regarded as a set of direct, unanalyzed associations between visual word forms and their pronunciations. As Figure 4-1 indicates, if reading takes place by this route, access to meaning is achieved by the feedback loop from OWR to semantic representations (SR). It follows that this part of the system is unable to distinguish semantically between homophones such as *ail* and *ale* or *grate* and *great*. The same incapacity is apparent when reading by the phonic route. Here semantic interpretation takes place through feedback from RB to OWR and thence to semantic interpretation in SR. Returning to the direct route, the output of OWR, a phonetic string that can direct the vocal tract's pronunciation of the word, is placed in RB to await instructions to articulate the word overtly.

The Lexical Route

Whole word representations (WWR) is also input to morphological decomposition (MD). The latter component takes the visual gestalt, or holistic word form, and segments it into morphemic constituents (base form and affixes). Thus the word *insubstantial*, for example, will be decomposed into *in* + *substan*(ce) + (t)*ial* (see Bradley [8] and Taft [43]. Morphological decomposition does not have access to a full lexicosemantic knowledge base; hence *mother* will be incorrectly segmented as *moth* + *er*, the correct analysis mode for such words as *taller* (= *tall* + *er*); *insect* will be incorrectly segmented as *in* + *sect*, the correct analysis for such words as *indecision* (= *in* + *deci*(de)

+ (s)*ion*). The segmented form (potential base plus potential prefixes and suffixes) is then passed to SR. In this component, the segmented string receives a full syntacticosemantic interpretation. If the segmentation is correct (e.g., *unpleasantness* = *un* + *pleasant* + *ness*), this interpreted form is then passed to OWR, where the appropriate phonology is assigned to the string. On some occasions, however, the morphological parsing will be incorrect (e.g., *instant* → *in* + *stant*). In this case, output will be blocked when *stant* cannot be assigned a semantic representation. At this point, the combined form, *instant*, will be recirculated to MD for an alternative parsing (in this example, as a nondecomposable base). In other cases, the initial morphological analysis will produce an analysis in which all segments are attested items of the language (e.g., *instance* → *in* + *stance*), but the decomposition is nonetheless incorrect. Such items will block at OWR, where no pronunciation that corresponds with the lexical decomposition *in* + *stance* is available. Once more, the form will be recirculated to MD where an alternative parsing can be assigned. Correctly segmented forms (and, variously, base forms, such as *chair*) are input to OWR, where they receive a phonological interpretation prior to being placed in the response buffer.

Acquired and Developmental Disorders of Reading

Our approach to both the acquired and the developmental dyslexias has been to conjecture that particular components of the schema outlined in Figure 4-1 can be perturbed while leaving the rest of the system relatively intact. In the acquired dyslexias, components are damaged or functionally disconnected from each other by demonstrable brain damage; in the developmental dyslexias, particular components and their interconnections fail to mature normally, throwing the burden of performance on the remaining, unimpaired parts of the functional architecture. To the extent that neither brain injury in the adult nor development lag or malformation in the child distort *qualitatively* the normal functional architecture shown in Figure 4-1, we should be able to discover strict parallels between the acquired and developmental dyslexias. Let us see if this is so.

Reading by the Phonic Route

Assume that brain damage in an adult has rendered the direct and lexical routes inoperative. Access to "sight" vocabulary, represented by WWR in Figure 4-1, is impaired, and reading must accordingly take place primarily by the phonic route. Patients with this pathology (e.g., J.C. reported in Holmes [23] and Marshall and Newcombe [31]) will have great difficulty when attempting to read words that contain complex consonant clusters, silent consonants, vowel digraphs, and highly "ambiguous" letters, such as *s*, *f*, *c*, *g*, *p*, and *r*, whose phonic value depends heavily on their graphemic context. Both words and nonwords with regular phonological correspondences (e.g., *maid*, *taid*) will be read aloud more accurately than irregular words (e.g., *plaid*). Errors will consist, in large part, of "regularizations"; that is, the vowel digraph in *plaid* will be given its normal pronunciation [ei], and the word will therefore be read as "played." Semantic interpretation is then determined by the phonological representation that the patient has constructed. Thus in the studies cited, J.C. assigns phonetic value to silent consonants and accordingly interprets *listen* as referring to the onetime holder of the world heavyweight boxing championship Sonny Liston. Such patients also have considerable difficulty with homophones even when the stimuli can be read aloud correctly. J.C., for example, reads *maid* correctly but interprets it as "made"; *billed* is read correctly but interpreted as "build". *Pair* is read correctly but glossed as, "It's either two of a kind or it's the one for eating. I don't know which." On substantial numbers of words, phonic regularization will result in a neologistic response. For example, J.C. assigns a standard pronunciation of *s* in *island*, a word in which *s* is nonstandardly silent. This produces a neologism that the patient recognizes as such: "It doesn't mean anything . . . there's no such word."

All of these phenomena can be found in a subset of children with developmental dyslexia who have failed to build up a normal sight vocabulary [11, 23, 24]. Holmes [23] reported four dyslexic boys who made such regularization errors as *of* → "off," *shoe* → "show," and *ceiling* → "selling." Silent consonants were pronounced so that, for example, *bristle* was read and interpreted as "Bristol." Homophone confusions were in evidence, as when *mare* was interpreted as "mayor" and *caught* as "court."

The syndrome of phonic-route reading is known as surface dyslexia, and it would seem that the behavioral manifestations of the condition are essentially identical across acquired and developmental cases.

Reading by the Direct Route

Patients with acquired dyslexia who read by the direct route, that is, by associating whole word representations with their output phonology, should be able to read irregular words aloud with the same facility that regular words can be read. However, the semantic interpretation of homophones should cause problems, as this route gains access to meaning only through feedback from oral word representations to the semantic system. There is evidence that this route is sometimes used by patients with surface dyslexia (i.e., who usually read by the phonic route). For example, J.C. reads *mown* correctly but often misinterprets it as "moan," "to cry or complain." Had this word been read by the phonic route, it would have been regularized to the neologism [maun]; that is, the standard phonic representation of *ow* is [au], as in *how*, *now*, *cow*, *crown*, *town*, or *gown*. The word cannot have been read by the lexical route, for if it had, the *correct* semantic interpretation would have been given. Similar arguments apply to *some*, which J.C. interpreted as "money" (i.e., "sum"), *bury*, interpreted as "a hat, headgear" (i.e., "beret"), and *four*, interpreted as "for you, for me, or for anyone else." In all cases, the words were read aloud correctly [34].

The most striking example of direct route reading, however, is seen in patient W.L.P., reported by Schwartz, Saffran, and Marin [40]. This woman presented with presenile dementia in which language difficulties, originally of an anomic type, were prominent against a background of generalized, progressive memory impairment. Despite a severe and progressive impairment of semantic knowledge (or access), she retained, for a considerable time, the ability to read aloud single words. She could read accurately such irregular words as *tortoise*, *leopard*, *climb*, *both*, *own*, and *flood* at a time when the evidence from her poor performance on semantic categorization, classification, and matching tasks strongly suggested that there was little or no comprehension of the meaning of the words read.

The ability to read without semantics (i.e., without access to the lexical route) immediately calls to mind the developmental pathology of "hyperlexia." Silberberg and Silberberg [41] described children whose ability to read words aloud was far superior to their comprehension of either the written or the spoken word. Silberberg and Silberberg proposed the designation "hyperlexia" for these children, and many subsequent reports have confirmed its existence in populations as diverse as the mentally retarded, the autistic, idiot savants, and otherwise basically normal children [20]. Clearly, these children have failed to acquire the central syntacticosemantic component of the lexicon. Granted that deficit, however, it is possible that their successful oral reading could be mediated solely by the phonic route. In this event, their reading aloud would have many of the characteristics of surface dyslexia, albeit without semantic access. Yet if the children were relatively successful at reading "exception" words, the direct route must be implicated in their performance.

Although the extensive literature on hyperlexia has sometimes implied that these children have advanced "word-calling" skills that extend to complex words, the first investigation of this issue was by Aram, Rose, and Horwitz [1]. Their patient, M.D., is a developmental hyperlexic, who is now in his late 30s. He has relatively intact grapheme-phoneme correspondence skills, as witnessed by his good performance when reading neologisms aloud. But in addition, he must "have established a considerable store of word-specific print to sound associations," for his ability to read irregular words aloud is also good, despite seriously impaired semantic access. Further study of the parallels between acquired direct dyslexia and developmental hyperlexia is obviously called for.

Reading by the Lexical Route

There are two well-studied pathologies of reading by the lexical route: acquired phonological dyslexia [2] and acquired deep dyslexia [30]. In both conditions, the phonic route and the direct route are seriously impaired. Consequently, patients cannot read neologisms aloud; attested words are read by the assignment of lexical and semantic structure.

In both conditions, there is impairment of the process of morphological analysis. Multimorphemic words with inflectional or derivational morphology are frequently misread. The misreadings consist of the addition, deletion, or substitution of prefixes and suffixes. Representative errors from A.M., a patient with acquired phonological dyslexia reported by Patterson [36], include *recent* → "recently," *solve* → "absolve," *disposal* → "dispose," and *ineradicable* → "eradicate." Similar errors from G.R., a patient with acquired deep dyslexia reported by Marshall and Newcombe [30], include *wise* → "wisdom," *truth* → "true," and *birth* → "born." Some patients with phonological dyslexia also experience difficulty reading individual function words, a phenomenon found in all deep dyslexics. Errors are typically failure to respond or substitutions of function words (e.g., from G.R., *for* → "and," *the* → "yes," *in* → "those"). Additionally, in deep dyslexia, but not phonological dyslexia, frank semantic substitutions are made when the patient reads aloud individual, unrelated words without time pressure or stimulus degradation. Representative examples from G.R. [30] include *sick* → "ill," *bush* → "tree," *act* → "play," *uncle* → "cousin," *ancient* → "historic," and *tall* → "long." When reading monomorphemic words, performance in phonological dyslexia can be relatively unimpaired. Small numbers of visual misidentifications may be made (e.g., *metamorphosis* → "metaphorical," *contemplate* → "compensate," from A.M.). These visual errors are also found in deep dyslexia (e.g., *stock* → "shock," *crocus* → "crocodile," from G.R.).

Can these conditions be found in developmental disorders of reading? Temple and Marshall [44] have recently described a 17-year-old dyslexic girl, H.M., who is of at least average intelligence and has an above average oral vocabulary. She is grossly impaired at nonword reading in comparison to word reading; her responses to nonwords are frequently real words that bear a reasonable visual similarity to the stimulus (e.g., *gok* → "joke," *hib* → "hip"). When she reads words, a high proportion of her errors are either visual or derivational paralexias. Representative examples include *bouquet* → "boutique," *cheery* → "cherry," *high* → "height," and *appeared* → "appearance." H.M. makes no semantic errors and no regularizations of the type seen in surface dyslexia. On all the dimensions studied, the features of H.M.'s performance are consistent with reported cases of acquired phonological dyslexia.

Is there also a developmental analogue to deep dyslexia? In the past, research on semantic paralexias reported in children with severe reading problems has not been explicit about whether such errors occurred in single-word reading or only when continuous text was read. If semantic errors occur only in sentence reading, they are diagnostic of deep dyslexia. Such errors are a common finding when normal adults read text aloud under time pressure, and they are also found in normal children who are *good* readers in the sense that they are using contextual information to predict words that will be syntactically and semantically coherent with the preceding discourse.

However, experienced clinicians do report having seen developmental dyslexics who make semantic paralexias on single-word reading [7, 35]. Moreover, Johnston [26] has recently described an adolescent girl, C.R., without known brain damage but of somewhat low intelligence, whose extremely poor reading shows many of the features of acquired deep dyslexia. C.R. is incapable of reading even the simplest nonwords. When reading individual words aloud, she makes semantic paralexias (*chair* → "table"), function word substitutions (*down* → "up"), derivational errors (*child* → "children"), and visual errors. The pattern of performance is clearly that of acquired deep dyslexia. One's principal reservations concern the very small proportions of semantic and derivational errors, approximately 3 percent and 2 percent respectively, given that there must be a nonzero "chance" rate of stimulus and response having lexical or semantic features in common [16]. Nonetheless, the case is an important demonstration of a parallel with acquired deep dyslexia and raises the hope that subsequent cases will be found among developmental dyslexics with higher IQs and larger reading vocabularies.

Conclusions

Some progress, then, has been made in describing the phenomenological characteristics of acquired and developmental dyslexias within a common framework. Furthermore, the basic observations can at least be conveniently summarized by fairly simple flow diagrams of the type shown in Figure 4-1. Future advances will, in my view, crucially depend on more detailed study of the behavioral features of impaired reading and on the construction of precise models of the mechanisms implicit in the all too black boxes of our current flow charts [33]. Only then will it make sense to inquire whether some of these mechanisms play a role in other aspects of linguistic and visuospatial skill. By following such a strategy we may eventually hope to discover which, if any, of the symptoms that are often associated with reading impairment, acquired or developmental, are causally implicated in the reading disorder.

References

1. Aram, D. M., Rose, D. F., and Horwitz, S. J. Hyperlexia: Developmental reading without meaning. Presented to the NATO Advanced Study Institute on Dyslexia: A Global Issue. Maratea, Italy, October 10–22, 1982.
2. Beauvois, M. F., and Dérouesné, J. Phonological alexia: Three dissociations. *J. Neurol. Neurosurg. Psychiatry* 42:1115, 1979.
3. Benson, D. F. The third alexia. *Arch. Neurol.* 34:327, 1977.
4. Benson, D. F. Alexia and the Neuroanatomical Basis of Reading. In F. J. Pirozzolo and M. C. Wiltrock (Eds.), *Neuropsychological and Cognitive Processes in Reading.* New York: Academic, 1981.
5. Benton, A. L., and Pearl, D. (Eds.), *Dyslexia: An Appraisal of Current Knowledge.* New York: Oxford University Press, 1978.
6. Boder, E. Developmental dyslexia: A diagnostic approach based on three atypical reading-spelling patterns. *Dev. Med. Child Neurol.* 15:663, 1973.
7. Boder, E. Personal communication, 1982.

8. Bradley, D. Lexical Representation of Derivational Relation. In M. Aronoff and M. L. Kean (Eds.), *Juncture*. Saratoga, Calif.: Anma Libri, 1980.
9. Clairborne, J. H. Types of congenital symbol amblyopia. *J.A.M.A.* 47:1813, 1906.
10. Coltheart, M. Lexical Access in Simple Reading Tasks. In G. Underwood (Ed.), *Strategies of Information Processing*. London: Academic, 1978.
11. Coltheart, M., et al. Surface dyslexia. *Q. J. Exp. Psychol.* 35A:469, 1983.
12. De Massary, J. L'Alexie. *Encephale* 1:53, 1932.
13. Dejerine, J. Sur un cas de cécité verbale avec agraphie, suivi d'autopsie. *Mém. Soc. Biol.* 3:197, 1891.
14. Dejerine, J. Contribution a l'étude anatomopathologique et clinique des différences variétés de cécité verbale. *C. R. Soc. Biol.* (Paris) 4:61, 1892.
15. Denckla, M. B. Childhood Learning Disabilities. In K. M. Heilman and E. Valenstein (Eds.), *Clinical Neuropsychology*. New York: Oxford University Press, 1979.
16. Ellis, A. W., and Marshall, J. C. Semantic errors or statistical flukes? A note on Allport's "On knowing the meaning of words we are unable to report." *Q. J. Exp. Psychol.* 30:569, 1978.
17. Fisher, J. H. A case of congenital word-blindness (inability to learn to read). *Trans. Ophthalmol. Soc. U.K.* 30:216, 1910.
18. Foerster, R. A propos de la pathologie de la lecture et de l'ecriture (cécité verbal congénitale chez un débile). *Rev. Neurol.* (Paris) 12:200, 1904.
19. Geschwind, N. The Anatomy of Acquired Disorders of Reading. In J. Money (Ed.), *Reading Disorders*. Baltimore: Johns Hopkins Press, 1962.
20. Healy, J. M. The enigma of hyperlexia. *Read. Res. Q.* 17:319, 1982.
21. Hinshelwood, J. *Letter-, Word- and Mind-Blindness*. London: Lewis, 1900.
22. Hinshelwood, J. A case of congenital word blindness. *Br. Med. J.* 2:1303, 1904.
23. Holmes, J. M. *Dyslexia: A neurolinguistic study of traumatic developmental disorders of reading*. University of Edinburgh, Ph.D. Thesis, 1973.
24. Holmes, J. M. "Regression" and Reading Breakdown. In A. Caramazza and E. B. Zurif (Eds.), *Language Acquisition and Breakdown: Parallels and Divergencies*. Baltimore: Johns Hopkins Press, 1978.
25. Ingram, T. T. S., Mason, A. W., and Blackburn, I. A. A retrospective study of 82 children with reading disability. *Dev. Med. Child Neurol.* 12:271, 1970.
26. Johnston, R. S. Developmental deep dyslexia? *Cortex* 19:133, 1983.
27. Kerr, J. School hygiene, in its mental, moral, and physical aspects. *J. R. Statist. Soc.* 60:613, 1897.
28. Lichtheim, L. On aphasia. *Brain* 7:433, 1885.
29. Low, A. A. A case of agrammatism in the English language. *Arch. Neurol. Psychiatry* 25:556, 1931.
30. Marshall, J. C., and Newcombe, F. Syntactic and semantic errors in paralexia. *Neuropsychologia* 4:169, 1966.
31. Marshall, J. C., and Newcombe, F. Patterns of paralexia: A psycholinguistic approach. *J. Psycholinguist. Res.* 2:175, 1973.
32. Mattis, S., French, J. H., and Rapin, I. Dyslexia in children and young adults: Three independent neuropsychological syndromes. *Dev. Med. Child Neurol.* 17:150, 1975.
33. Morton, J. Word Recognition. In J. Morton and J. C. Marshall (Eds.), *Psycholinguistics Series*, Vol. 2. Cambridge, Mass.: MIT Press, 1979.
34. Newcombe, F., and Marshall, J. C. On psycholinguistic classifications of the acquired dyslexias. *Bull. Orton Soc.* 31:29, 1981.

35. Newton, M. Personal communication, 1982.
36. Patterson, K. E. The Relation Between Reading and Phonological Coding: Further Neuropsychological Observations. In A. W. Ellis (Ed.), *Normality and Pathology in Cognitive Functions*. London: Academic, 1982.
37. Pringle Morgan, W. A case of congenital word-blindness. *Br. Med. J.* 2:1378, 1896.
38. Schmandt-Besserat, D. The envelopes that bear the first writing. *Technol. Culture* 21:357, 1980.
39. Schmidt, J. De oblivione lectionis ex apoplexia salva scriptione. *Miscellanea curiosa medico-physica Academiae naturae curiosorum* 4:195, 1676.
40. Schwartz, M. F., Saffran, E. M., and Marin, O. S. M. Fractionating the Reading Process in Dementia: Evidence for Word-Specific Print-to-Sound Associations. In M. Coltheart, K. Patterson, and J. C. Marshall (Eds.), *Deep Dyslexia*. London: Routledge and Kegan Paul, 1980.
41. Silberberg, N., and Silberberg, M. Hyperlexia: Specific word recognition skills in young children. *Except. Child.* 34:41, 1967.
42. Starr, A. The pathology of sensory aphasia. *Brain* 12:82, 1889.
43. Taft, M. Prefix stripping revisited. *J. Verbal Learn. Verbal Behav.* 20:298, 1981.
44. Temple, C. M., and Marshall, J. C. A case study of developmental phonological dyslexia. *Br. J. Psychol.* 74:517, 1983.
45. Venezky, R. L. *The Structure of English Orthography*. The Hague: Mouton, 1970.
46. Wernicke, C. *Der aphasische Symptomencomplex*. Breslau: Cohn and Weigert, 1874.

5 Patterns of Infant Behavior: Analogues of Later Organizational Difficulties?

Heidelise Als

Reading disabilities are purported to be related to patterning and organizational deficits involving perceptual disorders or difficulties. It is hypothesized that such organizational problems do not just arise when the child is exposed to formal education but have been part of the child's neuro-integrative makeup potentially from birth. It is well-known that premature and small for gestational age infants are at greater risk for many problems, including learning disability. Recent studies that followed large groups of prematurely born infants into school age have found that for those children who enter the regular school system, the incidence of school problems (i.e., poorer functioning than the tested IQ would cause one to anticipate), learning dysfunctions such as dyslexia [30, 43, 44], and behavior problems [28, 35, 40] is 40 to 50 percent, with a disproportionate number accounted for by those premature infants born too small for their gestational age. This high figure cannot be explained by social class alone, although in all studies low social class is shown to exacerbate the potential risk [28]. While these figures are disconcerting, looked at from the positive side, it means that approximately half the prematurely born infants, even the very young and very small ones, if they have survived the immediate newborn period and have entered regular school, are functioning comparably to their full-term peers. Who are these infants who, despite often extraordinary medical complications, are able to overcome a hazardous, traumatic start in extrauterine life? And who are the ones who are prone to organizational and processing disturbances that can form a major barrier to a fully productive and fulfilling existence? Can we identify early organizational analogues of later functioning that could provide a basis on which to seek and institute early preventive and therapeutic measures to alleviate or ameliorate the later difficulties?

When one reviews the literature over the last decade to seek support for predictability of functioning, that is, for intrinsic continuity of development of each organism, one finds that evidence abounds to support the opposite view. The discontinuities of early development and the unpredictability of later behavior and functioning from earlier behavior have received much attention. This might be attributable to the use of overly simplistic indices of functioning. The disillusionment with linear prediction models that looked for simple behavioral stabilities [36, 37, 38] led to the formulation of two alternative models: the transactional model [46, 51] and the transformational model [34, 36, 38, 41].

The transactional model postulates that predictions that do not take into account the ongoing transactions between child and environment are bound

---

The work presented was supported by grants HD10899 from the National Institute of Child Health and Human Development and by grant 3122 from the Grant Foundation, New York. Parts of this work were carried out at the facilities of the Mental Retardation Center, The Children's Hospital, Boston. The author is indebted to Braintech, Inc., for a grant supporting the use of the TICAS analysis system.

to be weak, since early diagnosis is complicated by the responsiveness of the environment and the adaptability of the human infant. The transformational model expands on the postulations of the transactional model by adding the formulation of the changing nature and composition of the infant's capacities with age, which is said to account for the negligible correlations between infant tests and subsequent performance. Competence in infancy is said to consist of a different combination of abilities than competence at later ages. The transformational model argues for the existence of a symptomatic gap [20, 42, 45] that is thought to be due to the human's inherent discontinuities of development. It is claimed that complex capacities that may reveal themselves as impaired later are not called upon earlier, and therefore, an impairment may not manifest itself until later ages. An expanded version of this model is the argument of continuity of discontinuity, which is espoused, among others, by Emde [29] and Brazelton [22]. This view perceives the continuity characteristic of the human in the nature of individual discontinuity and change of behavior.

This chapter, in contrast, proposes a synactive theory of development for the human, stressing the continuity of development that becomes apparent when one attends to the integrative differentiation and modulation of the human's functioning at each developmental stage.

Synactive Theory of Development

I am proposing a synactive model of development [5, 7] that outlines the degree of differentiation and of modulation of behavioral functioning as main parameters of the human's individuality and uniqueness recognizable over time. The conceptualization of development presented here focuses on the way the individual infant appears to handle his experience of the world around him rather than on the assessment of skills per se.* The infant's functioning is seen in a model of continuous intraorganism subsystem interaction, and the infant, in turn, is seen in continuous interaction with his environment. I have termed this view of development *synactive,* since at each stage in development and at each moment of functioning the various subsystems of functioning are existing side by side. These are often truly interactive, but also in a relative, mutually supportive holding pattern, as if providing a steady substratum for one of the systems' current differentiations (syn-action). These systems include:

1. The autonomic system
2. The motor system
3. The state organizational system
4. The attention and interaction system
5. A self-regulatory, balancing system

---

*For convenience, we have generally used the masculine pronoun to represent the infant and the feminine to represent the caregiver.

The functioning of all these systems is reliably observable without technical instrumentation. The autonomic system is behaviorally observable in the pattern of respiration, color changes, tremulousness, and visceral signals such as bowel movements, gagging, and hiccoughing. The motor system is behaviorally observable in the posture, tone, and movements of the infant. The state organizational system is behaviorally observable in the kind and range of states of consciousness available to the infants, from sleeping to aroused states, and in exhibited patterns of state transition. The attention and interaction system is exemplified in the infant's ability to come to an alert, attentive state and to utilize this state to take in cognitive and social-emotional information from the environment and in turn elicit and modify the inputs from the world around him. The regulatory system is behaviorally exemplified in the observable strategies the infant utilizes in maintaining a balanced, relatively stable and relaxed state of subsystem integration or in returning to such a state. If the infant's own regulatory capacity is exceeded at the moment and he is unable to return to an integrated, balanced subsystem state, a further parameter of functioning is identifiable in the kind and amount of facilitation from the environment that is necessary to aid the infant's return to balance.

Consequently, the questions posed regarding the infant in this synactive model of development are always the following: How well differentiated and modulated are the various subsystems in their functioning and mutual balance, given varying demands placed on the infant and varying developmental tasks attempted by him as a result of his intrinsic biological developmental motivation? Where are the thresholds of functioning beyond which smoothness and balance become strained or stressed and coping behaviors become costly, bare subsistence protections or even counterproductive maladaptations? Which subsystem is differentially vulnerable at which level of environmental and endogenous demand? How severe is its infringement on and kindling of other systems' imbalance by virtue of its own current disorganization? How much or how little does it take in terms of environmental modification to induce the reinstitution of a more balanced, integrated state?

The Developmental Task of the Newborn

From my work with healthy full-term newborns examined with the Brazelton Neonatal Behavioral Assessment Scale [21] and from direct observation of newborns with their mothers over the first 3 months [2, 3], I have learned that the differentiation of the attentional-interactive system is the most rapidly changing, apparently newly emerging, salient agendum of the human organism [4, 5]. Autonomic stability in terms of, for instance, respiratory control, temperature regulation, and digestive visceral functioning is relatively quickly restabilized after the birth process, as are smoothness of movements and adaptation of well-regulated, smooth balance between flexor and extensor posture [24]. The same holds true for state organization in terms of the range of states available and their transitions [47, 48]. Most healthy full-term newborns have no difficulty achieving a robust, lusty crying state and can return to a sleep state relatively readily. The functional issue most newborns seem to attempt to control in the first several weeks after birth is the increasing stabilization of the alert state in their movement from sleep to aroused, crying states and back down to sleep state. While in the 2-day-old infant the alert periods are still very difficult to attain and are embedded in long stretches of sleep and episodes of crying, by 2 to 3 weeks these periods of alertness have become increasingly reliable and solidified. By 1 month to 6 weeks, many infants achieve more easily and spend an hour at a time in an alert, socially and cognitively available state.

The Social Environment of the Newborn

It appears that the newborn is not the only one grappling to solidify these periods of alertness. His social partners, from the very first postnatal contact with him, tend to be keen and sensitive to aiding the newborn in stabilizing these periods. On the very first contact, mothers, and presumably fathers, will prod their newborn vocally and tactilely to open his eyes, even at the cost of eliciting crying. Once the newborn opens even one eye, the mother will typically acknowledge this initial connection and mutual recognition by an affectively positive, heightened vocal pattern accompanied by an animated facial expression, praising and encouraging the newborn for his accomplishment: "Hi! There you are—that's right—I knew you were in there! Hi!" she may say over and over again in a drawn out, loving manner [1]. Her behavior, in turn, appears to facilitate and support the newborn's alertness, and from a brief initial glance, he may go on to widen his eyes, raise his eyebrows, soften and raise his cheeks, and shape his mouth into an "ooh" configuration. The partners mutually support and drive each other to prolong this episode. One of them will then reset or break the intensity. For instance, the infant may avert his gaze and move into a yawn or a sneeze, thus resetting the intensity of the interaction at a lower level by utilizing subtle attentional regulation strategies. Or he may move into a fussy, crying, or drowsy state, thus utilizing state shifts to reset the interaction. He may not avert his gaze but may stay locked on the mother's face, become tense and perhaps spit up, begin to hiccough or gag, or even strain to have a bowel movement, thus reacting at an autonomic visceral level in resetting the interaction. If the infant is able to sustain his alertness for a substantial period, keeping his respective subsystems of functioning in balance, the mother may be the one who resets the intensity of the interaction by pulling the baby close and nuzzling and kissing him or by stroking and patting him, thus changing the cyclical attentional interchange.

It is curious that such emphasis appears to be placed on these early attentional episodes of the infant, embedded in affectively supportive and highly positive inputs from the parent, given that later this alertness will be much more available. From a species-evolutionary perspective, this early valuing of the attentional-interactive connection gains an added dimension. It appears that it is uniquely human and takes on significance as researchers have identified a correlation between an increasingly complex and simultaneously flexible social system in primates with an increasingly complex affective communication system. This has been established in comparative studies of the nocturnal prosimians via the old and new world monkeys to great apes and man [18, 19, 23, 32]. The essence of humanness and, in fact, of human species survival appears to be man's enormously complex social and emotional interaction capacity, which is the prerequisite for the virtual supersystem of material culture, that is, technology, that we have constructed and are dependent on for our survival as humans. Highly differentiated capacities for collaboration and cooperation of species members are necessary to make such a complex adaptation workable. It appears that from the very beginning of extrauterine life, the newborn is already launched onto the species-specific, interactive, collaborative-communicative track and is in turn supported and affectively rewarded by his caregivers for this capacity as social interactor. The attentional-interactive capacity of the newborn and young infant therewith becomes a salient characteristic of newborn functioning. It appears to be in current ascendancy and is highly valued and supported by those around him.

The Newborn's Attentional-Interactive Capacity and the Functioning of Other Systems

Not all newborns are equally able to build up this attentional-interactive capacity. For some, as we learned in a study of thin-for-height newborns [13], this is a very difficult task, which impinges on the infant's other functional subsystems. These thin infants showed great reluctance to come into alertness, instead moving into hypertonic, flexed, high guard arm position with fisted hands while becoming pale, having tachypneic and irregular respirations, and showing pained, drawn facial expressions. With slow, calm support, they would gradually open their eyes, but then the hypertonic, high guard fisted defendedness would shift abruptly into motoric flaccidity and tuning out, the color paling further, and breathing becoming slow and irregular. The mustered attention was of a glassy-eyed, strained, barely focused kind, which came at great cost to the automonic and motoric regulation. The identification of this pattern of subsystem "syncresis" and relatively poor respective subsystem differentiation—where, as one system attempts to accomplish a task, the other systems are drawn into the reaction in a generalized manner, exemplifying the relative cost to the total system on many levels—is one avenue toward understanding the current standing of the infant on the developmental lines of subsystem differentiation.

Assessing the Infant's Functioning from a Synactive Perspective

On the basis of my observations of this subsystem interaction and synaction, I have formulated the following parameters to be identified when assessing an individual infant's functioning:

1. The infant's current, newly emerging developmental agendum and a situation to test the degree of ascendancy of this agendum

2. The infant's current level of subsystem balance and smoothly integrated subsystem functioning, regardless of the agendum identified as in ascendancy
3. The threshold of disorganization indicated in behaviors of defense and avoidance at varying subsystem levels of functioning as the developmental agendum is in ascendancy
4. The degree of relative modulation and regulation of the various subsystems in accomplishing a new task
5. The degree of differentiation and effectiveness in rebalancing the subsystems in the accomplishment of the new task
6. The degree of environmental structuring, support, and facilitative aid necessary to bring about optimal implementation of the new task
7. The degree of environmental structuring, support, and facilitative aid necessary to bring about return to smooth, well-integrated, baseline functioning

This approach to the assessment of organism functioning is thought to be appropriate throughout the life span of the human. At each stage of development, newly salient agenda are being negotiated on the backdrop of previously accomplished subsystem differentiation and modulation. Figure 5-1 is a schematic attempt to visualize the conceptualization of the synactive perspective of development, applied to the fetal and neonatal stages.

Fig. 5-1. Model of the synactive organization of behavioral development. (From H. Als [7]).

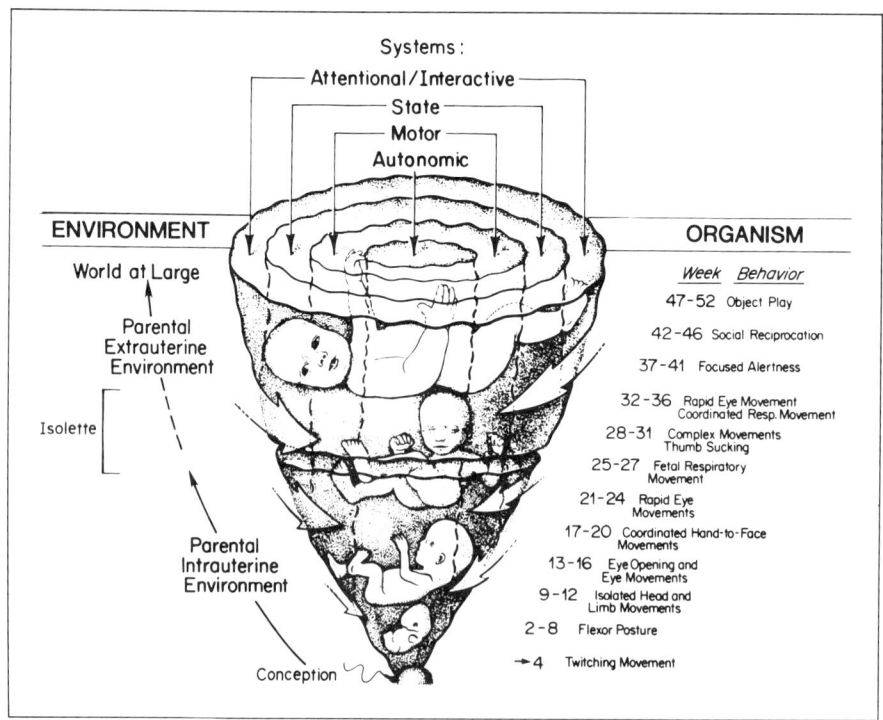

Looked at from above, four concentric circles or cones are seen, the innermost representing the autonomic system in its basic position supporting the organism's baseline functioning. Around it, as it were, is the motor system, unfolding from very early embryonic stages with recognizable flexor posture, limb, and trunk movements and becoming increasingly differentiated in its explication. Around it, as a third cone, lies the state organizational system, the unfolding of distinct states of consciousness from a diffuse quasi-sleep to increasingly differentiated sleep, wake, and aroused bands of consciousness. Finally, around this cone lies the gradual differentiation of the awake state into more and more elaborated, subtly branched, and finely tuned nuances of affective and cognitive receptivity and activity, shaping the social and inanimate world and in turn negotiating the organism's own developmental progression in the process of so doing. These cones are continuously in simultaneous contiguity, if not interaction, with one another, influencing and supporting one another or infringing on one another's relative stability. The within-subsystem differentiation for which each system is striving depends on the other subsystems' support and relative intactness. The whole organism with its intraorganism subsystem synaction is at all stages surrounded and embedded in an environment it has evolved to expect for its species-appropriate ontogenesis. At all times it is actively shaping and selecting from this environment as it is also actively challenged and impinged upon by this environment [33, 41].

The Preterm Infant Seen in a Synactive Developmental Perspective

I shall use the preterm infant as an example to further explain this synactive formulation of development. From 24 to 27 weeks' postconceptual age and thereafter, the human fetus can be kept alive in an extrauterine environment due to the advances of material culture, that is, medical technology. In trying to understand the preterm infant's functioning, our first questions must be, what is the species-appropriate adaptation with which the organism is equipped, and what is the environment (from the perspective of the central nervous system and other systems) he is adapted for? He is biologically expecting 13 to 16 more weeks of in utero existence, with respiratory, cardiac, digestive, and temperature control aided by maternal blood flow and placental functioning. He is expecting total cutaneous somesthetic input from the amniotic fluid. He is expecting motoric kinesthetic input from the contingently reactive amniotic sac, which prevents full extensor patterns and assures flexor inhibition and flexor maintenance for the typical adjustments and movements of softly modulated limbs, trunk, and head, so vividly described by Milani-Comparetti [39] and Birnholz [17]. He is expecting maternal diurnal rhythms presumably entraining his own gradually differentiating states of consciousness, and he is expecting presumably muted sensory inputs to his primary senses of vision and audition, readying himself for the experience of the extrauterine world. The preterm fetus is not an inadequate or deficient full-term infant, but rather a well-equipped, competently adapted organism appropriately functioning at his stage and in his environment.

Suddenly, the preterm newborn finds himself in a vastly different environment, the passage to which has irreversibly triggered his subsystem functioning in an environment only poorly matched to his expectations. Instead of the maternal organism, medical technology attempts to take care of respiratory, cardiac, digestive, and temperature control functions. The motor system, the state organizational system, and sensory functioning, intimately dependent on an adaptive environment, are largely left to their own devices. The center in our schematic model of Figure 5-1, autonomic functioning, is currently the primary focus of medical care. As the preterm infant reactivates himself after a period of "shut down" and "holding," trying to get back on track with his earlier accomplished developmental differentiation, we need to ask with what supports and in which situations the infant is already able to bring about the smooth and balanced functioning that will be critical for his realization of new pathways. The emerging strands of the next developmental agenda must be freed up on the background of well-integrated functioning. This establishes and maintains the path of development in a positive direction and avoids the unwitting reinforcement of only the disturbing, distorted, defense behaviors that are all too ready concomitants of the discrepant organism environment match and that all too easily lead to a vicious cycle of increasing and reverberating distortion and disorganization [31], possibly mediated neurosynaptically. From this perspective, it is not surprising that a disproportionately high number of autistic children and children with organizational, impulsivity, and attention deficits [25] were born prematurely. The developmental agendum that we have identified for the full-term newborn, namely increasingly to free up his ability to maintain an alert state, may not as yet be the appropriate issue for the preterm infant. The mutual regulation of autonomic functioning with motoric balance and equilibrium in a well-defined sleep state may well be the salient agendum for a while, before further state differentiation functioning becomes possible.

Description of the Assessment of Preterm Infant's Behavior (APIB)

In an attempt to identify systematically the infant's relative standing in terms of differentiation and modulation of behavioral subsystems, I have formulated the Assessment of Preterm Infants' Behavior (APIB) [12], which is appropriate not only for preterm infants but also for otherwise at-risk infants and well full-term infants. It is a substantial refinement and extension of the Brazelton Neonatal Behavioral Assessment Scale (BNBAS) [21] in that it provides an integrated subsystem profile of the infant, identifying his current level of smooth, well-balanced functioning in the face of varying developmental demands. Toward this goal, in the APIB, the maneuvers of the BNBAS are used as graded sequences of increasingly vigorous environmental inputs or packages, moving from distal stimulation presented during sleep to mild tactile stimulation, to medium tactile stimulation paired with vestibular stimulation, to more massive tactile stimulation paired with vestibular stimulation. The social interactive-attentional package is administered whenever in the course of the examination the infant's behavioral organization indicates his availability for this sequence. It receives priority in the examiner's attempts to facilitate the infant's organization. The system sheet of the assessment, which appears as Score Sheet I, permits one to read off which tasks are already handled with ease by the infant in terms of maintaining a well-regulated, balanced functioning of all subsystems, which tasks begin to stress the infant and trespass the balance and modulation of various subsystems yet can be handled with enough environmental facilitation, and which tasks are clearly inappropriate for the infant. In this fashion, developmentally appropriate goals can be established for the individual infant and developmentally supportive facilitations can be instituted in his care so that he is not continuously overtaxed or, less likely, underchallenged.

Aside from the system sheet, the APIB provides detailed information on each individual item of the tasks presented, as is the case in the BNBAS, yet the scales are expanded to document the behavior of the immature and dysmature as well as the mature full-term infant. Moreover, particular attention has been given to the reliably readable body language of the developing infant. A catalogue of specific regulation behaviors has been established that can be helpful in understanding the infant's current functioning. The signals can be classified as signals of stress or signals of stability and can be grouped into autonomic-visceral stress signals, motoric stress signals, and state-related stress signals on the one hand and signals of autonomic-visceral stability, signals of motoric stability, and signals of state organizational stability on the other hand. The concept underlying this approach is that stimulation, if inappropriately timed or inappropriate in its quality and intensity, will cause the infant to defend himself against it; if properly timed and appropriate in its quality and intensity, stimulation will cause the infant to seek it out and move toward it, while maintaining himself at a balanced level [26, 27, 49, 50].

The formulation of this dual antagonist integration of avoidance and approach as applied to the newborn infant can be helpful in identifying the infant's current thresholds of balanced, well-modulated functioning and can in turn facilitate the individualization of caregiving and interaction with the infant. Figure 5-2 shows a poorly integrated, withdrawn, and flaccid infant at 1 month postterm in optimal interaction with a social partner. Figure 5-3 shows a well-integrated, robust, and animated infant at the same age in social interaction. The difference of flexibility and modulation is quite apparent.

Exploratory Group Comparisons

The usefulness of the APIB in identifying relative behavioral organizational issues in preterm and full-term infants is demonstrated when one examines data from a subsample consisting of 10 preterm and 10 full-term infants of a larger longitudinal study [6]. The preterm infants selected were born before 34 weeks' postconceptional age, were free of known congenital anomalies or

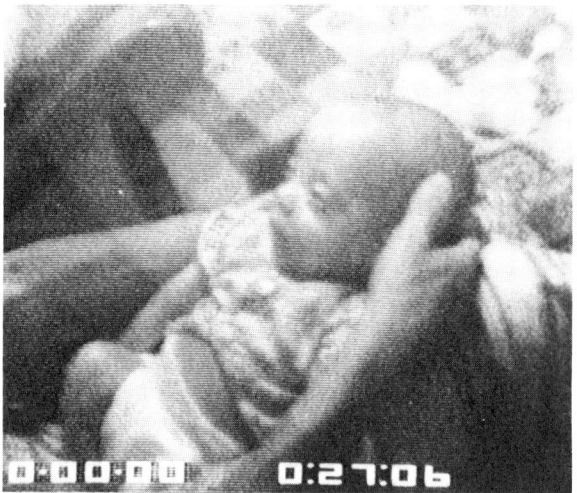

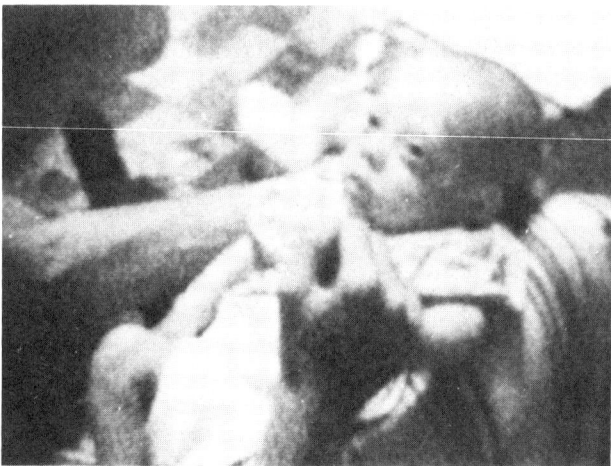

Fig. 5-2. Optimal alerting during social interaction (at 1 month postterm) of a poorly integrated infant (withdrawn and flaccid).

central nervous system insults, and were examinable by at least 36 weeks' postconceptional age. The full-term infants selected were free of any known complications.

All preterm infants were examinable by at least 36 weeks' postconceptional age, indicating their relative robustness. Interrater reliability in administration and scoring of the APIB was maintained in accordance with the criteria spelled out elsewhere [6, 7]. Figure 5-4 shows the APIB system sheet scores for the 10 preterm and 10 full-term infants at 40 and 44 weeks' postconceptional age. Presented is the median score as a measure of central tendency and the twenty-fifth and seventy-fifth percentiles as indicators of sample variability. The lower the score, the more well differentiated and well organized was the performance.

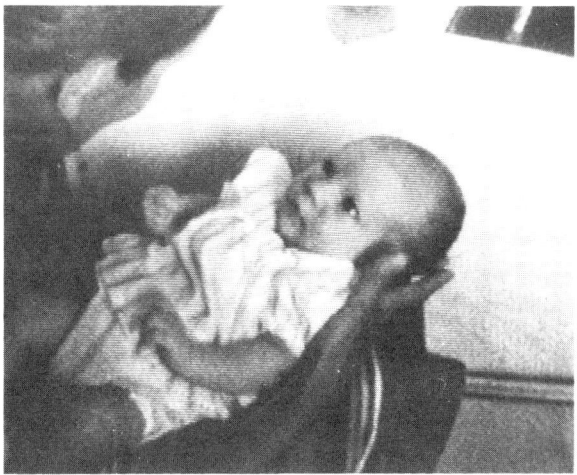

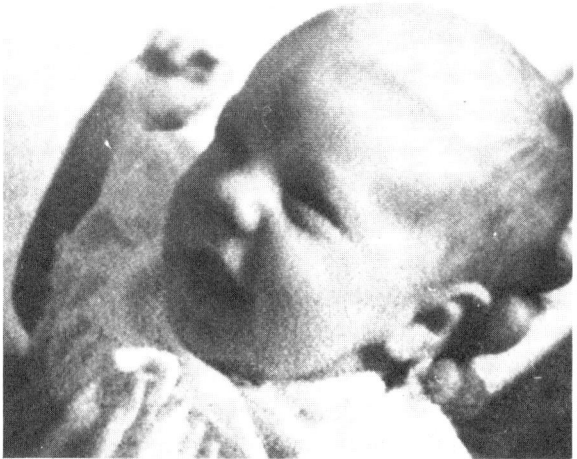

Fig. 5-3. Optimal alerting during social interaction (at 1 month postterm) of a well-integrated infant (animated and motorically modulated).

The preterm infants appear still more poorly organized than the full-term infants at term equivalent and at 1 month postterm in all systems. Inspection of Figure 5-5 indicates that all packages of manipulation also appear consistently more taxing to the 10 preterm infants in terms of system organization than to the 10 full-term infants, both at 40 weeks' postconceptional age and 1 month postterm.

Figure 5-6 indicates that the amount of examiner facilitation necessary to maintain and support the preterm infants in the course of the package manipulations is consistently higher than that necessary for the full-term infants, especially at 44 weeks.

It appears, then, that the APIB System and Package Sheet scores differentiate the organizational abilities of the 10 preterm infants from those of the 10

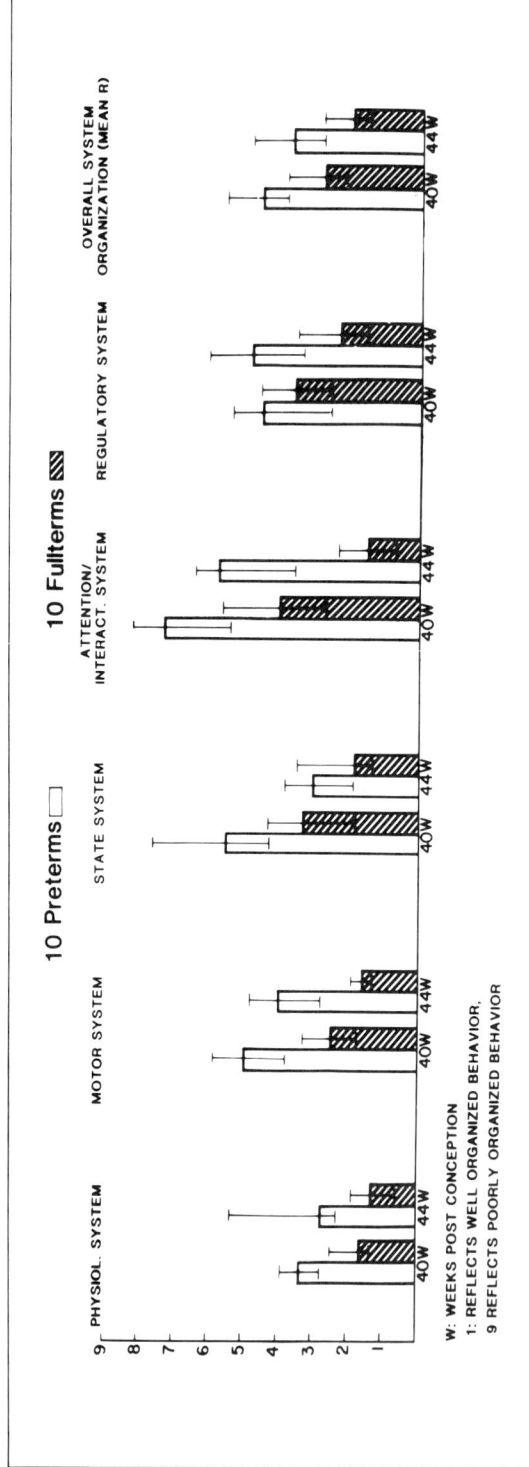

Fig. 5-4. APIB system scores (25th, 50th, and 75th percentiles) for 10 preterm and 10 full-term infants examined at 40 weeks (*40 W*) and 44 weeks (*44 W*) postconceptional age. A score of 9 reflects poorly organized behavior; a score of 1 reflects well-organized behavior. (From H. Als and F. H. Duffy, The Behavior of the Fetal Newborn: Theoretical Considerations and Practical Suggestions for the Use of the APIB. In A. Waldstein et al. [Eds.], *Issues in Neonatal Care*. Produced by WESTAR [Monmouth, Ore.] and TADS [Chapel Hill, N.C.], 1982. Pp. 21–60.)

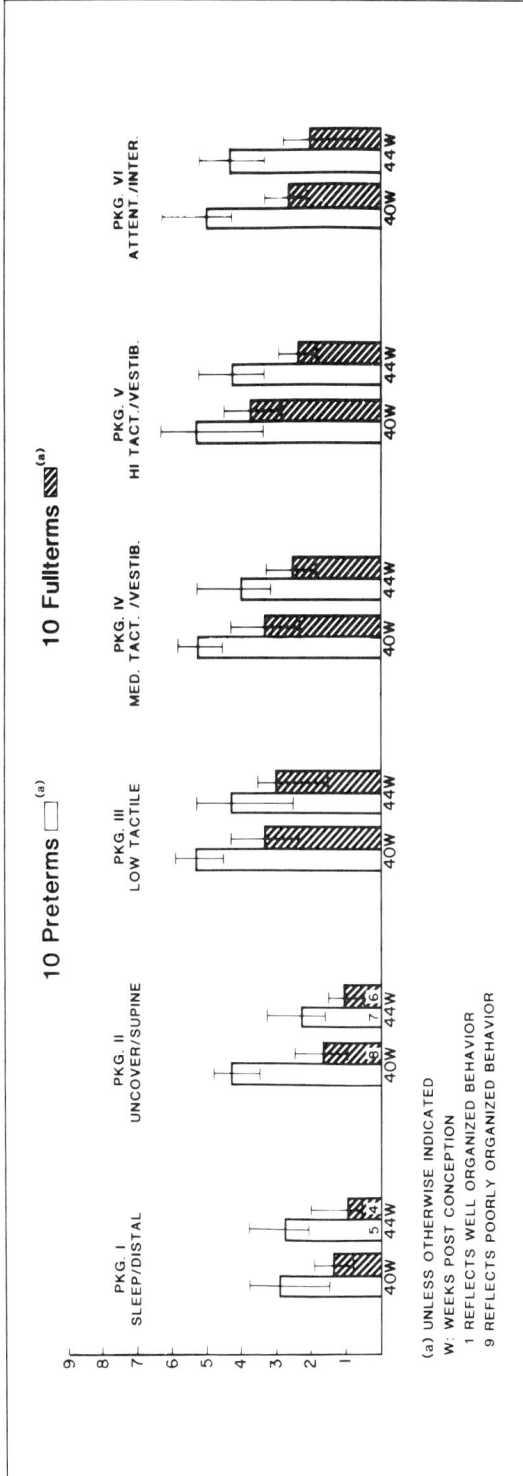

Fig. 5-5. APIB package scores (25th, 50th, and 75th percentile) for 10 preterm and 10 full-term infants examined at 40 weeks (*40 W*) and at 44 weeks (*44 W*) postconceptional age. A score of 9 reflects poorly organized behavior; a score of 1 reflects well-organized behavior. (From H. Als and F. H. Duffy, The Behavior of the Fetal Newborn: Theoretical Considerations and Practical Suggestions for the Use of APIB. In A. Waldstein et al. [Eds.], *Issues in Neonatal Care*. Produced by WESTAR [Monmouth, Ore.] and TADS [Chapel Hill, N.C.], 1982. Pp. 21–60.)

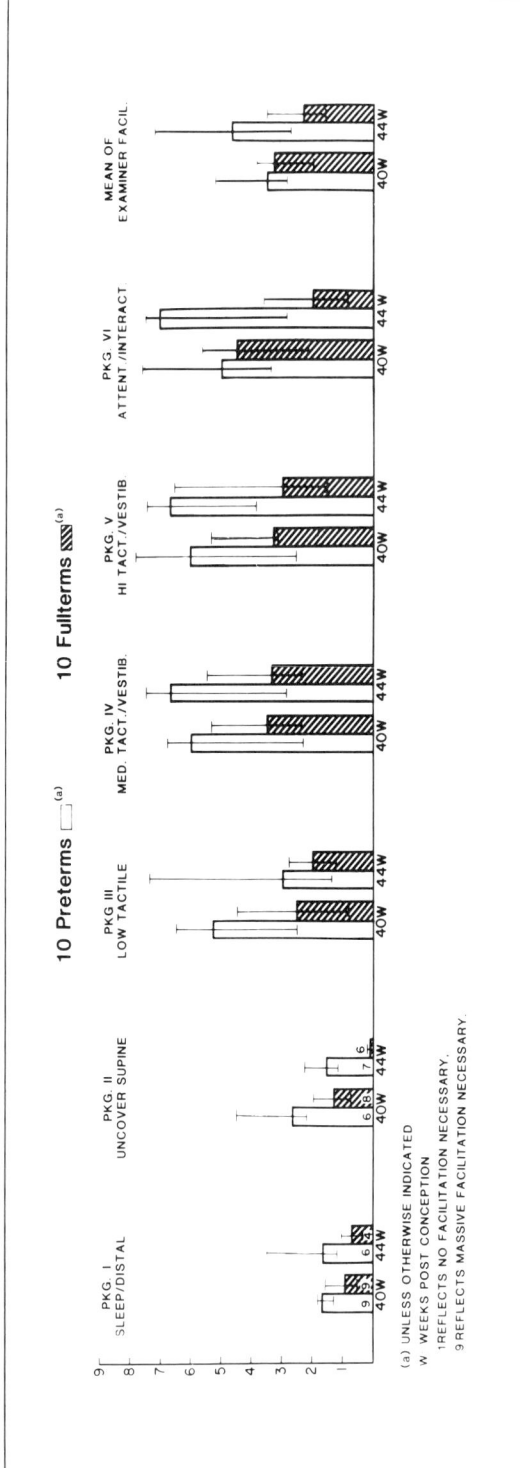

Fig. 5-6. APIB examiner facilitation scores (25th, 50th, and 75th percentiles) for 10 preterm and 10 full-term infants at 40 weeks (*40 W*) and 44 weeks (*44 W*) postconceptional age. A score of 9 reflects massive facilitation necessary; a score of 1 reflects no facilitation necessary. (From H. Als and F. H. Duffy, The Behavior of the Fetal Newborn: Theoretical Considerations and Practical Suggestions for the Use of the APIB. In A. Waldstein et al. [Eds.], *Issues in Neonatal Care.* Produced by WESTAR [Monmouth, Ore.] and TADS [Chapel Hill, N.C.], 1982. Pp. 21–60.)

full-term infants during manipulations at 40 and 44 weeks postconceptual age. Overall, the preterm infants emerge as more highly sensitive and readily overreactive to environmental inputs, more easily stressed and overstimulated, and necessitating more finely tuned, sensitive environmental structuring and support in order to free up maximally differentiated performance. Although individual capacities, such as visual tracking, are quite comparable by 44 weeks' postconceptional age, the behavioral organization embedding the capacities is consistently different.

Individual Patterns of Organization

The next issue is how to identify systematic patterns of behavior that allow one to group infants on the basis of similar behavioral configurations rather than on the basis of their prematurity or full-term status. The identification of such patterns would then permit one to classify any individual infant into one of these clusters and would provide a benchmark for prediction [10, 11]. To this end, we have explored the possibility of applying a clustering analysis system called the Taxonomic Intracellular Analytic System (TICAS), which was developed by Bartels and Wied [14, 15] for the detection of groups of cancerous lymphocytes within a group of normal lymphocytes.

On an a priori basis, 17 features were selected from the APIB that were thought to contribute to the differentiation of groups of infants on the basis of behavioral configuration. Eight of these were taken from the system sheet and are thought to represent comprehensive individual subsystem and overall system organization. Only the R scores, referring to systems organization during the administration of a package, were considered, since they are the most comprehensive scores. The baseline (B) and postpackage status (P) scores were not considered at this point. One feature was taken from the specific package and maneuver scales of the APIB (Score Sheet II) and eight from the Behavioral Summary Scales (Score Sheet III). For our study of the 10 preterm and 10 full-term infants examined at 40 and 44 weeks, the mean of each of the 17 features described from the 40- and 44-week examination was used.

Four clusters of infants were identified with the TICAS method [10]. They were ranked on the basis of their relative goodness, and it was found that the cluster with the highest rank contained seven full-term and no preterm infants, and the cluster with the lowest rank contained only preterms and, surprisingly, one full-term infant. The wider distribution of the preterm group among the clusters suggests, as one might expect, that it is a behaviorally more heterogeneous population.

Figure 5-7 shows the centroid values of the three best features by cluster or nimbuloid of infants. In nimbuloid one are infants whose motor capacity scores, attentional capacity scores, and overall subsystem organization scores are very good. Seven full-term infants achieved this nimbuloid status. In nimbuloid two are infants whose motor capacity scores, attentional capacity scores, and overall subsystem organization scores are in the midrange. Four preterm and one full-term infant achieved this nimbuloid status. In nimbuloid three are infants whose motor capacity scores are above average but whose

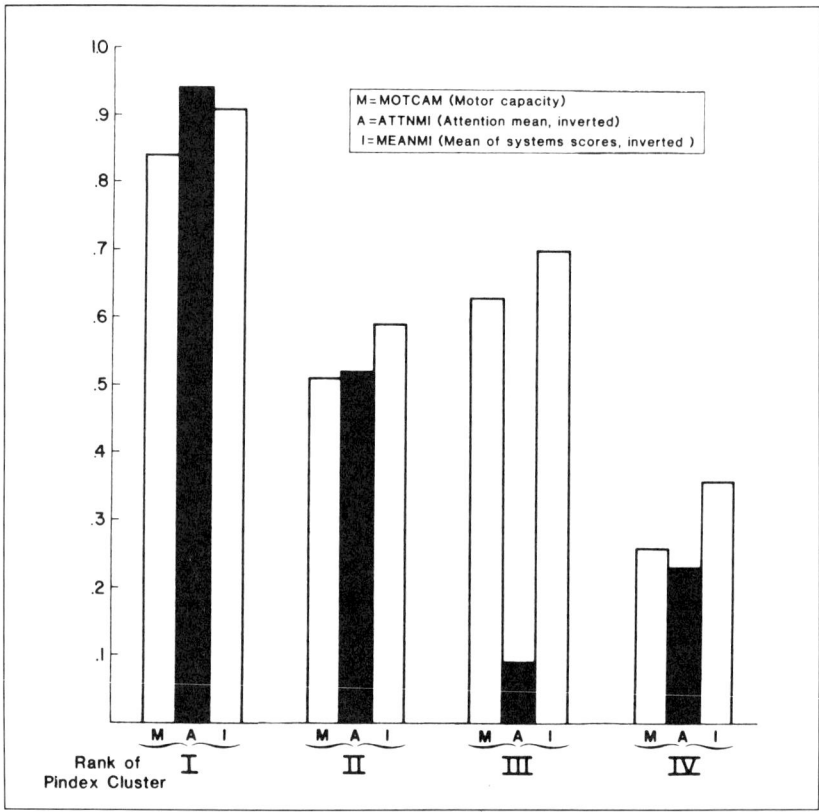

Fig. 5-7. Cluster centroids of four nimbuloids derived from the three best APIB features (n = 20). (From H. Als and F. H. Duffy, The Behavior of the Fetal Newborn: Theoretical Considerations and Practical Suggestions for the Use of the APIB. In A. Waldstein et al. [Eds.], *Issues in Neonatal Care.* Produced by WESTAR [Monmouth, Ore.] and TADS [Chapel Hill, N.C.], 1982. Pp. 21–60.)

atentional capacity is still very poor. One preterm and one full-term infant are in this nimbuloid.

In nimbuloid four are infants whose motor capacity, attentional capacity, and overall subsystem organization scores are low. One full-term and five preterm infants are in this nimbuloid. It is encouraging to find that nimbuloid membership cuts across the medical classifcation of preterm and full-term status and appears to yield conceptually meaningful, behaviorally distinct subgroups of infants.

Behavioral Organization of the Older Infant (Kangaroo-Box Paradigm)

Our next concern was that of consistency of classification over time. If the theoretical model of behavioral organization with the key parameters of differentiation and modulation is to be useful in identifying individuality over time, then a paradigm designed to assess the infant's status along these pa-

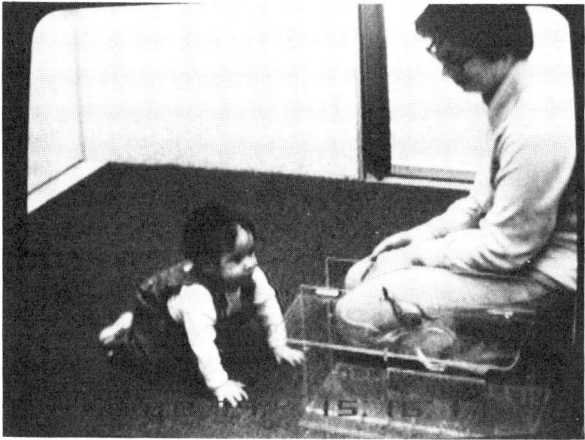
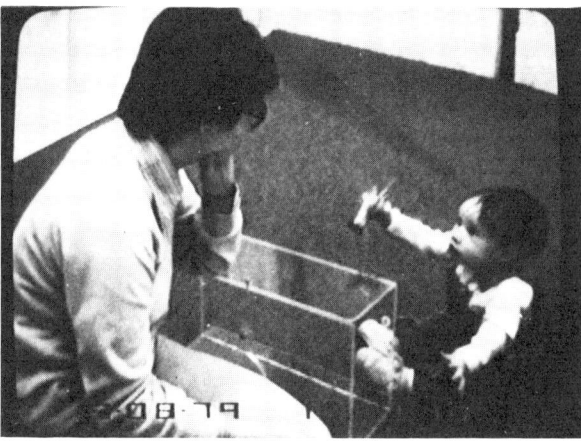

Fig. 5-8. K-Box "play episode" photographs taken from a videotape of a 9-month-old infant who has just attained the kangaroo and wants to give it to her mother. (From H. Als and F. H. Duffy, The Behavior of the Fetal Newborn: Theoretical Considerations and Practical Suggestions for the Use of the APIB. In A. Waldstein et al. [Eds.], *Issues in Neonatal Care*. Produced by WESTAR [Monmouth, Ore.] and TADS [Chapel Hill, N.C.], 1982. Pp. 21–60.)

rameters at a later age should yield a similar cluster membership distribution as found earlier. We focused as the next step on the prelinguistic 9-month age point.

The newly developed paradigm, applicable at 9 and 18 months postterm [6, 7, 9, 10], involves a toy task consisting of a transparent plexiglass box accessible through a transparent mobile porthole latch door and containing a hopping, windup kangaroo. The box is placed on the floor of a playroom. If the infant can walk, it is placed on a specially constructed stand. This makes the kangaroo-box (K-Box) paradigm appropriate from the time the infant is able to begin to move on the floor to approximately 2 years of age. We have recently developed and piloted a more complex and larger version of this paradigm appropriate for the 5- to 7-year-old child.

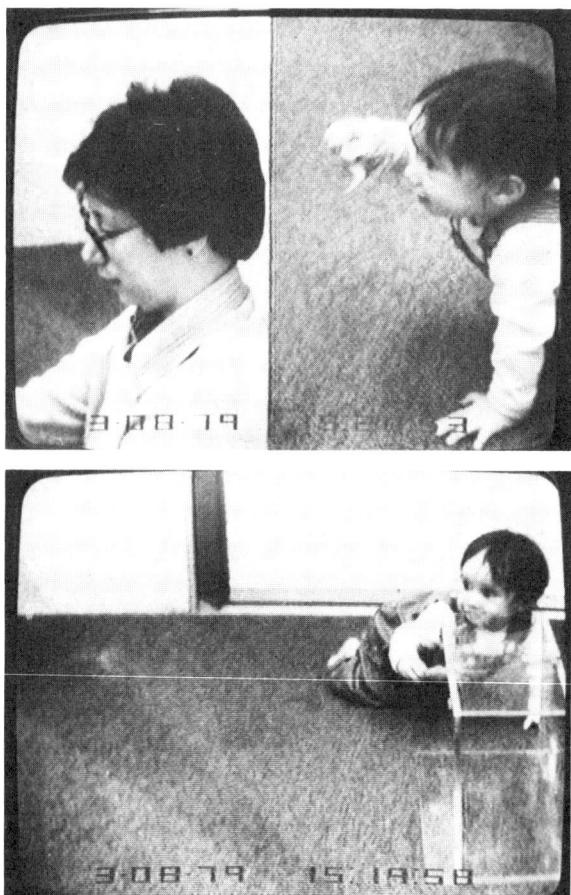

Fig. 5-9. K-box "still-face episode" photographs taken from a split-screen videotape of a 9-month-old infant who is attempting to engage her mother in play. The mother is instructed to maintain a still face. (From H. Als and F. H. Duffy, The Behavior of the Fetal Newborn: Theoretical Considerations and Practical Suggestions for the Use of the APIB. In A. Waldstein et al. [Eds.], *Issues in Neonatal Care.* Produced by WESTAR [Monmouth, Ore.] and TADS [Chapel Hill, N.C.], 1982. Pp. 21–60.)

During the observation, all other distractions (e.g., pictures, chair) are removed, and the mother and infant are asked to go into the room and play with the toy in whatever way they have the best time (Fig. 5-8). The mother and infant are observed and videotaped with a two-camera split-screen system through one-way mirror walls for 6 minutes. Then the mother is asked to place the kangaroo back into the box, close the latch door, and sit against the wall of the room looking at the infant but not interacting with or reacting to him (Fig. 5-9).

The infant is observed in this "still-face" situation for 6 minutes. Then a 3-minute reunion is observed in which the mother is again allowed to play with the infant. The kangaroo-box paradigm challenges the infant's cognitive, gross and fine motor, social, and affective capacities, and for some more stressed infants, even their autonomic physiological regulation as the infant attempts to retrieve the kangaroo from the box. Furthermore, it provides an opportunity to observe the mother's strategies in facilitating and expanding the infant's competence. Some mothers simplify the task for the infant by taking the kangaroo out for him, then winding it up, and playing only with the kangaroo in that way. If the infant wants to explore the box, he may use the box alone as a toy but not combine the kangaroo and box. Other mothers will aid the infant in figuring out how to open the latch door and then winding the kangaroo up. They may then restart the sequence for or with the infant and develop a complex, turn-taking cooperative game. The still-face situation highlights the infant's ability to negotiate this challenging task on his own, yet in the presence of the mother. Some infants become assertive and competent in the absence of the mother's enveloping them. Others will try to call on the mother for help once their initial efforts alone have failed. Others will become very intense and frustrated, focus on the task, be unable to solve it, and simultaneously be unable to move away from it. The more well-modulated infant typically takes some time out, explores the room, and then returns to the task.

The infant's capacities are scored during the play episode along 12 dimensions on a scale from 1 (minimal) to 5 (optimal), yielding a total score ranging from 12 to 60. The dimensions scored include autonomic organization, gross and fine motor organization, symmetry of tonus, movement and posture, apparent cognitive functioning, language and vocal organization, affective organization, social-interactive organization, competence in play with the object, competence in combining object play and social interaction, degree of self-regulation, degree of facilitation and structure necessary, and degree of pleasure and pride displayed by the infant. Attention is paid to the infant's autonomic reactions, movements, tone, vocalizations, and facial expressions in their interplay. The parent is scored on eight parallel dimensions, also on a scale from 1 (minimal) to 5 (optimal), yielding a total score ranging from 8 to 40. The dimensions scored include quality of parent's motoric input, social input, facilitation, ability to regulate toy task, affective organization, pleasure and pride, acknowledgment and praise, and degree of effort. Three summary interactive items—degree of playful turn-taking, overall synchrony of the interaction, and overall quality of the interaction—are also scored. From the still-face episode, 11 infant scores are derived, yielding one total infant score and one parent score. There is one summary reunion score [8]. The K-Box scales are developed to be directly related to the assessment scales of organizational capacities on the APIB.

We have investigated the possibility of identifying clusters of infants at the 9-month age point with the TICAS system [10] on the basis of competence as derived from the K-Box paradigm. We have available a total group of 20 preterm and 19 full-term infants observed at 9 months after expected due date, measured on the kangaroo-box paradigm and also tested on the Bayley Scales of Infant Development. Tapes on all 39 were scored by a trained but "blind" scorer who was not familiar with the infants as newborns. The 10 preterm and 10 full-term infants discussed previously are a subsample of this group.

It is of great interest that, as we had hypothesized on an a priori basis from our model of development, the degree of flexibility in integrating social and object play was the strongest feature in developing clusters and that several of the affective range features had good differentiation power, with pleasure and pride being the third best, after self-regulation and fine motor coordination and flexibility contributing to the differentiation. Pleasure and pride is conceived as the ability to set a goal for oneself, attain it, realize the attainment, and take pleasure and pride in this attainment. It thus reflects the closing of an intraorganism feedback loop, which we postulate is a key feature of integrated, autonomous development. It makes the attained achievement available over time to be called on more and more readily until it is part of the person's basic repertoire, thus freeing up energies for the next level of goals.

When we added the Bayley Mental Development Index of the Bayley Scales of Infant Development [16], a standard infant assessment score, which significantly differentiated the 20 preterm infants from the 19 full-term infants, the features from the K-Box paradigm appeared to add important dimensions of competence in identifying clusters of infants. The four resultant clusters of infants are shown in Figure 5-10.

Again, cluster or nimbuloid membership cuts across the medical classification of preterm and full-term status and appears to yield conceptually meaningful, behaviorally distinct subgroups of infants. That the Bayley Scale scores are modified by distinct configurations of behavioral parameters encourages us to hypothesize that potentially the predictability of the Bayley Scale can be improved by these functional differentiation and modulation measures.

Correspondence of Newborn Status and 9 Months Status

When we investigated the cluster classification stability from the newborn period to the 9-month point for the 20 initial subjects who are a subsample of the 39 subjects studied at 9 months, we saw, as Figure 5-11 shows, that there was a highly significant rank order relationship of behavioral competence cluster membership from the newborn period to 9 months. Only two outlying infants were identified, one who moved from "newborn status four" to "9 months status one," and one who moved from "newborn status one" to "9 months status three."

We are very encouraged by these results from our pilot work, since they indicate that it is indeed possible to identify behavioral patterns of competence that have continuity and that cut across medical variables such as prematurity and full-term status. We anticipate that the identification of such patterns will make the diagnosis of an individual infant's developmental functioning more succinct and will help in structuring appropriate early support and intervention and in measuring the effect of such support and intervention.

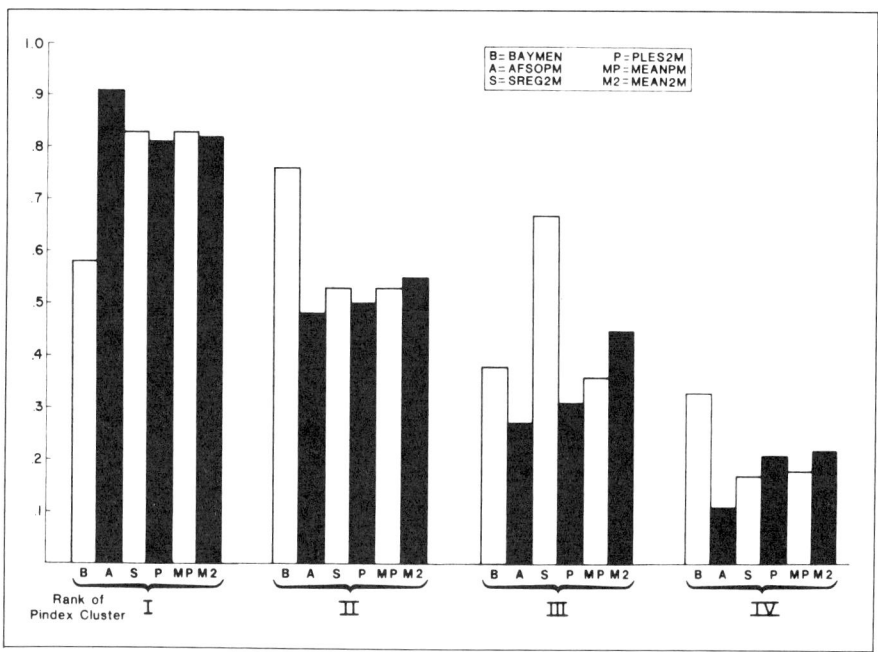

Fig. 5-10. Cluster centroids of four nimbuloids derived from the six best K-Box and Bayley Scale features at 9 months (n = 39). (From H. Als and F. H. Duffy, The Behavior of the Fetal Newborn: Theoretical Considerations and Practical Suggestions for the Use of the APIB. In A. Waldstein et al. [Eds.], *Issues in Neonatal Care.* Produced by WESTAR [Monmouth, Ore.] and TADS [Chapel Hill, N.C.], 1982. Pp. 21–60.)

Fig. 5-11. Correspondence of newborn and 9-month-old nimbuloid membership—APIB to Bayley Scale with K-Box. (From H. Als and F. H. Duffy, The Behavior of the Fetal Newborn: Theoretical Considerations and Practical Suggestions for the Use of the APIB. In A. Waldstein et al. [Eds.], *Issues in Neonatal Care.* Produced by WESTAR [Monmouth, Ore.] and TADS [Chapel Hill, N.C.], 1982. Pp. 21–60.)

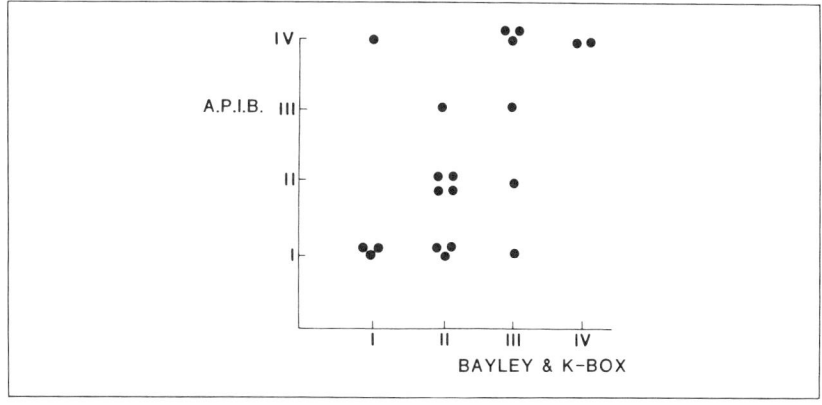

Conclusions

From my considerations and studies, I have arrived at the formulation of a synactive theory of development, postulating that at any stage in development there is a drive for modulation and integration of subsystem functioning fueled from within the human and impinged upon, facilitated, or potentially hindered from the environment. From fetal development onward, the goal of the human appears to be actively to structure his environment to allow him successive reintegrations following expansion and differentiation. The degree of human differentiation and the degree of openness of the band of modulation as newly emerging developmental agenda are being negotiated become the main dimensions of individuality.

My current work is concerned with the replication of these results on a larger sample. I am extending the assessment of infants to the 18-month and 3-year age points and eventually the 5-year and school-age points; and am engaged in the exploration of brain electrophysiological correlates of these behavioral patterns. It appears from the work with newborns and young infants that we can improve the degree of modulated functioning by our provision of more appropriate environmental inputs. This is possible when we take seriously the infant's thresholds of integration and his strategies of reorganization and self-regulation at each level and when we allow him to develop and practice his own, self-instituted return to modulated balance, autonomously closing the hierarchical feedback loops of goal setting, goal accomplishment, and the realization of goal attainment, thus making them increasingly easy to institute. If we give the grappling infant as much help as he needs, not to prevent this grappling, but to accomplish a goal he is trying to attain, accomplishing as much on his own strength as he can, we assure the gradual and open progression of increasingly modulated differentiation.

We are all familiar with the preterm infant in an Isolette who struggles and grasps and moves until finally he is tucked into the corner of the Isolette, shoulders, back, and head pressed against the wall, actively seeking help with motor inhibition and reflexion. As he achieves it through the physical barrier of the Isolette, his struggle finally ceases; he relaxes his frantic movements; they become smooth and subside; his respiration becomes modulated, and he can fall into a well-organized sleep state. How often have we then moved him back into the center of the mattress, forcing him to go through the whole rebalancing process over and over again? If we recognize his active efforts and respect his competence, we can help him accomplish his current goals by utilizing his own emerging skills and putting them increasingly at his service. If we do not respect his competence and do not understand his active self-organization efforts at each stage, we may continuously overload him or mistreat him and force him to expend his energies on costly shutting-out mechanisms, limiting his experience of increasing self-regulation and differentiation and forcing him to fall back again and again on poorly modulated, bare subsistence mechanisms. The extent to which the demise of the preterm infant is induced by our unwitting overriding of his own active efforts and how much is therefore preventable as we become better at identifying and supporting him in his own efforts at autonomic, motoric, state, and attentional regulation in their interplay are only beginning to become apparent, as we are allowing ourselves to see the integrative complexity of the human at every stage. In a fuller appreciation of the interactive complexities of intraorganism subsystems and organism-environment synaction lies the possibility of much prevention and the opportunity for much support and for models to be developed for the better understanding of neurointegrative functioning over time.

Acknowledgments

I wish to acknowledge my indebtedness to Dr. T. B. Brazelton, Chief of the Child Development Unit at Children's Hospital Medical Center, Boston; my former colleagues, Dr. B. M. Lester and Dr. M. Yogman, coinvestigators on a project of preterm infant development; and Dr. F. H. Duffy for his continued guidance and collaboration from a neurologist's perspective as well as his assistance in the use of the TICAS analysis system. Special thanks go to the infants and their families who make our observations and studies possible and who have contributed so generously to our understanding of the early developmental process.

References

1. Als, H. The human newborn and his mother: An ethological study of their interaction. University of Pennsylvania, Doctoral Dissertation, 1975.
2. Als, H. Autonomous state control: The first stage in successful negotiation of parent-infant interaction. Presented at the Meetings of the American Academy of Child Psychiatry, Toronto, 1976.
3. Als, H. The newborn communicates. *J. Commun.* 27:66, 1977.
4. Als, H. Assessing an assessment: Conceptual considerations, methodological issues, and a perspective on the future of the neonatal behavioral assessment scale. In A. J. Sameroff (Ed.), Organization and Stability of Newborn Behavior: A Commentary on the Brazelton Neonatal Behavioral Assessment Scale. *Monogr. Soc. Res. Child Dev.* 43:14, 1978.
5. Als, H. Social Interaction: Dynamic Matrix for Developing Behavioral Organization. In I. C. Uzgiris (Ed.), *Social Interaction and Communication in Infancy: New Directions for Child Development,* Vol. 4. San Francisco: Jossey Bass, 1979.
6. Als, H. Infant Individuality: Assessing Patterns of Very Early Development. In J. Call, E. Galenson and R. L. Tyson (Eds.), *Frontiers of Infant Psychiatry.* New York: Basic Books, 1983. Pp. 363–378.
7. Als, H. Toward a synactive theory of development: Promise for the assessment of infant individuality. *Infant Ment. Health J.* 3:229, 1982.
8. Als, H., and Berger, A. *Scoring Manual for Kangaroo Box Paradigm.* Boston: Child Development Unit, Children's Hospital Medical Center, 1980.
9. Als, H., and Brazelton, T. B. A new model of assessing the behavioral organization in preterm and fullterm infants: Two case studies. *J. Am. Acad. Child Psychiatry* 20:239, 1981.

10. Als, H., and Duffy, F. H. The Behavior of the Premature Infant: A Theoretical Framework for a Systematic Assessment. In T. B. Brazelton and B. M. Lester (Eds.), *New Approaches to Developmental Screening of Infants*. Amsterdam: Elsevier, 1983. Pp. 153–173.
11. Als, H., and Duffy, F. H. Quantifying the Quality of Infant Behavior. In L. Lipsitt (Eds.), *Monographs in Infancy*. Hillsdale, N.J.: Lawrence Erlbaum. In preparation.
12. Als, H., et al. Manual for the Assessment of Preterm Infants' Behavior (A.P.I.B.). Appendix to H. Als et al. Towards a Research Instrument for the Assessment of Preterm Infants' Behavior (A.P.I.B.). In H. E. Fitzgerald, B. M. Lester, and M. W. Yogman (Eds.), *Theory and Research in Behavioral Pediatrics*, Vol. I. New York: Plenum, 1982.
13. Als, H., et al. The behavior of the fullterm yet underweight newborn infant. *Dev. Med. Child Neurol.* 18:590, 1976.
14. Bartels, P. H., and Wied, G. L. Extraction and Evaluation of Information from Cell Images. In C. R. Richmond et al. (Eds.), *Proceedings of the First Los Alamos Life Science Symposium: Mammalian Cells, Probes and Problems*. Washington, D.C.: Technical Information Center, Office of Public Affairs, U.S. Energy Research and Development Administration Conference, 731007, 1973.
15. Bartels, P. H., and Wied, G. L. Computer analysis and interpretation of microscopic images: Current problems and future directions. *Proc. Inst. Electrical Electronic Engineers* 65:252, 1977.
16. Bayley, N. *Manual for the Bayley Scales of Infant Development*. New York: The Psychological Corporation, 1969.
17. Birnholz, J. C., Stephens, J. C., and Faria, H. Fetal movement patterns: A possible means of defining neurologic developmental milestones in utero. *Am. J. Roentgenol.* 130:536, 1978.
18. Bolwig, N. A study of the behavior of the chacma baboon, Papio Ursinus. *Behavior* 14:136, 1959.
19. Bolwig, N. Observations and thoughts on the evolution of facial mimic. *Kodoe* 2:60, 1959.
20. Brandt, I. Patterns of Early Neurological Development. In F. Faulkner and J. M. Tanner (Eds.), *Human Growth: A Comprehensive Treatise*, Vol. 3. New York: Plenum, 1973.
21. Brazelton, T. B. The Neonatal Behavioral Assessment Scale. *Clinics in Developmental Medicine*, No. 50, London: Heinemann, 1973.
22. Brazelton, T. B. Assessment techniques for enhancing infant development. Paper presented at the Meetings of the National Center for Clinical Infant Programs, Washington, D.C., December 6–7, 1979.
23. Buettner-Janusch, J. *Origins of Man*. New York: Wiley, 1966.
24. Casaer, P. Postural Behavior in Newborn Infants. *Clinics in Developmental Medicine*, No. 72. London: Heinemann and Philadelphia: Lippincott, 1979.
25. Denckla, M. B. Minimal Brain Dysfunction. In *Education and the Brain*, 77th Yearbook of the National Society for the Study of Education. Chicago: University of Chicago Press, 1978.
26. Denny-Brown, D. *The Cerebral Control of Movement*. Springfield, Ill.: Thomas, 1966.
27. Denny-Brown, D. *The Basal Ganglia and Their Relation to Disorders of Movement*. London: Oxford University Press, 1972.
28. Drillien, C. M., Thomson, A. J. M., and Bargoyne, K. Low birth weight children at early school-age: A longitudinal study. *Dev. Med. Child Neurol.* 22:26, 1980.

29. Emde, R. N. Commentary to organization and stability of newborn behavior. In A. J. Sameroff (Ed.), Organization and Stability of Newborn Behavior: A Commentary on the Brazelton Neonatal Behavioral Assessment Scale. *Child Dev.* 43:135, 1978.
30. Francis-Williams, J., and Davies, P. A. Very low birth weight and later intelligence. *Dev. Med. Child Neurol.* 16:709, 1974.
31. Herzog, J. M. Attachment, attunement, and abuse, and occurrence in certain premature infant-parent dyads and triads. Presented at the American Academy of Child Psychiatry Meetings, Atlanta, 1979.
32. Huber, E. *Evolution of Facial Musculature and Facial Expression.* Baltimore: Johns Hopkins Press, 1931.
33. Hunt, J. M. *Intelligence and Experience.* New York: Ronald, 1961.
34. Kagan, J., Kearsely, R. B., and Zelazo, P. R. *Infancy, Its Place In Human Development.* Cambridge, Mass.: Harvard University Press, 1978.
35. Kitchen, W. H., et al. A longitudinal study of very low birthweight infants: I. An overview of performance at eight years of age. *Dev. Med. Child Neurol.* 22:172, 1980.
36. Lewis, M. Infant intelligence tests: Their use and misuse. *Hum. Dev.* 16:108, 1973.
37. McCall, R. B. Toward an epigenetic conception of mental development in the first three years of life. In M. Lewis (Ed.), *Origins of Intelligence: Infancy and Early Childhood.* New York: Plenum, 1976.
38. McCall, R. B., Hogarty, P. S., and Hurlbert, N. Transitions in infant sensorimotor development and the prediction of childhood IQ. *Am. Psychol.* 27:728, 1972.
39. Milani-Comparetti, A. Fetal movement. First E. Zausmer Lecture, Children's Hospital Medical Center, Boston, 1980.
40. Neligan, G. A., et al. Born too soon or born too small: A follow-up study to 7 years of age. *Clinics in Development Medicine,* No. 61. London: Heinemann, 1976.
41. Piaget, J. *The Origins of Intelligence in Children.* New York: Norton, 1963.
42. Prechtl, H. F. R. Strategy and Validity of Early Detection of Neurological Dysfunction. In C. P. Douglas and K. S. Holt (Eds.), *Mental Retardation, Prenatal Diagnosis and Infant Assessment.* London: Butterworth, 1972.
43. Rubin, R. A., and Balow, B. Perinatal Influences on the Behavior and Learning Problems of Children. In B. B. Lahey and A. E. Kazdin (Eds.), *Advances in Child Clinical Psychology,* Vol. 1. New York: Plenum, 1977.
44. Rubin, R. A., and Balow, B. Infant neurological abnormalities as indicators of cognitive impairment. *Dev. Med. Child Neurol.* 22:336, 1980.
45. Saint-Anne D'Argassies, S. Long-term neurological follow-up study of 286 truly premature infants: I. Neurological Sequelae. *Dev. Med. Child Neurol.* 19:462, 1977.
46. Sameroff, A. J., and Chandler, M. Reproductive Risk and the Continuum of Caretaking Casualty. In F. D. Horowitz (Ed.), *Review of Child Development Research,* Vol. 4. Chicago: University of Chicago Press, 1975.
47. Sander, L. W. Issues in early mother-child interaction. *J. Am. Acad. Child Psychiatry* 1:141, 1962.
48. Sander, L. W. Adaptive relationships in early mother-child interaction. *J Am. Acad. Child Psychiatry* 3:232, 1964.
49. Schneirla, T. C. An Evolutionary and Developmental Theory of Biphasic Processes Underlying Approach and Withdrawal. In M. R. Jones (Ed.), *Nebraska Symposium on Motivation.* Lincoln: University of Nebraska Press, 1959.

50. Schneirla, T. C. Aspects of stimulation and organization in approach/withdrawal processes underlying vertebrate behavioral development. *Adv. Stud. Sci.* 1:1, 1965.
51. Sigman, M., and Parmelee, A. H. Longitudinal Evaluation of the Preterm Infant. In T. M. Field et al. (Eds.), *Infants Born at Risk*. New York: Spectrum, 1979.

6 Should So-Called Modality Preferences Determine the Nature of Instruction for Children with Reading Disabilities?

Isabelle Y. Liberman

The sensory modalities have figured importantly for many years in the thinking of educators and clinicians concerned with the learning problems of children. It goes without saying that sensory deficits can interfere with learning efficiency. Any sensory deficits a child has should certainly be assessed and remediated to the extent possible. Children undoubtedly learn better when they can see the book or blackboard and can hear the teacher.

Recently, however, the sensory modalities have been used educationally in a different way, one that I have serious misgivings about. That is, children's deficiencies in test performance have been used to classify them as "visual" or "auditory learners," or as having a "visual" or "auditory learning style." Questions about whether a child is deficient in one or the other modality have, in many places in this country and abroad, become central in the diagnosis of learning disabilities generally and reading disabilities in particular.

Moreover, methods of reading instruction have themselves been characterized as visual or auditory, and the child's relative proficiency in the so-called visual or auditory tasks has then been used to determine the appropriate method of instruction for that child. Thus, for example, children who do better on visually presented tasks than on those auditorily presented are said to be visual learners, requiring a different method of instruction from their auditorily inclined classmates. Since most educators believe in teaching to the strengths of the child, the reading instruction they will offer such a child will emphasize "visual" approaches such as memorization of whole words by their visual configurations, reading for meaning by guessing from the context, and little or no analysis of the phonological structure of the word. If, on the other hand, the child is better on auditorily presented tasks and is therefore considered to be an auditory learner (a relatively small number qualify), a so-called auditory approach will be offered instead. An auditory method customarily means one in which phonic analysis is stressed. In either case, then, the determination of what to do about the child's reading problem is made on the basis of a purported modality difference.

As I see it, there is, for most children, no reasonable basis for espousing a visual approach to reading. In addition, the so-called auditory approach is badly misnamed and, what is more critical, perhaps misunderstood. Finally, the visual-auditory contrast, as usually conceived, may indeed be irrelevant to the problems of reading acquisition.

The work presented was supported by grant HD-01994 from the National Institute of Child Health and Human Development to Haskins Laboratories. Parts are adapted from papers presented at the annual conference of the New York Academy of Sciences, New York, May 7, 1982, and at the 33rd annual conference of the Orton Dyslexia Society, Baltimore, November 5, 1982.

The characterization of children as visual or auditory learners is typically determined by means of various measurement procedures carried out during the testing required prior to special education placement. A recent comprehensive review of modality preference studies [15] concluded that most such measurement devices in current use do not demonstrate the reliability required for differential assignment of children to instructional programs by modality. But even if we set aside this objection, we must still ask, what is the evidence that the children's reading problems are actually due to deficits in these modalities?

Reading Disability and Visual Deficits

Review after review of all available research year after year to the present [2, 6, 34, 35, 36] has concluded that most reading disabilities are not associated with deficits in visual discrimination. A number of studies by our Haskins Laboratories reading research unit are also relevant here. Our first group of studies examined the reading errors of beginning readers [10, 11, 33]. Reading errors were selected for study because it was considered that they could provide a window through which to view the special problems of learning to read. In this research, we found that the errors made by beginning readers and older children with reading disabilities tend to be linguistic, not optical, in nature; that is, they relate to the phonological structure of words and not their optical shapes. Thus, we found that the frequency of errors on consonants, but not on vowels, depends on their position in the syllable (errors on final consonants are more frequent than on initial consonants, whereas vowel errors occur with equal frequency in every position). Errors on consonants, but not on vowels, tend to be similar to the target letter in terms of phonetic features. Finally, when errors are tallied with respect to opportunities for error, vowel errors are much more numerous than consonant errors. There is surely no way to account for such an error pattern on a visual basis. After all, the difference between the sets of consonants and vowels is linguistic, not visual.

In emphasizing the importance of the linguistic nature of their reading errors, we do not mean to imply that poor readers never make visually based errors. They do, of course, on occasion. The most commonly remarked error that can be counted as visually based is the reversal of the reversible lowercase letters (e.g., *b, d, p, q*). However, we have found in our research [23] that while reversal errors do occur, they represent a very small proportion of the total number of errors that are made, even by second graders who are having the greatest difficulty with reading. We found that of all the errors made by these children, reversals of letter orientation accounted for only 15 percent of the total errors as compared with 32 percent for other consonants and 43 percent for vowels. Transposition errors (e.g., *from* → *form*) accounted for the remaining 10 percent.

Thus, visual-type errors appear to account for relatively few of the errors made by poor beginning readers. Moreover, in other experiments we have shown, as others have, that poor readers actually do very well on visual tasks that are nonverbal. For example, we have found that when the task requires children to hold in memory visually presented forms that are hard to code verbally, like the Kimura nonsense figures, or photographs of faces in which all easily describable elements have been masked, poor readers have no more difficulty (and in fact may do somewhat better) than their good-reading peers. In contrast, despite a procedure identical in every way except for the nature of the items presented, poor readers do significantly worse than good readers when the items to be held in memory are simple, three-letter printed nonsense syllables [26]. Similarly, we have found that poor beginning readers have no trouble with a sequential memory task like the Corsi blocks, where the sequence does not lend itself to linguistic coding, but are easily distinguished from good readers in the ability to hold strings of words or even meaningful sentences in working memory [28, 29].

Space does not permit me to describe the numerous studies by other investigators that have come to similar conclusions by means of many other experimental procedures (see references 34 and 35 for reviews). However, I should like to mention two that seem to be particularly cogent here. Several years ago, Rozin, Poritsky, and Sotsky [32] found that when Chinese-like characters were used to represent words, learning-disabled children who were essentially nonreaders readily learned to identify the visually complex optical patterns of those characters. More recently, House, Hankey, and Magid [13] have shown that retardates with a mental age of 5 years or less, who had also never been able to learn to read, could be taught to identify 200 or more of these complex visual forms.

In view of this sort of evidence, it would be unlikely to find that the problem of poor readers lies in a purely visual deficit, that is, in an inability to discriminate the 26 letters of the alphabet as visual forms. Of course, some might say that they did not mean to imply that the visual deficiency of the poor readers has to do only with the discrimination of shapes. In this connection, we have seen references to a visual deficiency of 90 percent of poor readers that purportedly includes signs of nystagmus and difficulties in visual tracking [16]. As far as I know, such findings have not been replicated by other experimenters nor have there been comparisons with normal controls. Moreover, neurologists have reported patients with nystagmus who have learned to read well in spite of it [31]. As for the tracking behavior of poor readers, it is well-known that reading is not carried out by tracking movements of the eyes but rather during the fixations between saccadic movements. How efficiently or poorly children can track moving objects may be of interest for other reasons; if a child wished to become a ball player or airplane spotter, for example, one would want to evaluate and train that ability. But I cannot see it as pertinent to the reading process. In conclusion, it is certainly fair to say that the number of poor readers with visual problems is relatively small [2, 4, 9, 30, 35].

Reading Disability and Auditory Deficits

What is the evidence that poor readers have auditory problems? We know that the deaf do have difficulties in learning to read, but the poor readers we are discussing are not deaf. In fact, most research studies of disabled readers make the point that their subjects are carefully screened to have no hearing loss. A commonly held view, however, is that although these children have no hearing deficits, they do have an auditory perception problem. What is the evidence for that view? I would suggest that some of the evidence is based on tests that tap abilities beyond simple perception of an acoustic stimulus.

A widely used auditory test, the Wepman Test of Auditory Discrimination [38], for example, as with others of similar format, appears to be misnamed, since it tests more than either auditory or discrimination abilities. To be sure, it is auditory with respect to its mode of presentation and does require discrimination of word pairs, but it places other demands on the child as well. It requires, in addition, an understanding of the concept of same-different and, more important still, requires the ability to make a phonemic analysis of the word pairs. The child not only must be able to discriminate between auditorily presented word pairs, as the title of the test implies, but also must be able to stand back from the word pairs and consider their formal structure, to determine whether their phonemic structure is the same or differs in one phonemic element. As Blank and Bridger [3] demonstrated years ago, children might have no difficulty in repeating the individual words of the pairs correctly, thus showing adequate auditory discrimination, and nonetheless do poorly on the test. I propose that the reason for this is that their problem may not be auditory at all—indeed, they may be deficient in the ability to do that kind of phonological analysis.

Nonetheless, there *are* hints that reading-disabled children may indeed have deficits in the perception of auditorily presented material. However, the deficit appears to be specific to phonological perception rather than relating to auditory perception generally. Consider the recent findings by Brady, Shankweiler, and Mann [5] at Haskins Laboratories, who carried out an experiment in which good- and poor-reader groups were tested on two auditory perception tasks, one involving words and the other nonspeech environmental sounds. The identification tasks were each presented under two conditions: with favorable and with unfavorable signal-to-noise ratios. The findings were that the poor-reader group did show a deficit, but it was specific to the speech stimuli and occurred only in the noise-masked condition. That is, the poor readers made significantly more errors than did the good readers when listening to speech in noise; they did not differ from the good readers in the perception of nonspeech environmental sounds, whether noise-masked or not.

It has been suggested [40] that poor readers tend to require higher quality information for adequate performance in perceptual tasks. Note that the poor readers in the Brady, Shankweiler, and Mann study [5] did need a higher quality of signal than did the good readers for error-free performance, but only with speech, *not* with nonspeech (environmental) sounds. Their results suggest that the poor reader's perceptual deficit may be related not to auditory perception in general, as people have assumed, but rather to the apprehension of the phonetic and phonological structure of words. Put another way, the perceptual difficulty of the poor reader may not be auditory in some general sense but may be best characterized as a difficulty with language.

Reading as a Language-Based Skill

There has been ample demonstration that poor readers do have difficulty in apprehending language structures [37, 39]. I do not find this surprising because my conception of the reading process is based on the assumption that an orthography is a communication system that is language-based and not primarily visual in its organization. The orthography is more than simply a set of visually perceived forms composed of ascenders, descenders, and diagonals. It is more even than combinations of such forms. Instead, the orthography transcribes a language. Therefore, if we want to understand what reading requires of a child, and particularly why those requirements are so hard for so many children, we must understand just how our orthography represents the language and why, given that particular kind of representation, it might be hard for the child to make the connection. Such considerations have led our research group to pay particular attention to what we believe to be two critical aspects of the reading process. The first has to do with the reading (and understanding) of words: given a printed word, how do readers find in their lexicon the real word that the printed word represents? The second part has to do with the reading and understanding of sentences: given that readers have apprehended the words, how do they hold the words until the meaning has been extracted from the constituent structures [22, 24]?

We have taken as given, as others have [12], that in understanding language, whether written or spoken, one gets to the meaning by dealing in distinctly linguistic ways with the units of the language (e.g., the phonologically represented words) and the larger syntactic structures they form (the phrases and sentences). Surely, in order to comprehend language, both the reader and the listener must carry out some kind of linguistic processing, however automatic it may be. Readers are not going to get the meaning directly from the optical forms of the orthography any more than listeners can get meaning directly from the auditory patterns of the acoustic signal. The processes that extract meaning from language are different in important ways from those that extract meaning from other visual representations, like pictures, or from auditory stimuli like automobile horns or cowbells. Perhaps one can go directly from a picture to one or another of its typically many meanings or from the sound of an automobile horn to some idea of what it signifies. But whatever the processes by which we get meaning from a picture or from a nonlinguistic pattern of sound, the processes by which we derive meaning from language are different.

Words and sentences are uniquely linguistic things, processed in special ways in the brain [7]. A word is a string of abstract, meaningless phonological units, and its relation to meaning is arbitrary; there is nothing about the acoustic form of a spoken word nor about its visual representation that can possibly give its meaning directly. As for a sentence, its meaning is even less directly available; it is certainly not to be reached by a simple sum of the meanings of its constituent words. In an important sense, the meaning of a sentence, whether spoken or written, is in its structure, and to get to that meaning we must depend on the use of uniquely grammatical devices—word inflections, word order, and grammatical words (e.g., *of, a*). In my view, if they are to understand either spoken or written language, both the listener and the reader would do well to take account appropriately (and, in the ideal case, automatically) of the constituent phonological and syntactic structures and devices of the language (see reference 21 for a detailed discussion).

To sum up, I would suggest that reading and listening to language are both cognitive-linguistic activities. Whether language comes in through the ear or the eye, by an auditory or visual route, it is processed in a different mode than are other stimuli, one that relates to the structures of language. The perception of speech is only peripherally auditory; it involves, in addition, specific processes in the language mode, both phonological and syntactic, that are different from the perception of nonspeech sounds [17, 18].

Reading and the Apprehension of Phonological Units

As for the reading of print, it is, of course, also only peripherally visual; that is, the letters of the orthography are not simply optical displays to be apprehended visually like a Mondrian painting. They also represent the units of language and have been developed to fit its phonology. It is clear that the letter patterns are not totally arbitrary with respect to the language. For example, they never represent a phoneme and a half, or a syllable and a quarter, or a word and a third. Instead, they represent phonemes, syllables, and words. And because they do, normal readers can, at an early stage, make contact with those structures of the phonology and syntax that already exist in their heads and are perfectly natural to all human beings. Normal readers can thus invoke their normal and natural language processes to reach the message that the orthography conveys. Conversely, a would-be reader with deficits in those language-processing abilities might well have difficulties.

One of the reasons why this field is so vexed may be that there is so much misunderstanding about language processing and, particularly, about what phonology and the phonological units are. Many think of the phonology and its units as sounds. Instead, the phonology is an abstract linguistic scheme that provides a structure for the language process. It allows us to have a huge vocabulary of tens of thousands of words with the use of a very small number of signal elements. The phonological units thus are neither primarily auditory nor primarily visual. Rather, they are to varying degrees abstractly linguistic [12, 14, 21].

A phenomenon discovered by McGurk and MacDonald [27] illustrates what this might mean. It shows, quite dramatically, that when optical and acoustic signals convey information about the same *linguistic* event, they cannot be distinguished from each other.

The phenomenon is easily described. The subjects watch a talking head on a television screen. In one variation, produced at Haskins Laboratories, the head articulates /dee/ /dee/ /dee/ while a voice says /ba/ /ba/ /ba/. That is, the video is producing /dee/ over and over and the audio is producing /ba/ over and over. Although the voice the subjects hear is actually saying /ba/, what the subjects perceive is not /ba/ but /da/. In other words, their percept takes the *consonant* from what they *see* and the *vowel* from what they *hear*. But they are not at all aware of a mismatch between what they saw and what they heard. They do not realize that their percept was formed from a combination of optical information (the face on the screen mouthing /dee/) and acoustic information (the voice on the tape saying /ba/). If they look away from the screen for a moment, they hear /ba/ /ba/ /ba/; but when they look at the screen again, they again perceive /da/ /da/ /da/. Thus the distal object that the subjects are perceiving is neither auditory nor visual—it is a linguistic event.

One has to experience this remarkable phenomenon to appreciate how compelling it is. Subjects report that even with the most careful introspection, it is virtually impossible to be aware of any mismatch between what they heard and what they saw. This is as clear an illustration as I can find* of the fact that whereas phonetic information does, of course, have to come in through some normal sensory channel, the phonetic percept itself is neither auditory nor visual, but a distinctly linguistic thing.

Implications for Instruction and Remediation

What I should like to emphasize, then, is that if our concern is with how well or how poorly a child can process language, whether written or spoken, we should consider the *linguistic* requirements of the task and understand that those requirements are something apart from the general requirements of the auditory and visual input channels. Of course, if a child has peripheral deficits in hearing or vision, that is another matter. Such deficits need to be corrected, if possible. It is assuredly difficult to learn language by ear if you cannot hear or by eye if you cannot see.

But, as I have said, most poor readers do not have nonlinguistic, purely sensory deficits. For that reason, I deplore methods of teaching reading that are adapted to the child's purported sensory learning style. I think they are based on misconceptions of what reading and language are all about and may in some cases prevent rather than promote learning.

As I see it, the instruction customarily recommended for the child dubbed an auditory learner may actually not be too harmful, though perhaps misnamed and motivated by the wrong reasons. As I have noted earlier, children are

---

*The author is indebted to Alvin M. Liberman for suggesting this illustration.

frequently classified as auditory learners because they do relatively well on verbal/analytical tests that are, to my mind, only superficially auditory and that, in addition, require some appreciation of linguistic structures. If children show this pattern of strengths, they may be assigned to a teaching method (commonly misnamed auditory) that emphasizes the language structure and the constituent elements of words, a method that I would consider to be fundamentally linguistic or language-based. Although some versions of this method may be preferable to others, the children assigned to any of them are, in my view, more fortunate (other things being equal) than their peers who have been dubbed visual learners.

What about the visual learner? Here I would question both the procedure by which the purported learning style is determined and the instruction that is tailored to that designation. As I have pointed out, children are called visual learners largely on the basis that they do relatively poorly on tasks that have been misnamed auditory but that are really verbal/analytic, since they require the subjects to comprehend linguistic structures or to hold linguistic information in memory. Accordingly, these children are not necessarily visual learners at all, but are instead individuals with deficits in language processing. Therefore, it would be unfortunate to provide a so-called visual teaching procedure for such children, that is, one that emphasizes whole-word learning, nonanalytic memorization of visual configurations, and guessing from context. Such a method, to my mind, must effectively delay or even prevent a child's understanding of the structure of the language and of how the orthography transcribes it, and it may well leave him functionally illiterate, unable to read new words that he has not already seen and memorized.

In short, I would argue that the question of the place of the sensory modalities in the diagnosis and remediation of reading disabilities badly needs reassessment in view of what we know about language and the reading process. I would emphasize once again, as I have for many years [19, 20], that because the particular segment represented by an alphabetic orthography is sublexical and difficult to isolate, the cognitive demands on all beginners will be considerable (and the task of the teacher correspondingly difficult). English, of course, further compounds the difficulty for beginners by the highly abstract way in which it often represents the language [14, 21]. It is important for those planning reading instruction to understand that learning to read may be hard for beginning readers of English. It will be harder, at least, than for beginners in writing systems like the Chinese, where the segment to be extracted from the speech stream is the easily isolable word and where any subsequent analysis of the phonological structure of the word is minimal. For writing systems of that kind, simple paired-associate memory of symbol and word is sufficient for mastery, but such an approach is not sufficient in an alphabetic system.

Beginners in an alphabetic orthography *can*, of course, ignore the alphabetic nature of the writing system and approach reading the same way the Chinese child does, as if it were a simple paired-associate memory task. That is precisely what the learning-style advocates would have the beginner do when they classify him as a visual learner. But if beginners are taught that way, if they are taught to adopt a simple strategy in which they try to associate a given string of optical shapes with a particular word, they will lose the remarkable benefits of the alphabetic system. They will not be able to use the alphabet in the way it was intended, that is, to help them to apprehend new words. Like the Chinese children learning logograms, they will begin to amass a collection of memorized graphic patterns and their associated words. Because logographies are not productive, a new word for such learners will then be a new graphic pattern to be paired with an associated word, memorized, and added to an ever increasing collection of memorized symbol-word associations. As their collection of memorized words grows larger, what small advantage there was in starting out that way would certainly begin to be lost.

Ironically, their problem will actually be much greater than that of the Chinese child, because our alphabet orthography, unlike the Chinese, was not designed to be used that way. Unlike the logographic characters, the strings of letters that form our written words are very poorly suited to be apprehended by overall shape or indeed by any means that does not take account of the distinct and distinctive letters and what they represent. Consider as logographic entities such words, for example, as *hit, hut, bit, but, bet, hot, bat, hat,* and *dot*. Methods of instruction that emphasize the visual configuration of the whole word can surely end only in the bafflement of the beginner.

I think it is likely that most children who have difficulty learning to read are probably those who have been using a whole-word strategy already, never managing to see the alphabetic principle on their own, and thus falling farther and farther behind their more insightful classmates. To lead them back again to the same strategy, as the learning-style advocates would do, seems to me quite indefensible. To make the best use of an alphabetic orthography, the reader, whether he is skilled or a beginner, had best go beyond visual shape to apprehend the internal structure of the word. The skilled reader does it quite automatically, and beginners, though it may be difficult for them, should, in my view, be given instruction directed toward that goal from the very beginning.

Elsewhere [22, 25] my colleagues and I have described detailed guidelines for preventive and remedial instruction that take into account the principles discussed in this chapter. We can recommend them with confidence, since reading curricula based on similar general principles have been consistently found to be effective since the seminal work of J. Chall almost 20 years ago [1, 8].

References

1. Beck, I. L. Reading Problems and Instructional Practices. In G. E. MacKinnon and T. G. Waller (Eds.), *Reading Research: Advances in Theory and Practice.* New York: Academic, 1981.
2. Benton, A., and Pearl, D. (Eds.). *Dyslexia: An Appraisal of Current Knowledge.* New York: Oxford University Press, 1978.

3. Blank, M., and Bridger, W. H. Deficiencies in verbal labeling in retarded readers. *Am. J. Orthopsychiatry* 16:840, 1966.
4. Boder, E. Developmental dyslexia: A diagnostic approach based on three atypical reading-spelling patterns. *Dev. Med. Child Neurol.* 15:663, 1973.
5. Brady, S., Shankweiler, D., and Mann, V. Speech perception and memory coding in relation to reading ability. *J. Exp. Child Psychol.* 35:345, 1983.
6. Calfee, R. C. Assessment of Independent Reading Skills: Basic Research and Practical Applications. In A. S. Reber and D. L. Scarborough (Eds.), *Toward a Psychology of Reading.* Hillsdale, N.J.: Erlbaum, 1977.
7. Calvin, W. H., and Ojemann, G. A. *Inside the Brain.* New York: New American Library, 1980.
8. Chall, J. *Learning to Read: The Great Debate.* New York: McGraw-Hill, 1967.
9. Denckla, M. B. Clinical syndromes in learning disabilities. *J. Learn. Disabil.* 5:401, 1972.
10. Fowler, C. A., Liberman, I. Y., and Shankweiler, D. On interpreting the error pattern in beginning reading. *Lang. Speech* 20:162, 1977.
11. Fowler, C. A., Shankweiler, D., and Liberman, I. Y. Apprehending spelling patterns for vowels: A developmental study. *Lang. Speech* 22:243, 1979.
12. Gleitman, L. R., and Rozin, P. The Structure and Acquisition of Reading: Relation Between Orthographies and the Structure of Language. In A. S. Reber and D. L. Scarborough (Eds.), *Toward a Psychology of Reading: The Proceedings of the CUNY Conference.* Hillsdale, N.J.: Erlbaum, 1977.
13. House, B. J., Hankey, M. J., and Magid, D. F. Logographic reading by TMR adults. *Am. J. Ment. Defic.* 85:161, 1980.
14. Klima, E. How Alphabets Might Reflect Language. In J. F. Kavanaugh and I. G. Mattingly (Eds.), *Language By Ear and By Eye: The Relationships Between Speech and Reading.* Cambridge, Mass.: MIT Press, 1972.
15. Larrivee, B. Modality preference as a model for differentiating beginning reading instruction: A review of the issues. *Learn. Disabil. Q.* 4:180, 1981.
16. Levinson, H. N. *A Solution to the Riddle Dyslexia.* New York: Springer, 1980.
17. Liberman, A. M. On finding that speech is special. *Am. Psychol.* 37(2):148, 1982.
18. Liberman, A. M., and Studdert-Kennedy, M. Phonetic Perception. In R. Held, H. W. Leibowitz, and H. L. Teuber (Eds.), *Handbook of Sensory Physiology: Perception.* New York: Springer, 1978. Vol. VIII, pp. 143–178.
19. Liberman, I. Y. Basic research in speech and lateralization of language: Some implications for reading disability. *Bull. Orton Soc.* 21:71, 1971.
20. Liberman, I. Y. Segmentation of the spoken word and reading acquisition. *Bull. Orton Soc.* 23: 65, 1973.
21. Liberman, I. Y. A Language Oriented View of Reading and Its Disabilities. In H. Myklebust (Ed.), *Progress in Learning Disabilities,* Vol. V. New York: Grune & Stratton, 1982.
22. Liberman, I. Y., and Shankweiler, D. Speech, the Alphabet, and Teaching to Read. In L. B. Resnik and P. A. Weaver (Eds.), *Theory and Practice of Early Reading.* Hillsdale, N.J.: Erlbaum, 1979. Vol. 2, pp. 109–134.
23. Liberman, I. Y., et al. Letter confusions and reversals of sequence in the beginning reader: Implications for Orton's theory of developmental dyslexia. *Cortex* 7:127, 1971.
24. Liberman, I. Y., et al. Orthography and the Beginning Reader. In J. F. Kavanagh and R. Venezky (Eds.), *Orthography, Reading, and Dyslexia.* Baltimore: University Park Press, 1980.

25. Liberman, I. Y., et al. Steps Toward Literacy. In P. Levinson and C. Harris Sloan (Eds.), *Auditory Processing and Language: Clinical and Research Perspectives.* New York: Grune & Stratton, 1980.
26. Liberman, I. Y., et al. Children's memory for recurring linguistic and non-linguistic material. *Cortex* 18:367, 1982.
27. McGurk, H., and McDonald, J. Hearing lips and seeing voices. *Nature* 264:746, 1976.
28. Mann, V. A., and Liberman, I. Y. Phonological awareness and verbal short-term memory: Can they presage early reading problems? *J. Learn. Disabil.* 17:592, 1984.
29. Mann, V. A., Liberman, I. Y., and Shankweiler, D. Children's memory for sentences and word strings in relation to reading ability. *Memory Cognition* 8:329, 1980.
30. Mattis, S. Dyslexia Syndromes: A Working Hypothesis that Works. In A. L. Benton and D. Pearl (Eds.), *Dyslexia: An Appraisal of Current Knowledge.* New York: Oxford University Press, 1979.
31. Reuben, R. Neurological assessment of a child with a reading problem. Paper presented at a meeting of the Institute for Research in Behavioral Neuroscience on Neuropsychology of reading disorders: Recent research and clinical implications, New York University Medical Center, October 16, 1982.
32. Rozin, P., Poritsky, S., and Sotsky, R. American children with reading problems can easily learn to read English represented by Chinese characters. *Science* 71:1264, 1971.
33. Shankweiler, D., and Liberman, I. Y. Misreading: A Search for Causes. In J. F. Kavanagh and I. G. Mattingly (Eds.), *Language By Ear and By Eye: The Relationship Between Speech and Reading.* Cambridge, Mass.: MIT Press, 1972.
34. Stanovich, K. E. Individual differences in the cognitive processes of reading: 1. Word decoding. *J. Learn. Disabil.* 15(8):449, 1982.
35. Vellutino, F. R. *Dyslexia: Theory and Research.* Cambridge, Mass.: MIT Press, 1981.
36. Vernon, M. *Backwardness in Reading.* Cambridge, Engl.: Cambridge University Press, 1960.
37. Vogel, S. A. Syntactic abilities in normal and dyslexic children. *J. Learn. Disabil.* 7:47, 1974.
38. Wepman, J. M. *Auditory Discrimination Test.* Los Angeles: Western Psychological Services, 1973.
39. Wiig, E. H., and Semel, E. M. *Language Assessment and Intervention for the Learning Disabled.* Columbus, Ohio: Merrill, 1980.
40. Wolford, G., and Fowler, C. A. The Perception and Use of Information by Good and Poor Readers. In P. Tighe and B. Shepp (Eds.), *Perception, Cognition, and Development: Interactional Analysis.* Hillsdale, N.J.: Erlbaum, 1983.

7 Brain Electrical Activity Mapping (BEAM): The Search for a Physiological Signature of Dyslexia

Frank H. Duffy and Gloria B. McAnulty

Topographic mapping of electroencephalographic (EEG) and sensory evoked potential (EP) information promises to be a valuable tool for the investigation of brain function in learning-disabled children. In this chapter, we shall describe our method known as brain electrical activity mapping (BEAM) and demonstrate some interesting results of its application to a study of a group of 10- to 12-year-old dyslexic boys. To understand BEAM, however, it is necessary to have an appreciation of the strengths and weaknesses of the EEG and EP data that underlie it.

Electroencephalography

Electroencephalography began with the report by Hans Berger [3] in 1929 that a 10-hertz (Hz) electrical rhythm could be recorded from the occipital scalp of humans. Moreover, he noted its presence only on eye closure, with absence on eye opening. The observation by Gibbs, Davis, and Lenox [21] in 1935 that clinical epilepsy was accompanied by a unique electrical rhythm known as the spike and wave advanced EEG into the forefront of neurodiagnostic techniques. Thus, by 1940, the view was widely held that it would only be a matter of time before careful inspection of polygraphic tracings would reveal unique signatures for many clinical abnormalities and/or normal variations of mental state. As we know, of course, the major contribution of EEG has remained in the epilepsies, and only a few additional diagnostic signatures have been demonstrated. Regrettably, for many entities including the learning disabilities, the EEG abnormalities found were too nonspecific to form useful diagnostic constellations [27]. For some time, we have held the belief that EEG data contain too much information to be easily assimilated by unaided visual inspection of polygraphic tracings. It is for this reason, not because of an inherent insensitivity to underlying brain function, that EEG has not completely realized its early optimistic expectations.

Figure 7-1 demonstrates a typical clinical EEG and the formidable task of its intepretation by visual inspection. Initial evaluation involves a visual search for obvious discontinuities in the otherwise smooth flow of activities known as background. Two such discontinuities are shown: the first, a temporal lobe epileptic spike and the second, an eye blink. It is not a difficult task for the trained clinician to discriminate discontinuities, nor is it difficult to differentiate artifactual from brain-generated discontinuities. Indeed, few computerized programs perform spike recognition as well as does the human eye, and probably none do better. It is no surprise, therefore, that diseases most commonly diagnosed by EEG are those that produce recognizable discontinuities, such as the spike and wave of epilepsy.

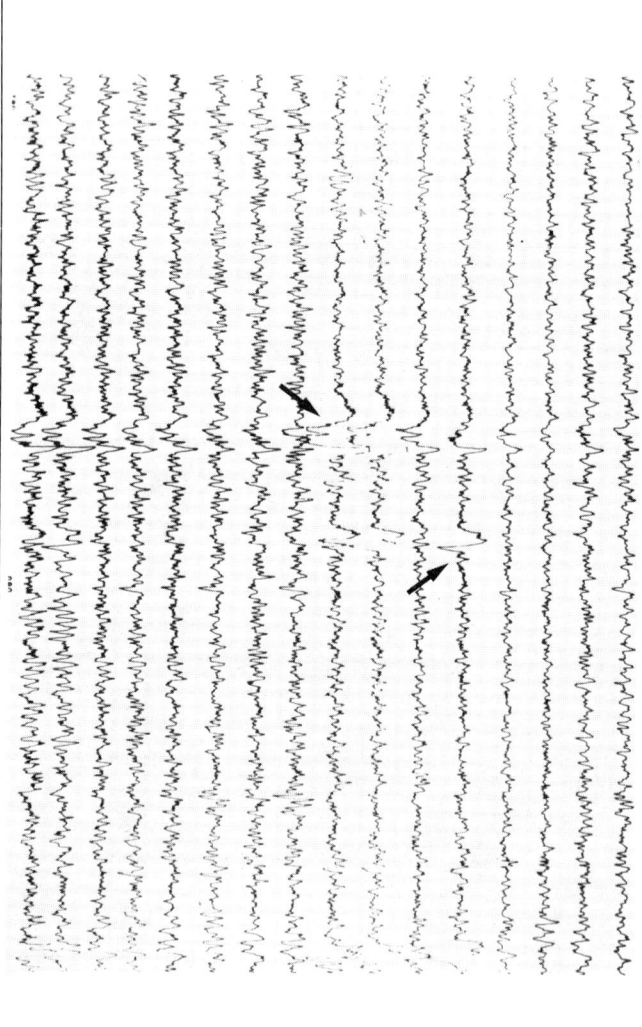

Fig. 7-1. Typical 20-second epoch from a clinical EEG showing 16 channels of information recorded from 16 electrodes placed in an array on the subject's head. Two "discontinuities" are demonstrated by arrows. The arrow on the left demonstrates a spike that is confirmatory of temporal lobe epilepsy. The right-hand arrow indicates an artifactual discontinuity, an eye blink. EEG discontinuities are easy to delineate by unaided visual inspection; moreover, the discrimination between the real and artifactual discontinuities is readily done by a trained electroencephalographer. Few computer programs do as well. The remainder of the tracing consists of classic EEG "background," which is more difficult to evaluate by simple inspection; computers have been most helpful in this effort (see text).

Assessment of brain function by inspection of EEG background is a more complex process. To a large extent, it involves four analytical phases: spectral, spatial, temporal, and statistical. Each EEG channel is visually analyzed for the relative amounts of activity in the four standard EEG frequency bands of delta (0–4 Hz), theta (4–8 Hz), alpha (8–12 Hz), and beta (>12 Hz). Next, the change in EEG spectral content is evaluated at different scalp electrodes (spatial locations). Pathology, for example, often manifests itself by augmented slow activity (delta, theta) and diminished fast activity (alpha, beta). A localized abscess might be differentiated from a generalized encephalopathic process by a finding of focal delta waves (abscess) as opposed to spatially generalized slowing (encephalopathy). Next, the stability of a finding over time is assessed. Typically, a consistent background abnormality suggests an anatomical lesion, whereas a fluctuating abnormality suggests a more functional lesion. Finally, all data observed are compared to past experience, and a decision is made as to the degree of abnormality present. Performance of these four analyses by simple visual inspection places a major burden on the electroencephalographer and potentially limits the information that can be extracted from such resting brain electrical activity. At the very least, information becomes a function of the skill of the electroencephalographer. As we shall see, similar problems beset the EEG's cousin, the evoked potential.

Evoked Potentials

The EEG may be considered the ambient electrical activity of the brain revealed by electrical "auscultation." By analogy, EPs may be considered the transient electrical activity of the brain in response to discrete sensory stimulation, that is, electrical response to sensorial "percussion." In animal preparations, well-formed EPs are recorded directly from primary cortex in response to single stimuli. In the intact human, however, little can be seen at the scalp in response to a single stimulus. The background EEG electrical signal is from 10 to 100 times as large as the EP and causes it to be obscured. This problem is partially obviated by signal averaging, an approach whereby the stimulus is repeated many times to improve the signal-noise (EP/EEG) ratio. Although many stimulations may be required to produce an EP, the resultant waveform is treated as if it were the response to just one. Diverse stimulus modalities, ranging from simple flashes, clicks, and shocks to more complicated ones such as spoken words or changes of visual patterns, have been used to produce EPs. The early components of the evoked response (the first 20 msec) are reproducible and are quite useful clinically in the assessment of subcortical brain function. With a few exceptions, the mid and late components, lasting up to 500 to 700 msec, have failed to achieve the clinical utility afforded the EEG and short-latency EP. The late components show considerable intra- and intersubject variability, which limits their value. One exception is the reliable 100-msec component produced by reversals of a checkerboard visual pattern.

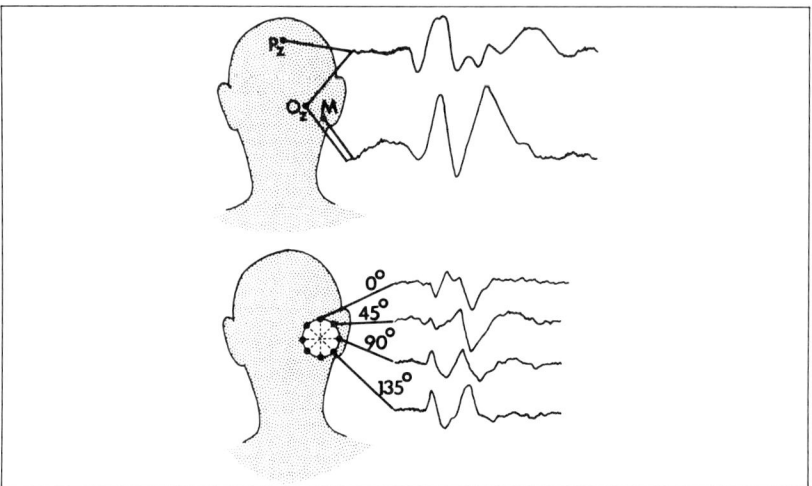

Fig. 7-2. Six averaged evoked response waveforms in response to stroboscopic flash simultaneously generated in one subject. In the upper tracing, wide electrode separation is employed. In the lower tracing, closely spaced electrodes are used over the right visual cortex (rosette pattern). Note the marked difference between these tracings despite the fact that they were simultaneously created. We hypothesize that such complex waveform morphology has until now prevented such long latency evoked potentials from achieving a high degree of clinical utility. Each tracing above represents 512 msec from time of stimulation.

Figure 7-2 illustrates the complex visual evoked response (VER) to stroboscopic flash by one subject. Note how the EP waveshapes differ as a function of electrode position. It has been our working hypothesis that EP, like EEG, contains not too little, but too much spatiotemporal information to be easily grasped by simple, unaided visual inspection. Rather than reducing the amount of EP data by examining just a few scalp locations, we have employed the full of EEG set of 20 electrodes, using subsequent topographic mapping to simplify an otherwise complex analysis.

Topographic Mapping Method

To assist assessment of the spatial distribution of EEG and EP data, we recently developed a method for topographic imaging known as brain electrical activity mapping, or BEAM [12]. It builds on the pioneering work of others in this area [2, 4, 5, 17, 22, 23, 26, 34, 36, 40, 41] using present-day computer hardware. The construction of a BEAM image from 20 channels of EP data is illustrated in Figure 7-3. Basically, the head is divided into 4,096 picture elements (pixels). A number is assigned to each pixel based on the three nearest real values (i.e., actual electrode output values) by linear interpolation. Such three-point linear interpolation gives more accurate numerical representation than four-point interpolation and polynomial approximation.

Each pixel is displayed in color, each particular color representing a range of numerical values. Current practice is to use a rainbow scale for data when all values are positive.

An example of this display technique as it has been applied to the present study of dyslexic children is provided in Figure 7-7. The first image represents the topographic distribution of spectral energy in the delta (0–4 Hz) frequency range. Like images are also produced for theta (4–8 Hz), alpha (8–12 Hz), and beta 1 (12-16 Hz) through beta 4 (24–28 Hz) frequency bands.

Analysis of EEG data begins by computerized spectral analysis of the data from each electrode by means of the fast Fourier transform (FFT) technique. The amount of spectral energy in each of the classic EEG frequency bands is then determined by integrating the resultant 20 spectral curve across the appropriate frequencies. This analysis, then, provides single numbers for each of the 20 electrodes that are the underlying numerical values for the topographic mapping procedure as illustrated in Figure 7-3. Finally, displays of the spatial distribution within each EEG band are created using each display to summarize from one second to 30 minutes of EEG data.

When data are expected to have both positive and negative values, shades of red are used for positive values, and shades of blue are used for negative values, such as those yielded by EP and certain statistical data. These display conventions have been interactively developed in collaboration with numerous clinicians who regularly read clinical BEAM images. Note that original BEAM images produced by an earlier system [12] did not have the rainbow capacity; hence, all displays were shaded red or white except for limited statistical displays.

For EP data, we visualize the dynamic change of electrical activity over time. The topographic mapping technique for evoked potentials is analogous to that used for the formation of EEG spectral maps. In the case of EP data, mean EPs are formed from each of the 20 recording sites. The entire EP spans 512 msec, which is divided into 124 four-msec intervals. The mean voltage value for each of these intervals is calculated and plotted as shown in Figure 7-3. The 512 msec before the stimulus is also sampled to act as baseline, a zero reference value for the EP. This prestimulus interval, itself, is always evaluated to determine the adequacy of averaging and to ensure that there is no time-locked anticipatory phenomena.

An example of the evoked potential display technique is illustrated in Figure 7-8 as it applies to the present study. The first 2 images represent the evoked response to an auditory discriminatory stimulus (computer generated speech sounds "tight" or "tyke") in a dyslexic child. The second 2 images represent the same interval in the evoked response, this time in a group of normal control children.

It is usual to view the 128 frames of the EP as a continuous movie. This is accomplished by computer controlled "cartooning" of the images. This sequential display technique produces an animation effect that highlights the spread of EP activity over the head.

These two methods summarize the spectral and spatiotemporal information obtained from multielectrode recordings and assist the clinician by providing immediate visual access to the data. Latency, amplitude, and frequency band

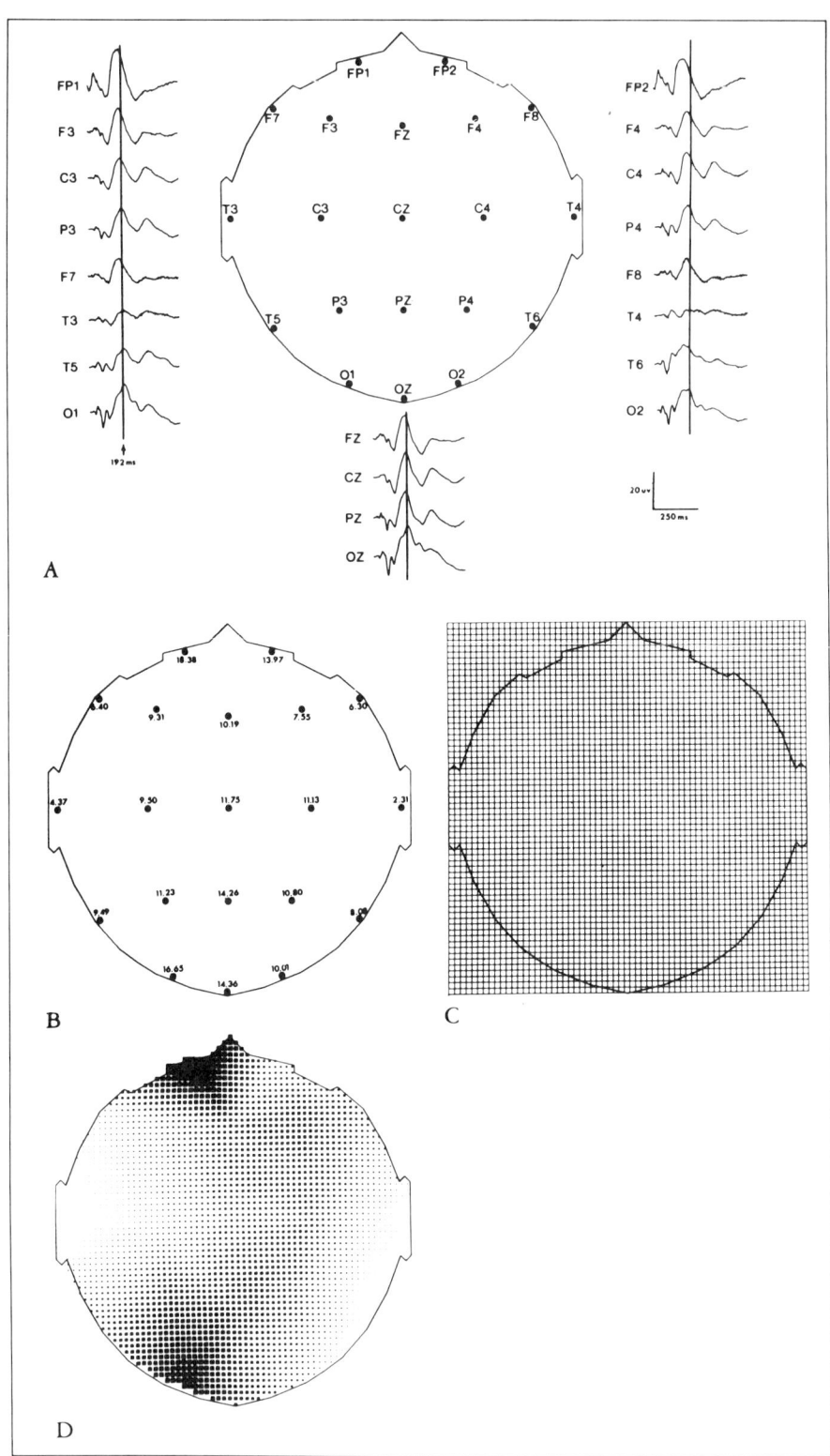

information accompany each image. Furthermore, the numerical matrices underlying each BEAM image are maintained for subsequent visual or statistical manipulation.

Brain electrical activity mapping is now a routine clinical neurophysiological test in the Seizure Unit at The Children's Hospital, Boston. The patient population studied using this technique ranges in age from the premature infant to the learning-disabled child to the adult with senile dementia.

The clinician relies on the fact that brain abnormalities produce regional changes in the topographic distribution of EEG activity that are readily visible and of an intuitive nature. For example, functionally inactive or deafferentated cortex manifests reduced electrical activity over all frequency ranges. On the other hand, irritative cortex, such as that found in epileptogenic regions or those adjacent to brain tumors, increases overall activity, especially in the higher frequency bands. Brain electrical activity mapping EP images demonstrate sequential activation over the entire cortex, presumably from activation of association cortices through short and long intrahemispheric tracts. As such, peripheral sensory stimulation "lights up" the brain. As is true for EEG, cortical atrophy reduces EP amplitude, and cortical irritability augments it. Analysis of EEG and EP data by BEAM has proved of great use in the clinical evaluation of patients at risk for neurological disease.

The technique of significance probability mapping (SPM) was developed to provide a display demonstrating the location and degree of abnormality of an individual subject when compared to a control group or the differences between groups [11]. The goal of SPM is to delineate regional topographic differences of brain activity using a statistical measure such as the z-statistic for individual subjects, t-statistic for two group comparisons, and F-statistic for multiple group comparisons. The results of SPM are displayed in the same manner as for BEAM images of raw EEG or EP data. Figures 7-4 and 7-5 illustrate the manner in which BEAM, computed axial tomography (CT), and neuropsychological data complement each other in the evaluation of central nervous system pathology. In the following sections, we demonstrate the utility of BEAM-SPM in the elucidation of electrophysiological differences between normal and dyslexic boys.

Fig. 7-3. Example of the construction of a topographic map for EP data. (A similar procedure is employed for the spatial map that ordinarily plots activity over a range of frequency bands.) Mean EPs are formed from each of 20 recording sites by dividing each EP into 128 four-msec intervals and calculating the mean voltage value for each interval. A. Individual EPs are shown for the electrode locations indicated on the head diagram. B. Mean voltage values at these locations are shown for the interval beginning 192 msec after the stimulus, indicated by the vertical line in A. Next, the head region is treated as a 64×64 matrix, resulting in 4,096 spatial domains (C). Each domain is assigned a voltage value by linear interpolation from the three known points. Finally, for display, the raw voltage values are fitted to a discrete-level equal-interval intensity scale (D). The images are displayed on a color television screen using the gray scale in "pseudocolor format." Sequential EP images can be viewed by computer-controlled cartooning of these images. (From Duffy et al. [11].)

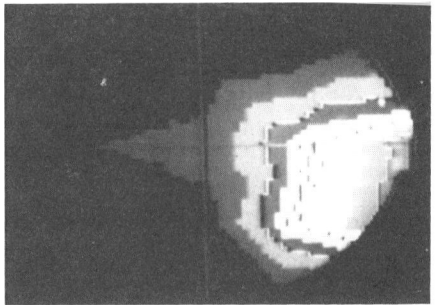
BEAM-SPM

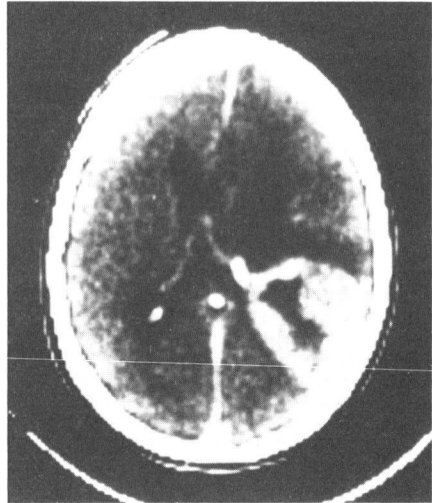
CT scan

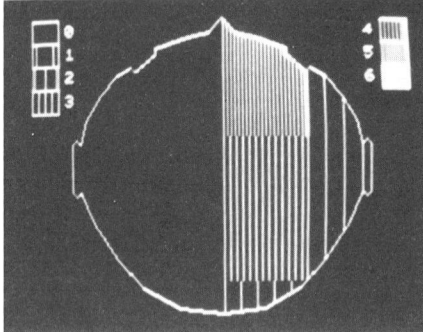
Structured report

Fig. 7-4. The relative value of three neuroimaging techniques is demonstrated in the diagnosis of a malignant tumor, glioblastoma multiforme, located to the right posterior temporal and parietal regions. For all images, the vertex view is employed with the right ear to the right and the nose above. The BEAM significance probability mapping, here (as in Fig. 7-5) reproduced in black and white from the color scale image (top), and the CT scan (middle) very accurately locate this classic anatomical lesion. The neuropsychological test scores, compiled and summarized for display in a structured report (bottom), implicate the right hemisphere but overemphasize the frontal abnormalities. (Compare Fig. 7-5.)

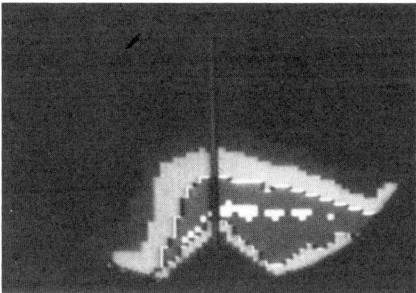

BEAM-SPM

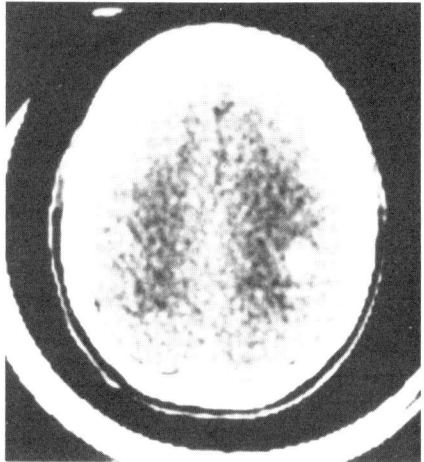

CT scan

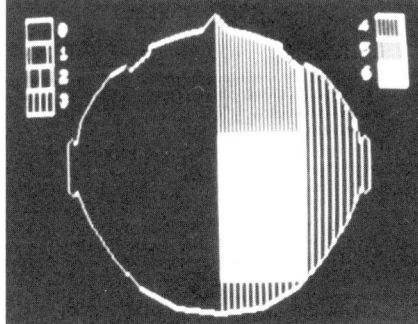

Structured report

Fig. 7-5. The combined use of BEAM, CT scan, and neuropsychological testing in clinical practice is illustrated here, using the same display conventions as in Fig. 7-4. Unlike the lesion seen in Fig. 7-4, this particular brain tumor is very small and is barely delineated by CT scan and barely detected by BEAM. On the other hand, the structured report, based on the neuropsychological test scores, clearly demonstrates the locus of abnormality in the right parietal lobe.

Dyslexia Study

Although community surveys have shown that 3.5 to 6.0 percent of school-aged children are dyslexic [35], theories as to dyslexia's physiological origins have generally lacked neuropathological confirmation. Indeed, only one histological analysis of a dyslexic brain has been reported [18, 19]. Microscopic abnormalities were seen in the left temporal lobe. Since the subject was also epileptic, the specificity of the findings regarding dyslexia await further confirmation. Complicating the paucity of pathological case material is the possibility suggested by clinical studies that dyslexia, even when apparently more or less "pure," may be a heterogeneous entity.

Accordingly, many authors have used or suggested the use of neurophysiological methods to delineate postulated abnormalities in dyslexia [6, 25, 27, 29, 37, 38, 39]. Regrettably, until recently, the EEG and EP abnormalities in children with dyslexia have been nonspecific. Moreover, with the exception of Hanley and Sklar [25], few have looked beyond the visual (occipital) or classical speech (temporoparietal) regions for abnormalities.

Two areas in which electrophysiological data may prove to be of importance in the study of dyslexia are (1) characterization and localization of the brain system components that are distinctively different in dyslexia and (2) establishment of a less culturally dependent criterion for objective diagnosis. Our previous research [14, 15] using the BEAM-SPM methodology suggests that physiological aberrations in the brains of dyslexics are more widespread than previously suspected. In the present analysis, we also summarize newer data demonstrating differences among subtypes of pure dyslexics.

Methods and Subjects

Our initial question was whether EEG and EP data could demonstrate physiologically meaningful differences between normal subjects and dyslexics. Accordingly, we felt it best to diminish sources of variation by limiting our subjects to boys aged 10 to 12 years with normal IQs. The subjects' dyslexia was not accompanied by emotional problems, epilepsy, neurological abnormalities, attentional deficits, or other learning difficulties. All boys exhibited the cognitive aptitude/reading achievement discrepancy outlined by the World Federation of Neurology in their definition of dyslexia. In addition, the selected subjects were free from the behavioral symptom complex associated with the attention deficit disorder as defined in the third edition of the *Diagnostic and Statistical Manual of Mental Disorders (DSM-III)*. This set of characteristics corresponds to the "dyslexia-pure" category of Hughes and Denckla [27]. All dyslexics and controls came from suburban Boston schools. Dyslexia was defined as being 1.5 years below expectation for reading [35].

We were not certain whether it would be possible to demonstrate EEG differences between dyslexics and normal readers at rest or whether complex test methodologies would be required. Accordingly, we chose to include some simple and some complex paradigms during EEG and EP recording. Electroencephalograms were recorded at rest under the following conditions:

1. Eyes open
2. Eyes closed
3. During tasks designed to activate the left hemisphere (reading and recall, listening to speech)
4. During right hemispheric tasks (geometric figure memorization and recall, listening to music)
5. During tasks designed to activate both hemispheres (forming associations between geometric forms and nonsense words)

Evoked potentials were created to simple flash and click stimulation as well as to more complex auditory stimuli (words *tight* and *tyke*). Evoked potentials were formed from 250 to 500 stimulus presentations. The details of these paradigms have been described in our earlier research [12].

For all EEG and EP states, data were recorded from 20 electrodes applied to the scalp with collodion in the standard 10–20 format done for routine clinical EEG (see Chap. 9 for a graphic presentation of these locations). Signals were tape-recorded after amplification by a Grass polygraph and replayed, off-line, into a PDP-12 or, more recently, PDP-11/60 computer (Digital Equipment Corporation). Filtering and analogue-to-digital sampling were performed to permit spectral analysis from 0.5 to 32.0 Hz without contamination by 60-Hz interference. Prior to spectral analyses, all EEG segments were visually inspected, and those containing eye blink, eye movement, muscle, or other artifacts were eliminated. Evoked potential segments containing eye blink were eliminated from the signal averaging process. This process was controlled by the comprehensive SIGSYS software system (Braintech, Inc.).

Differences Between Normal Readers and Dyslexics

Details of the following findings can be found in a previous publication [14]. Inspection of BEAM data on individual subjects revealed the following:

1. Normal readers showed considerable between-state variability in their EEG and EP topographic distributions.
2. Dyslexics tended to show less state variance in their BEAM plots.
3. Dyslexics seemed to show more EEG alpha activity overlying the left hemisphere.
4. Dyslexic EP readings tended to be less complex, showing fewer transient asymmetries than those of normal readers.
5. Simple visual inspection of individual images failed to yield accurate classification as to reading status because of the additional factor of intersubject, as well as intergroup, variability.

The SPM did, however, demonstrate large and coherent regions of between-group differences (as measured by the t-statistic), summarized as follows:

1. The EP-derived between-group differences were largely posterior, whereas EEG differences were largely anterior.

2. Both EEG and EP differences were bihemispheric, although the left hemisphere was most prominently involved.
3. Although the classical left temporal and parietal speech regions were prominent as a locus of dyslexic versus normal difference, a between-group difference was also highlighted bilaterally in the frontal region.
4. Group differences were better demonstrated during activated EP and EEG states when stimuli requiring a behavioral response were presented than during the passive or resting states.
5. For the EEG activation states, speech, reading, and making visual-verbal associations evoked greater group differences than did listening to music or performing a geometric figure memory-recognition test. For EP, the "tight-tyke" paradigm produced more between-group differences than did simple flash or click stimulation.

The changes in brain electrical activity patterns in a normal reader as a function of two of these activation tasks is depicted in Figure 7-6. The t-SPM images topographically display regions where changes in alpha (8–12 Hz) activity occur when a child is asked to listen to 3 minutes of a recorded fairy tale (left frame) and 3 minutes of an instrumental musical piece (right frame) compared to 3 minutes at rest. Note that listening to speech results in a change in alpha primarily over the left central-parietal-posterior speech regions. Listening to music produces a change primarily over analogous regions in the right hemisphere, and to some degree on the left also. The resultant t-values in these comparisons were 2.74 for speech and 3.39 for music. In each case alpha was diminished over the changing region.

The findings are in accord with the traditional theory that speech activates left posterior areas while music activates right posterior areas. It is of interest, however, that not all normal subjects show these "classical" changes, an interesting finding under active investigation.

Figures 7-7 and 7-8 demonstrate the presence not only of a left posterior quadrant between-group difference, but also of right-sided differences by z-statistic SPM in the same 11-year-old dyslexic. In Figure 7-7, the two upper images demonstrate the topographic distribution of delta (0–4 Hz) activity during the Kimura figures testing phase. The top left BEAM display shows the topographic pattern of delta for the subject. Note the relatively symmetrical bifrontal maximum, a normal pattern. Note, however, the relative increase of delta in the right posterior quadrant. The top right image demonstrates the control group mean delta distribution. There is no obvious posterior asymmetry.

The lower image is a z-statistic SPM. For this example, the red color indicates the subject had more delta activity than the control group (blue would indicate less activity). The bright yellow color, in this case, indicates z-values in excess of 2.00. The maximum value was 2.46. Thus, for this subject there was an "abnormal" increase in right posterior quadrant slow activity (delta) during geometric figure testing (KFT).

Right posterior quadrant abnormalities in our dyslexic-pure boys were surprisingly common. This showed up in individual studies, such as this case

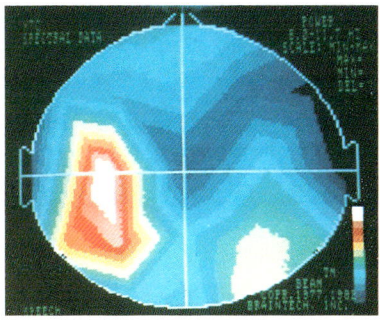
T-statistic SPM, speech × eyes open,
alpha 8–12 Hz

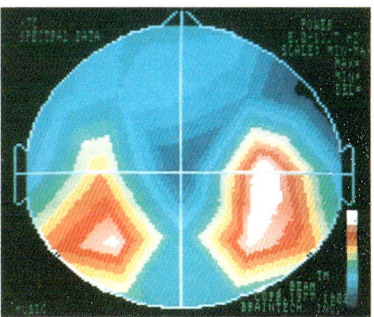
T-statistic SPM, music × eyes open,
alpha 8–12 Hz

Fig. 7-6. SPM-delineated regional differences resulting from listening to speech and music (see text).

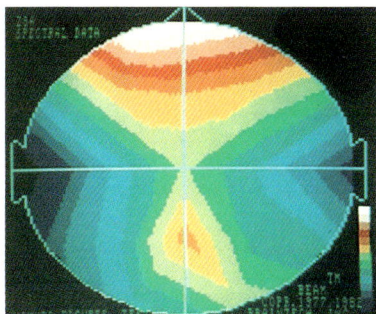
Subject, Kimura figures testing,
delta 0–4 Hz

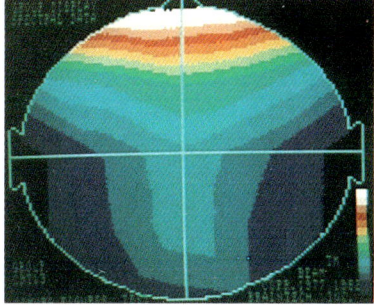
Control group, Kimura figures testing,
delta 0–4 Hz

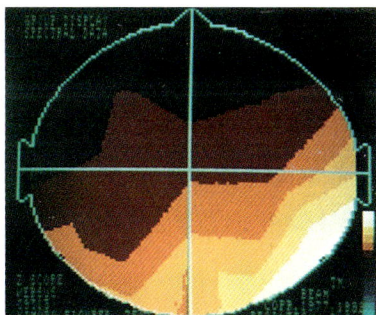
Z-statistic SPM

Fig. 7-7. BEAM images demonstrating unexpected right posterior quadrant abnormalities in an 11-year-old dyslexic (see text; compare Fig. 7-8).

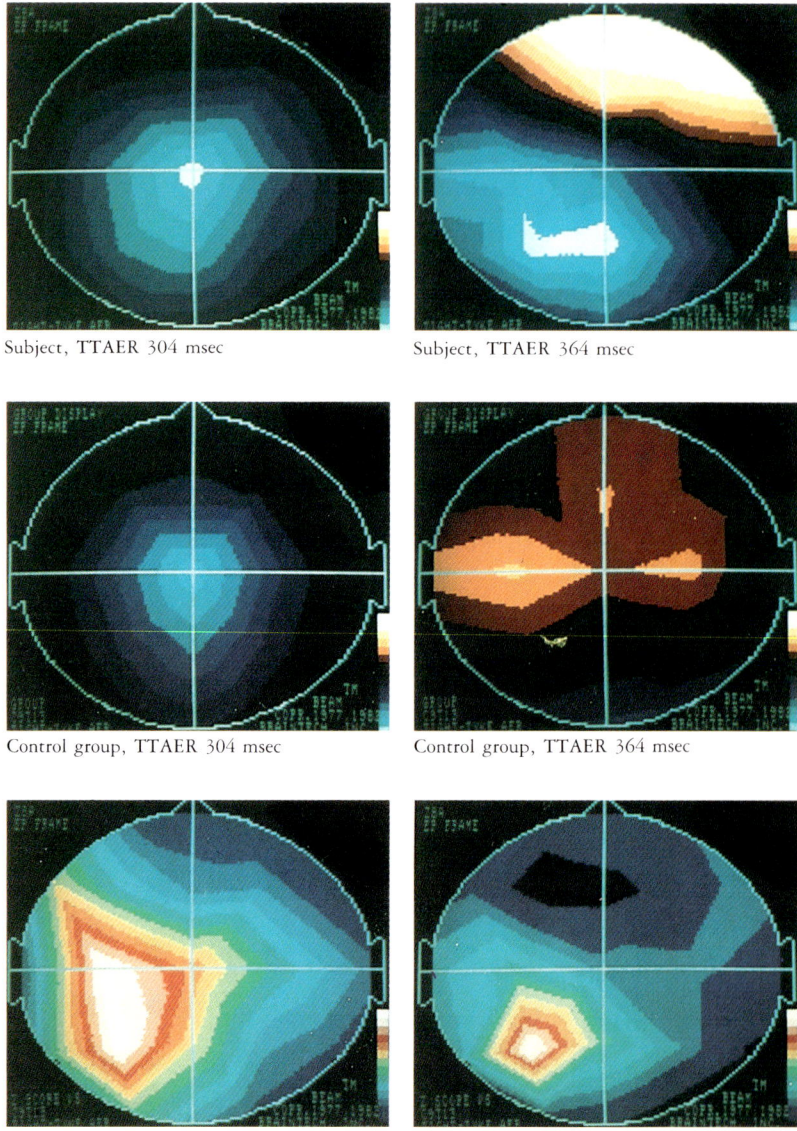

Fig. 7-8. BEAM images demonstrating localization of abnormality in the classical left hemisphere speech regions in an 11-year-old dyslexic (see text; compare Fig. 7-7).

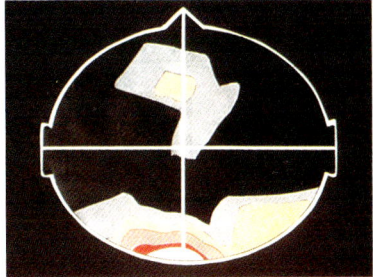

Anomic

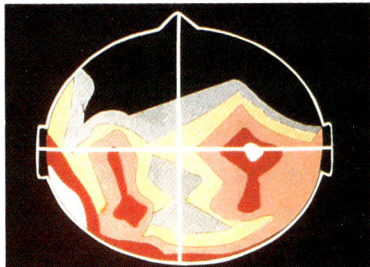

Dysphonemic

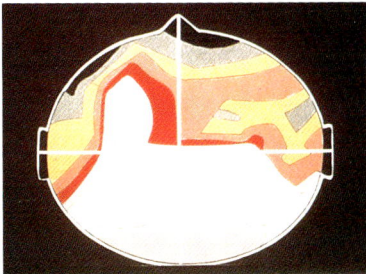

Global

Fig. 7-9. Composite t-SPMs summarizing preliminary findings of the dyslexia subgrouping study (see text).

study, and in the control group versus dyslexic group comparison t-statistic SPM.

Six BEAM images are shown in Figure 7-8. The top row of two represents single frames from the "tight-tyke" AER (TTAER). The middle row demonstrates corresponding frames from the grand control mean for the same latency period. The bottom row shows the z-statistic SPM produced by comparison of the individual subject with the control group data. To demonstrate the consistency of the displayed data, each SPM summarizes a full 20 msec of EP data, not just the 4 msec of data shown above.

The left-hand column represents that data at 304 msec latency of this subject's (and the control group's) TTAER. Note the slightly increased negativity of the subject's data, especially in the left posterior quadrant. By SPM, there is a marked deviation from the control group, centered about the left central and parietal electrodes. This difference reached a maximum t-value of 2.36. The range of colors from light pink through white shows the region above a t-value of 2.00.

The right-hand column represents the data at 364 msec of the same subject's TTAER. Note the striking difference from the control at the same latency. The z-statistic SPM reached a t-value of 5.16. Almost the entire head surpasses a t-value of 2.00, but the largest deviation is seen to be focal about the left parietal electrode.

As illustrated by this case, we have found z-statistic SPM to be of great value in delineating where the brain electrical activity of an individual subject differs from a normalized group. The findings of "abnormality" in the left central-parietal-posterior temporal region are characteristic of dyslexia.

Differences Within the Dyslexia-Pure Subgrouping

The following preliminary findings were based on a larger group of 44 boys, ages 10 to 13 years, who meet the criteria for dyslexia-pure. Neuropsychological test results, subjected to a multigroup statistical classification algorithm, generated assignment rules by which the children were segregated, with a probability of .75 or better, into one of three clinical subgroups: anomic-repetition disorder, dysphonemic-sequencing disorder, or globally language impaired. Thirty of the 44 children were clinically subgrouped at the .75 level. The linguistic deficit patterns for the dyslexic subtypes are as follows:

1. *Anomic-repetition disorder* is characterized by paraphasic errors and use of circumlocutions on confrontation naming, in spite of normal articulatory and comprehension skills. Repetition score (words or digits) is lower than normal. Thirteen children were assigned to this category.
2. *Dysphonemic-sequencing disorder* is characterized by the subject's loss of the sequential order of material in repetition tasks. While naming skills are within normal limits, errors of a phonemic nature are most common. Eight children met these criteria.
3. *Global or mixed language disorder* is defined by below-average performance on most or all language measures, including receptive language ability Nine children were categorized as globally or mixed language impaired.

We were guided by the observation by Denckla [9] that the parsimonious approach to categorization of clinical entities, in cases where the underlying cause is unknown, is on the basis of chief complaint or complaint clusters. Encouraged by the compatibility of these data to behaviorial subgrouping, we sought to assess whether these subgroups demonstrate significant differences in topographic organization of brain activity. Our hypothesis was that the observable differences in test performance within the dyslexia-pure group that allow clinically meaningful subgrouping could also be demonstrated in examinations of culture- and experience-free neurophysiological activity patterns. The implication, independent of the cause-effect issue, is that dyslexia is not a single etiological entity.

Figure 7-9 consists of three composite-feature maps delineating regions in which significant between-group differences were found across all states for comparison of each particular dyslexic subgroup with all other dyslexics taken as a group. The colored areas in the top image demonstrate regions where the brain electrical activity patterns of anomic children differed significantly from the nonanomic dyslexics (global and dysphonemic-sequencing dyslexics) across all features. Color scales indicate regions where t-values for the comparisons achieved a level of 2 or more (gray = 2.0–2.5, yellow/orange = 2.5–3.0, light red = 3.0–3.5, dark red = 3.5–4.0, pink = 4.0–4.5, and white = 4.5 and above). The regions that permitted the differentiation of the anomic children from the other dyslexics were the bilateral medial frontal and the occipital areas.

The composite-feature region map depicting areas where the dysphonemic-sequencing dyslexic subgroup differed from the other dyslexics (middle) demonstrates bilateral differences involving central and parietal areas and, to some extent, the left temporal lobe. Note also the more or less complementary regional involvement clearly indicating different patterns for the anomic and the dysphonemic comparisons.

The composite-feature map for comparison of the global dyslexic subgroup versus other dyslexics (bottom) is notable for the extent of cortical area in which significant differences were found. Once again both hemispheres were involved, with t-values reaching their maxima in the posterior quadrants and left frontal areas. Note the much greater overall involvement encompassing all regions involved in the anomics and dysphonemics.

To summarize these findings:

1. For all groups, areas in both hemispheres were usually involved.
2. The features indicating statistically significant differences for the anomic versus other dyslexics comparison involved very small amounts of cortical area, whereas the regions involved in the global–other dyslexics comparison were cortically pervasive.
3. The patterns of regional differences varied markedly for the three comparisons:
    a. Bilateral medial frontal and occipital involvement predominated for the anomic comparisons.

b. Bilateral central parietal and left temporal involvement were demonstrated in the dysphonemic-sequencing comparisons, with no frontal and minimal occipital involvement.
c. The globals showed extensive bihemispheric regional differences, with the left hemisphere somewhat more involved.

There is a clear and initially surprising lack of primary left hemisphere involvement for any of the three comparisons. It is likely that differences in these classically defined speech regions are shared by all the subgroups of dyslexics, with differences manifest in other regions being those that uniquely define the subgroups.

Implications for a Physiological Signature of Dyslexia

Topographic mapping procedures have demarcated regional differences between dyslexic boys and age-matched normal readers. These regions include the medial frontal lobes (supplementary motor area), the left anterolateral lobe (Broca's area), and the left posterior quadrant speech-associated areas (Wernicke's area, angular gyrus, posterior temporal lobe, and parietal lobe), with minor differences shown in the right parietal lobe.

It is reassuring that our study indicates that activity patterns in these classic posterior speech regions differentiate between normal readers and dyslexics. Concepts of dyslexia based on analogies to traditional aphasiology have implicated this area, as does the previously mentioned postmortem analysis [18, 19]. Moreover, other neurophysiological studies have implicated portions of this region as differing in dyslexics [25, 28, 37, 38, 39].

The frontal lobe areas involved in the between-group difference are more surprising and unpredicted. An explanation may stem from the work of Larsen, Skinhoj, and Lassen [30] and Lassen, Ingvar, and Skinhoj [31], who have identified, using xenon-labeled regional cerebral blood flow studies, the cortical regions that are activated during speech, oral reading, and silent reading in normal subjects. The locations identified with xenon mapping appear to be similar to all the regions demarcated by the SPM technique, including the bilateral medial frontal lobes. It has also been shown that electrical stimulation of these same cortical areas interferes with normal speech [33]. Thus, the regions shown to differ electrophysiologically between the brains of normal and dyslexic boys appear to coincide with the regions shown by blood flow studies to be active in normal subjects during speech and reading. One explanation may be that dyslexia represents dysfunction of the entire complex, bihemispheric system normally active in language-related tasks. More recent studies [13] have demonstrated similar findings in a larger group of dyslexic boys, as well as in 5-year-old preschool children considered "at risk" or "not at risk" for reading problems as predicted by preschool screening assessments [16].

Involvement of the supplementary motor area of the frontal lobe in linguistic tasks has been suggested by many observers. Focal seizures emanating from lesions in this region have been reported to interfere with speech [24, 25] or to produce palilalia [1]. Penfield and Roberts [33] have reported both speech arrest and vocalization from stimulation of this region. Masdeu, Schoene, and Funkenstein [32] reported aphasia and dysgraphia as a consequence of an infarction in this region. Thus, it may be that the medial frontal lobes, prominently demarcated by our SPM, play a previously underemphasized role in aphasia and in concepts of dyslexia and dysgraphia. Moreover, the known clinical and statistical association of dyslexia with the hyperactive syndrome [7] and attentional deficits [10] might be explained on the basis of some yet unspecified, perhaps more extensive, frontal lobe dysfunction than that found in our population of boys with dyslexia. That this region has not been previously implicated in neurophysiological investigaions results, in part, from the fact that electrodes are seldom placed in this area in current research. This emphasizes the importance of not limiting oneself, on the basis of a priori hypotheses, to a limited set of electrodes when attempting to correlate brain electrical activity with underlying brain function.

When anterior regions showed between-group difference, a greater mean EEG alpha activity was found in the dyslexic group. Many investigators interpret increases in alpha activity to represent relative inactivity or "idling" of underlying cortex [20]. Conversely, decreases in alpha activity are taken to represent cortical activation [8]. The increased anterior alpha activity in dyslexics may signify relative underactivation of frontal systems as compared to normal readers during states requiring active responses. A similar difference was found in these regions during the simple eyes open or closed state.

To some extent, it may appear contradictory that our findings implicate widespread and bihemispheric differences in dyslexia when the only neuropathological investigation of a dyslexic brain has demonstrated microscopic abnormalities (cortical heterotopias) primarily in the left posterior hemisphere. We suggest that these findings need not be considered discrepant. Indeed, the microanatomical lesions may be strategically placed so as to interfere with neural communication, thereby disrupting function over wide and distant areas. An alternative, of course, is the possibility that dyslexia may be the result of more than one etiology. A relevant recent finding is that behavioral subcategories of dyslexia-pure demonstrate specific regional differences by BEAM [16] (see Fig. 7-9).

Given the limited size of the study population, our specific findings should not necessarily be considered universally applicable to all dyslexics. Indeed, we have already uncovered additional evidence suggesting that the clinical heterogeneity of dyslexia may be associated with corresponding differences of brain electrical activity. What we do suggest is that topographic mapping of electrophysiological data may prove a useful adjunct to neuropsychological assessment and radiographic studies in the investigation of the aberrant physiology of the learning disabilities.

References

1. Alajouanine, T., Castaigne, R., and Sabourard, O. Palilalie paroxystique et vocalisations itératives au cours de crises epileptiques par lesion interessant de l'aire motrices supplémentaire. *Rev. Neurol.* (Paris) 101:685, 1959.
2. Allison, T., et al. The scalp topography of human visual evoked potentials. *Electroencephalogr. Clin. Neurophysiol.* 42:185, 1977.
3. Berger, H. Ueber das Elektrenkephalogramm des Menschen: I. Mitteilung. *Arch. Psychiatr. Nervenkr.* 87:527, 1929.
4. Bickford, R. G., et al. The compressed spectral array (CSA)—a pictorial EEG. *Proc. San Diego Biomed. Symp.* 11:365, 1972.
5. Bickford, R. G., et al. Application of Compressed Spectral Array in Clinical EEG. In P. Kellaway and J. Peterson (Eds.), *Automation of Clinical Electroencephalography*. New York: Raven, 1973. P. 55.
6. Connors, C. K. Cortical visual evoked response in children with learning disorders. *Psychophysiology* 7:418, 1970.
7. Connors, C. K. Psychological assessment of children with minimal brain dysfunction. *Ann. N.Y. Acad. Sci.* 205:283, 1973.
8. Davidson, R. J., and Schwartz, G. E. The influence of musical training on patterns of EEG asymmetry during musical and non-musical self-generation tasks. *Psychophysiology* 14:58, 1977.
9. Denckla, M. B. Minimal Brain Dysfunction and Dyslexia: Beyond Diagnosis by Exclusion. In M. E. Blau, I. Rapin, and M. Kinsbourne (Eds.), *Child Neurology*. New York: Spectrum, 1977.
10. Douglas, V. Perceptual and Cognitive Factors as Determinants of Learning Disabilities: A Review Chapter with Special Emphasis on Attentional Factors. In R. M. Knights and D. J. Bakker (Eds.), *The Neuropsychology of Learning Disorders*. Baltimore: University Park Press, 1976.
11. Duffy, F. H., Bartels, P. H., and Burchfiel, J. L. Significance probability mapping: An aid in the topographic analysis of brain electrical activity. *Electroencephalogr. Clin. Neurophysiol.* 51:455, 1981.
12. Duffy, F. H., Burchfiel, J. L., and Lombroso, C. T. Brain electrical activity mapping (BEAM): A method for extending the clinical utility of EEG and evoked potential data. *Ann. Neurol.* 5:309, 1979.
13. Duffy, F. H., McAnulty, G. B., and Badian, N. Unpublished data, 1983.
14. Duffy, F. H., et al. Dyslexia: Regional differences in brain electrical activity by topographic mapping. *Ann. Neurol.* 7:412, 1980.
15. Duffy, F. H., et al. Dyslexia: Automated diagnosis by computerized classification of brain electrical activity. *Ann. Neurol.* 7:421, 1980.
16. Duffy, F. H., et al. Unpublished data, 1983.
17. Estrin, T., and Uzgalis, R. Computer display of spatio-temporal EEG patterns. *I.E.E.E. Trans. Biomed. Eng.* 16:192, 1969.
18. Galaburda, A. M., and Eidelberg, D. Symmetry and asymmetry in the human posterior thalamus: II. Thalamic lesions in a case of developmental dyslexia. *Arch. Neurol.* 39:333, 1982.
19. Galaburda, A. M., and Kemper, T. L. Cytoarchitechtonic abnormalities in developmental dyslexia: A case study. *Ann. Neurol.* 6:94, 1979.
20. Gevins, A. S., et al. Electroencephalogram correlates of higher cortical functions. *Science* 203:655, 1979.

21. Gibbs, F. A., Davis, H., and Lennox, W. G. The electroencephalogram in epilepsy and in conditions of impaired consciousness. *Arch. Neurol. Psychiatry* 34:1133, 1935.
22. Goff, G. D., et al. The scalp topography of human somatosensory and auditory evoked potentials. *Electroencephalogr. Clin. Neurophysiol.* 42:57, 1977.
23. Gotman, J., Gloor, P., and Ray, W. F. A quantitative comparison of traditional reading of the EEG and interpretation of computer-extracted features in patients with supratentorial brain lesions. *Electroencephalogr. Clin. Neurophysiol.* 38:623, 1975.
24. Guidetti, B. Désordres de la parole associés a des lésions de la surface interhémisphérique frontale postérieure. *Rev. Neurol.* (Paris) 97:122, 1957.
25. Hanley, J., and Sklar, B. Electroencephalographic Correlates of Developmental Reading Dyslexias: Computer Analyses of Recordings from Normal and Dyslexic Children. In G. Leisman (Ed.), *Basic Visual Processes and Learning Disability*. Springfield, Ill.: Thomas, 1976.
26. Harris, J. A., Melry, G. M., and Bickford, R. G. Computer-controlled multidimensional display device for investigation and modeling of physiologic systems. *Comp. Biomed. Res.* 2:519, 1969.
27. Hughes, J. R., and Denckla, M. B. Outline of a Pilot Study of Electroencephalographic Correlates of Dyslexia. In A. L. Benton and D. Pearl (Eds.), *Dyslexia: An Appraisal of Current Knowledge*. New York: Oxford University Press, 1978.
28. Hughes, J. R., and Park, G. C. Electro-clinical correlation in dyslexic children. *Electroencephalogr. Clin. Neurophysiol.* 26:117, 1969.
29. John, E. R., et al. Neurometrics. *Science* 196:1393, 1977.
30. Larsen, B., Skinhoj, E., and Lassen, N. A. Variations in regional cortical blood flow in the right and left hemispheres during automatic speech. *Brain* 101:193, 1978.
31. Lassen, N. A., Ingvar, D. G., and Skinhoj, E. Brain function and blood flow. *Sci. Am.* 239:62, 1978.
32. Masdeu, J. C., Schoene, W. C., and Funkenstein, H. Aphasia following infarction of the left supplementary motor area: A clinicopathologic study. *Neurology* 28:1220, 1978.
33. Penfield, W., and Roberts, L. *Speech and Brain Mechanisms*. Princeton, N.J.: Princeton University Press, 1959.
34. Petsche, H. Topography of the EEG: Survey and prospects. *Clin. Neurol. Neurosurg.* 79:15, 1976.
35. Rutter, W. Prevalence and Types of Dyslexia. In A. L. Benton and D. Pearl (Eds.), *Dyslexia: An Appraisal of Current Knowledge*. New York: Oxford Unversity Press, 1978.
36. Shipton, H. W. A new frequency-selective toposcope for electroencephalography. *Med. Electron. Biol. Eng.* 1:483, 1963.
37. Sobotka, K. R., and May, J. G. Visual evoked potentials and reaction time in normal and dyslexic children. *Psychophysiology* 14:18, 1977.
38. Symann-Louett, N., et al. Wave form difference in visual evoked responses between normal and reading disabled children. *Neurology* 27:156, 1977.
39. Torres, R., and Ayers, F. W. Evaluation of the electroencephalogram of dyslexic children. *Electroencephalogr. Clin. Neurophysiol.* 24:281, 1968.
40. Vaughn, H. G., Jr., and Ritter, W. The sources of auditory evoked responses recorded from the human scalp. *Electroencephalogr. Clin. Neurophysiol.* 28:360, 1970.
41. Walter, W. G., and Shipton, H. W. A new toposcopic display system. *Electroencephalogr. Clin. Neurophysiol.* 3:281, 1951.

8 Sound-Film Microanalysis: A Means for Correlating Brain and Behavior

William S. Condon

This chapter deals with microbehavioral asynchronies and the observed occurrence of these asynchronies in the behavior of dyslexic children, autisticlike children, and children with other disorders. The method used to study patterns of microbehavior was sound-film microanalysis. The primary emphasis of this approach is based on the analysis of both normal and pathological behavior organization *as* organization—as patterns of change within change. The microanalysis revealed that for children with disorders, one side of the body moves in sound-induced organizations of change that are out of phase, that is, *a*synchronous, with those of the other side of the body. By contrast, normal children exhibit a synchronous organization of behavior. Analogously, studies of brain electrical activity in subjects with a variety of disorders also reveal asymmetries, whereas normal subjects exhibit symmetrical brain electrical activity.

Background

Motion pictures store the ongoing flow of events in the form of a series of still pictures, usually taken at 24 frames per second (fps). When these are played back through a motion picture projector at the same speed, the observer sees the event repeated and is not aware that he is seeing rapidly sampled segments of an originally continuous process. Sound is recorded by a different system and is essentially continuous, as opposed to the rapid, discrete series of pictures. The sound is synchronized with the visual events on a separate sound track running in parallel to the pictures and advanced 26 frames. When a gun fires or an object strikes a table, the observer hears the appropriate co-occurring sound. Film frames are numbered to provide a number to correlate speech and body motion at the same point of recorded action. Such films provide the data base for the microanalysis of behavior.

Films have been used in industry for many years to study complicated industrial and machine processes. The movie films store what processes have happened so that they can be viewed over and over. Events and the changing relationships among events that happen too fast or where many are occurring at the same time can be studied more carefully and described in detail. For example, two engineers from General Motors were interested in how the flame in the combustion chamber of an automobile burns [22]. They were seeking methods to save fuel through a more efficient burning process. They constructed a transparent piston chamber and filmed the firing process. The resulting film was studied frame by frame and the flow structure of the flame described from moment to moment. Another example involved two scientists who studied the suction method used by the angler fish to engulf its prey. They took films at 800 and 1,000 fps and found that the fish could engulf its prey in 4 msec [18]. It has recently been reported that a laser camera has been built that can take pictures at 2 million fps. It has also been found that a television camera aimed through a light microscope can improve the contrast, sensitivity, and resolution of images and can capture the movement and every microscopic aspect of living cells and minute organisms. Moving structures only 25 nm wide are made clearly visible. Films based on this technique can then be slowed down or speeded up for study. Thus, even very microscopic living events can be stored and reviewed over and over for analysis of patterns [24].

Human behavior, both normal and pathological, can be filmed and studied in the same frame-by-frame fashion, using frame-numbered sound film. Human speech and body motion are very rapid, complicated, and essentially continuous processes. Sound-film microanalysis, which can cover the range from $1/96$ second up to and including 2 or 3 seconds, provides a "microscope" to study the complicated organization of normal and pathological behavior. Films of human behavior can be viewed repeatedly as needed in the search for order and pattern. In going through a film once, the observer discerns certain details. Viewing the film a second time, he sees more. In time, complex and interpenetrating patterns of organization can be discovered that the observer could never have anticipated. Countless reviews of the same material by the same investigator are necessary for such hidden forms of *organization* to become apparent. The investigator himself has to store and work on the material over time. The major task of this application of sound-film analysis involves the identification and description of the nature of the "units" and organizations of units of both speaker and listener within the flowing stream of behavior at this very minimal level. When a normal person speaks, there are often many parts of the body moving at the same time. The arms, hands, and head may be moving simultaneously and almost constantly, and while this is occurring, speech is emerging. This *organized* complexity of ongoing speech and body motion, where several body parts are moving together at once and for varying lengths of time, must be faced by any investigator analyzing behavior at the microlevel. As indicated, behavior is fundamentally continuous, and the investigator's task is that of determining the "units" within that continuum. Natural human communication is composed of these microorganizational events, which had never really been carefully examined before.

Normal Human Behavior at the Microlevel

The Microanalysis of Natural Speech

When we listen to a person talking, we usually understand what is being said. We are aware of the words being spoken and can distinguish them from one another. The meaning of the individual statements and of the total conversation can be understood. But the empirical determination of where the sounds forming phone types (the minimal and very rapid units of speech), words, and phrases begin and end is not an easy matter. Human speech is a continuous phenomenon, thereby creating a problem for one attempting to locate the precise boundary points of the elements of speech as spoken sound. There is an overlap of features as one element transforms into another, with no exact point where one phone ends and another begins. There is a transitional moment of 15 to 20 msec in which a speech form exists that contains features of both the preceding and following form. This occurs at all levels where phone, syllable, word, phrase, and sentence are connected. There are usually no periods of silence between phones or between words in the normal flow of speech, except for occasional hesitation pauses [15]. Speech from a 24-fps frame-numbered sound film of a naturalistic dyadic interaction was played through an oscilloscope, and the resulting waveforms were filmed at 24 fps. The speech creating the waveform was simultaneously rerecorded on the film of its own oscilloscopic display so that the speech could be heard as well as seen. Each frame of the film was numbered. The slow decay time of the phosphoric image permitted the storage of information that occurred while the camera shutter was closed. This provides an image of the continuous flow of sound even though the camera takes discrete film frames. One can view in totality a waveform contour that begins in the middle of one frame and ends in the middle of another. This also provides an ability to analyze sound even at the one-half frame level.

Figure 8-1 shows enlarged photographs of the initial vocalization of the word *pressure* as taken from a 16-mm film of an oscilloscopic display of speech. The word lasts for 11 frames or slightly under ½ second. Only the first 7 frames of the word have been presented, with the full height of some of the framing having been cropped to conserve space. The camera is focused on a full face of the oscilloscope, and the sound wave travels from left to right. The camera shutter opens and closes three times, producing three pictures for each sweep of the scope. Each picture shows what is on the full face of the scope at a given moment, including some of the preceding portion (which is decaying) and the following portion (which is dark). The onset of the /p/ beginning *pressure* occurs in frame number 3337, the image occurring only in the middle of the scope. The small wavy line preceding the burst for /p/ is the decaying scope trace for silence on the preceding frame. The next frame, 3338, shows the sound /p/ continuing and reaching the end of the scope sweep. The part of /p/ that was on frame 3337 is seen decaying on frame 3338 directly below itself. The trace then begins a new sweep. Frame 3339 shows the /r/ and the beginning of /ɛ/. The /r/ sound can be seen just as the frame begins, and the valley between /r/ and /ɛ/ can be seen on the right. Frame 3340 shows the continuation of /ɛ/. The /s/ sound begins in frame 3341. It lasts for three frames and can be seen trailing off just prior to the onset of the concluding /r/, which is not shown. Comparable, accurate single-frame analysis can be done on any word or set of words. The word *pressure* is also seen and discussed in Figure 8-4. A great deal of precision is attainable in analyzing natural speech in this manner. Tests have been conducted with independent judges segmenting sound with high reliability at the one-frame level. Further, independent judges can also determine the onset point of both speech and inanimate sounds following silence with 98-percent accuracy at the one-frame level and 90 percent at the half-frame level. This finding has been replicated several times.

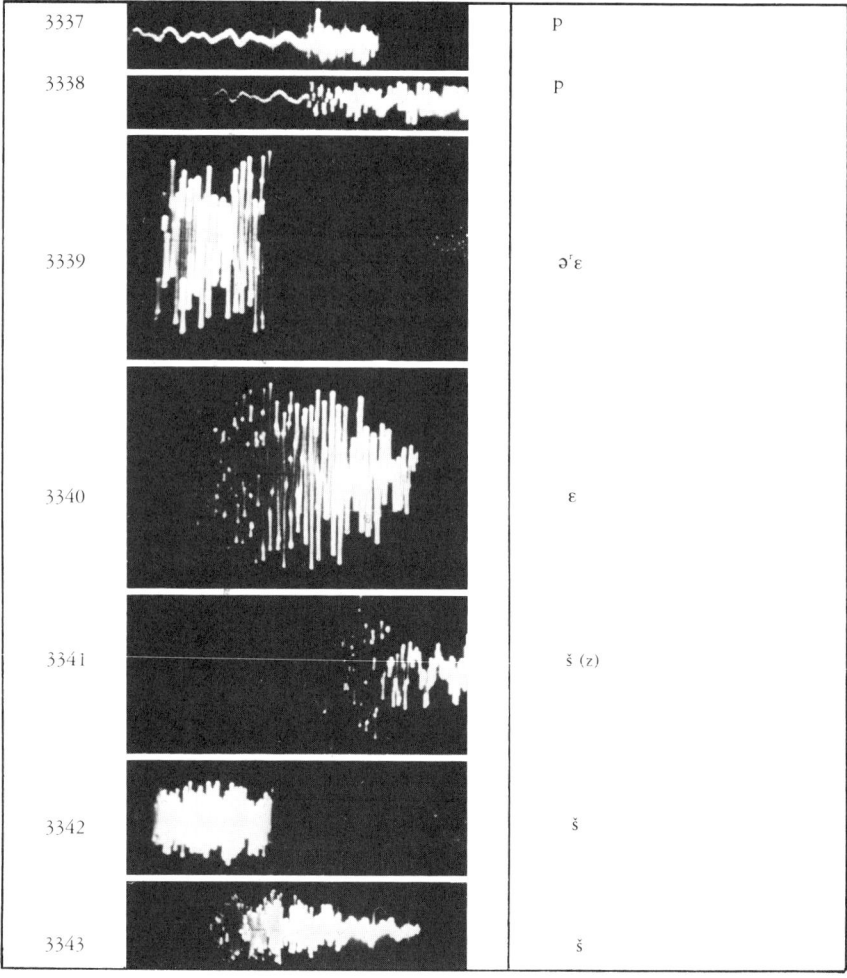

Fig. 8-1. Oscilloscopic display of the first part of the word *pressure,* illustrating the sound-film microanalysis of human speech.

The Microanalysis of Body Motion

When a person speaks, he typically accompanies his speech with gestures and movements of many different kinds. During speech, there are many movements occurring simultaneously and in an ongoing fashion so that body motion is continuous. As previously stated, the critical problem is the determination of what might constitute "units" within this organized flow of behavior. Intricate, systematic, and synchronous relationships have been found between speech and body motion across multiple levels. At the frame-by-frame level of analysis, body motion has been seen to be formed of "quanta" or "synchronized movement bundles," which are the building blocks of still wider forms of movement organization. These minimal units were called process units to emphasize their organizational nature. This is a new, basic hypothesis concerning the nature of the pulselike organization of human body motion at the microlevel [5]. Body motion is *already* organized at the most minimal level and is not composed of parts that are put together to form organized behavior. This may characterize much of animal motion. Figure 8-2 illustrates the great complexity of this self-synchronous, sustaining, and "changing together" of the body parts.

Figure 8-2 shows a sound-film microanalysis of a segment of speaker's speech and body motion from a film taken at 96 fps. While the figure contains excessive detail, it is useful for present purposes in that it demonstrates the great amount of behavior that can actually take place in a 1-second interval. The process units, which seem like pulses, are characterized by a "sustaining of a relationship together" for a brief period of time by whatever body parts happen to be moving at a given time. Behavior is the serial and continuous flow of such pulselike forms. Body motion is continuous; yet there are "discretelike" organizations of change within this ongoing process. A young woman approximately 25 years old is seated talking to a young man of the same age. As part of her conversation, she says, "an [sic] *so* I'd get put back in that way." Using the body movement co-occurring with the /s/ of *so* as an illustration, the pattern of change of motion at the microlevel has the following characteristics. There is a synchronous change of the body parts, where they alter direction and/or velocity. Not all body parts need change; some may sustain a given direction for a longer interval. The changes that initiate the beginning of a process unit always differ from the changes that indicate the ending of that process unit, this ending also being the beginning point of a new process unit. At the onset of the process unit co-occurring with /s/, there is a change of direction in the head, eyes, first and second fingers of the right hand, and right shoulder. There is a change in velocity of the right wrist and the right elbow. No change is detected in the extension of the right thumb, which continues to extend. That which forms the *content* of the process unit is the sustenance of the relationship between the moving body parts. That these quanta or pulses also co-occur isomorphically with the units of speech provides additional support for their existence.

Across the emission of /s/, the head moves left and slightly up, *while* the eyes move left and down, and the lids close, beginning a slight blink, *while* the right thumb continues to extend, *while* the first and second fingers of the right hand hold, *while* there is acceleration in the left wrist and elbow, and *while* the right shoulder rotates out and adducts. One can sweep back and forth across these five frames of film with the analyzing projector and discern a smooth flow of motion where all the body parts are sustaining their relationship of movement together. This "sustaining together" also illustrates the basic principle of the organization of normal speaking behavior across multiple levels. The emergent verbal phones are accompanied by a form of body motion, and the words are accompanied by forms of body motion, as are the phrases and sentences. It is this mutual sustaining of the units of speech and body motion across varying temporal durations that characterizes the hierarchical organization of speaker behavior. For example, the first and

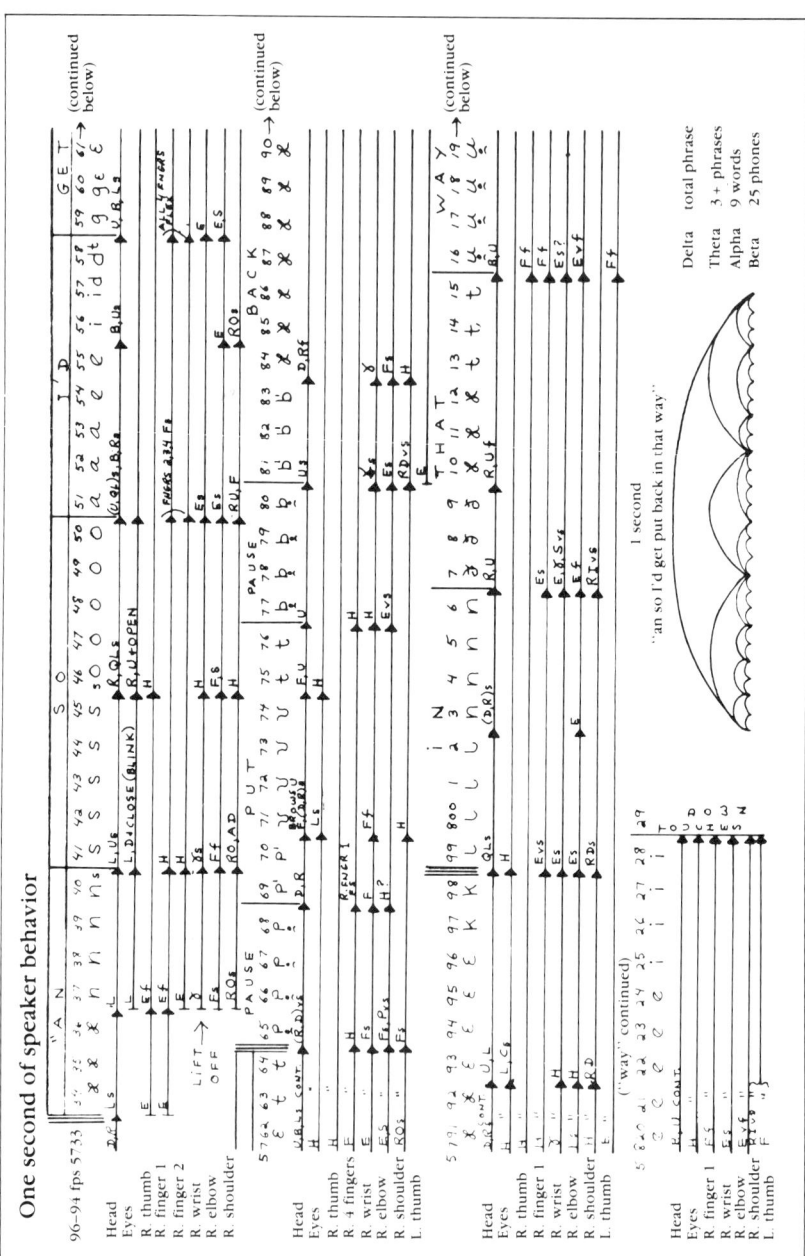

Fig. 8-2. Sound-film microanalysis of the hierarchically synchronized speech and body motion of a woman saying, "an [sic] so I'd get put back in that way." The film was taken at approximately 96 fps.

second fingers of the right hand cease moving at the end of the /n/ of *an,* hold their lack of movement exactly across the emission of the total word *so,* and then begin to flex at the beginning of *I'd.*

A behavioral model for speech where discrete lower parts or pieces are put together to form larger parts, which are, in turn, put together to form still higher parts, is inadequate to deal with its organization. All normal behavior studied thus far is similar in organizational principle to that presented in Figure 8-2. The process unit sustaining across /s/ differs from that sustaining across /o/. The /o/ process unit was not added to the /s/ process unit to create a larger /so/ body motion. There is no way the /o/ unit added to the /s/ unit could go back in time to create the hold of the first and second fingers that sustained across the entire word *so*. This principle also applies to the larger forms of body motion that accompany speech across wider forms such as phases. We seem to be dealing with a form of organization where multiple levels are emerging together simultaneously, where organization *as* organization is a structural principle. Behavioral organization is not "composed of" or "more than" these moving body parts and speech synchronized together; it is *in* all of them, at all levels simultaneously. The investigator begins with organized behavior, the living, talking people in the film, and discovers their behavior to consist of many forms of organization integrated together.

The precision with which the speaker's body accompanies his or her speech in a hierarchically organized fashion can also be seen in Figure 8-2. Most of the phone types have co-occurring process units. A speaker's speech at the minimal level appears to be formed of an ongoing flow of unified speech and body motion units. Both seem to be the product of a more basic neurological organization. The body motion process unit or pulse accompanying the /n/ of *an* has a sustained organizational integrity that is isomorphic with the articulation of /n/. This is different from a similarly sustained body motion organization accompanying /s/. This, in turn, is different from that accompanying /o/, and so on. This synchrony has been observed in films of all normal speakers, including speakers from many different cultures. As indicated in Figure 8-2, this synchrony also occurs hierarchically where body motion forms simultaneously accompany wider aspects of speech. Whatever organizes speech also appears to organize body motion simultaneously. The articulation of sound is a motor behavior, and its related body motion is also a motor behavior.

In our example, spoken words usually have body motion forms accompanying them. Across the vocalization of *an,* the head goes left, the first right finger extends, and the thumb extends. Across *so,* the first and second fingers do not move. Across *I'd,* the right elbow extends, the second, third, and fourth fingers flex slightly, and so on. There are three phrases that have co-occurring body motion forms. Her right arm, which is initially resting in her lap, sweeps up and right to shoulder height while she says, "an [sic] so I'd get." It sweeps left in front of her body during "put back" and then directly down to her lap across "in that way," reaching her lap just as the utterance ends. The utterance, as a totality which lasts approximately 1 second, is accompanied by the right arm's leaving and returning to the lap. As will be seen later, such 1-second movement forms are generally characteristic of speaker behavior. Behavior follows forms of structural organization. The study of pathological behavior also reveals forms of organization, but forms that differ from normal organization.

Reliability studies were conducted to determine the ability of independent judges to detect the process units of body motion. In determining that a process-unit boundary has occurred, 27 points of the body are evaluated at each frame using a manually operated 16-mm time-motion analyzing projector. These points are primarily at the joints where body movements such as extension/flexion, pronation/supination, and abduction/adduction occur. A detectable change at any one of these 27 decisional points of the body is considered to constitute the occurrence of a process-unit boundary. In most instances, however, there were several changes co-occurring in the same frame of film. Thus, for each frame analyzed in studies 1 and 2 following, there were 27 decisions on the part of each independent judge as to whether a change occurred. The frames at which any change occurred and the number of changes at those frames formed the basis of the reliability correlations.

The following constitutes a summary of study results demonstrating the reliability of independent judges in detecting body motion process units. I first summarize a number of observations from my own research and then include the results from three other studies.

1. Two independent judges performed a frame-by-frame analysis of 188 frames of 24-fps film showing the continuous behavioral body motions of a listener where several body parts were in constant motion. Since the data were skewed, a Spearman Rank Correlation was used. The results (correlation = .842) were statistically significant with $p < .001$.
2. A replication study by two independent judges was conducted using 48-fps film. This time, 211 frames of continuous movement were analyzed using the same procedure as the previous study. The Spearman Rank Correlation was again used, with significant statistical results ($p < .001$).
3. Independent judges detected the onset point of eye blinks with 90-percent agreement at the one-frame level using 24-fps film.
4. Independent judges were able to detect eye gaze changes (orienting responses) with 95-percent agreement in one study and 87 percent in another study at $1/15$ second.
5. Beebe, Stern, and Jaffe [4] detected head changes at the one-frame level using 24-fps film.
6. Peery [27], in discussing reliability, notes,

   One 60 second segment, which was scored by the first observer, was recorded by the second observer as an interrater reliability check. There was 99-percent agreement about the occurrence of a movement and 97-percent agreement about its duration, plus or minus one frame. High interrater reliability is the rule with film analysis.

7. Plooij [28], in speaking about self-synchrony, says,

   At certain moments (frames) in time, several body segments such as the head, a hand, a finger, or a foot change direction of movement. Condon calls these movements "process-unit-boundaries". Personally, I verified Condon's finding in newborn babies, although my study was not set up with this purpose in mind. Instead, I studied the development of preverbal communication in the human mother-infant interaction in a face-to-face situation. The main part of this study consisted of frame-by-frame analysis of filmed sessions. In doing so, one could not help noticing the self-synchrony. For instance, the eyes would blink and a foot would bend at the same time.

While more work needs to be done to demonstrate the ability of independent judges to segment behavior reliably at the microlevel, the work that has been done documents the ability to do so.

Overt Behavior as Wave Phenomena

The hypothesis is presented herein that speech and body motion are precisely synchronized across multiple levels in the normal speaker, suggesting that they are the product of a unitary neuroelectric process. This speech/body motion hierarchical organization can also be interpreted as wavelike, since it exhibits characteristic periodicities.

The following determinations were made from the previously described oscilloscopic film used to segment speech. In an analysis of phone type, the mean length of 1,055 consecutively analyzed phone types was 1.61 film frames (or 15 per second of 24-fps film) with a standard deviation of 0.88 and a standard error of 0.03. Short, rapidly spoken words would also fit this periodicity at times, depending on articulation. In the word-length analysis, the polysyllabic words were divided into their components. The mean length of 365 consecutive words, with pauses omitted, from the same film was 4.5 frames (5.3 per second), with a standard deviation of 2.22 and a standard error of 0.12. Utterances are seen very clearly in the body motion, where a marked, 1-second periodicity has been observed. Ninety-six consecutive speech sequences from both speakers were analyzed. It was observed that the 1-second rhythm form is usually manifested bodily by a head or arm (or, less frequently, another body part) movement ensemble sustaining a given direction during the utterance or by some aspect of the body's moving from a given position and then back to that position. Twelve of the 96 utterances were approximately ½ second in length, and the rest averaged 23.9 frames (24 frames = 1 second). The range was from 19 to 29 frames.

Another study was conducted to further explore the 1-second rhythm. In another 24-fps filmed dyadic interaction, 188 consecutive natural speech sequences from two speakers were analyzed. Of the 188 sequences, 30 consisted of one- or two-word replies of "yes" or "no" or "um hum" to questions; these were excluded. Thus, 158 sequences were examined. The major criteria for segmentation at this level were the sustained body motion forms occurring during a spoken sequence. The mean frame duration of the 158 sequences was 24 frames, with a range from 19 to 30 frames. Among the 158 sequences were 48 that occurred in relative isolation; that is, the speech sequence was preceded and followed by silence. All of these fell within the 19- to 30-frame range, so that the analysis of speech length alone (without the accompanying body motion forms) also demonstrated a marked 1-second periodicity. The number of words per utterance in the sequences ranged from 1 to 8 frames with a mean of 4.56 frames, a standard deviation of 1.61, and a standard error of 0.13. This would be in the theta periodicity and agrees well with the mean length of words obtained from the separate oscilloscope study.

These observations imply that there is an ongoing multilevel, organizational rhythm hierarchy in terms of which behavior behaves. Both speech and body motion obey this hierarchical rhythm structure and are simultaneously synchronized across multiple levels in their co-occurrence. The ongoing flowing and changing together of the body parts do so in terms of an underlying organizational template. It is somewhat of a departure from the traditional view of human behavior to conceptualize speech/body motion as wavelike, but in our analysis, the characteristic organizational flow of speaker behavior is particularly clearly revealed to be an ongoing process formed of several levels of waves emerging simultaneously. The behavior that forms the slower wave begins at the same moment that the faster (smaller) waveforms begin. The smaller waves are integrated with the slower wave but are not added together to form it. Metaphorically, it is as if the organism were constantly generating an integrated, multilevel wave hierarchy that behavior necessarily follows. All behavior appears to be integrated together as a function of a basic, organized rhythm hierarchy. The speaker's eye blinks, which might seem to occur randomly, actually occur synchronously with the rest of behavior. They tend to occur at articulatory change points, primarily at phone boundaries.

Behavior appears to be phenomenologically both discretelike *and* continuous simultaneously, without contradiction, providing an organizational form where the discretelike is fused into the continuous. The faster waveforms (carrying the words) may get integrated into the slower waveform (carrying the unitary meaning of the sentence in which the discretelike words result). The speech/body motion wave hierarchy of a normal speaker's behavioral self-synchrony appears to exhibit periodicities similar to the delta, theta, alpha, and beta (DTAB) waves of the brain revealed by electroencephalography. This may be only a coincidence, but the similarities are striking. The DTAB waves all occur together at the same time in the brain. This is also true of the body's behavioral waves. Brain waves are sequentially continuous, and so are the behavioral waves. The body motion organization accompanies the phone types, *while* it accompanies the words, *while* it accompanies the phrases and sentences. This is a simultaneous, multilevel accompaniment, as was seen in Figure 8-2. It is the periodic form of the behavioral waves that seems to be synchronous with the periodic form of the brain waves, the DTAB. The new hypothesis is that human speech/body motion behavior can be interpreted as behavioral waves characterized by continuous, hierarchically integrated series of waves. Analysis of behavior from $\frac{1}{96}$ second up to 1 or 2 seconds is revealing forms of order that appear to link brain and behavior. If the hierarchical organization of the behavioral waves is synchronous with, or a reflection of, the brain waves, sound-film microanalysis can contribute importantly to the study of how behavior reflects brain wave processes. For example, it would suggest

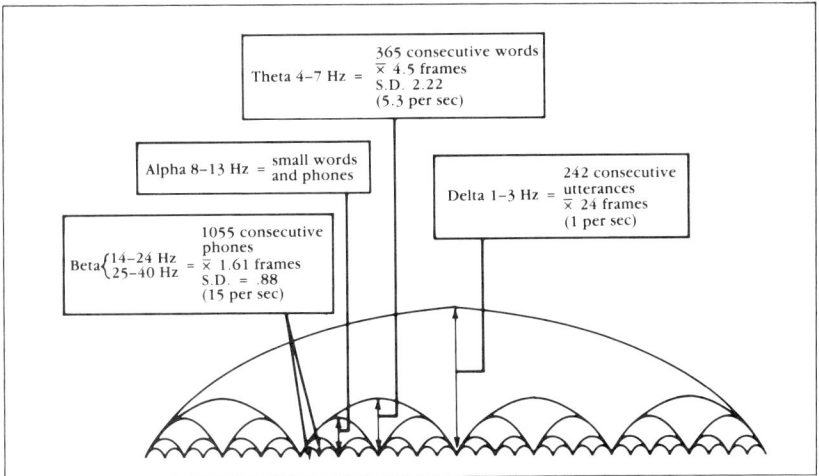

Fig. 8-3. Illustrative schema of behavioral wave periodicities compared to brain wave periodicities.

that the brain waves may be operating together synchronously and hierarchically like the behavioral waves. It would also suggest that brain wave organization may entrain with the structure of incoming speech. This will be seen in the following discussion of listener behavior. A view is emerging that everything may be organizationally linked together. Behavior and the brain processes that mediate it may not be separate systems but rather may constitute an organizational integrity across many levels.

Figure 8-3 presents a speculative schema of behavioral wave periodicities compared to brain wave periodicities based on the phone, word, and sentence length analyses.

Listener Entrainment to Speaker Speech

The previous section dealt with the synchronization and periodicities of speaker behavior observed by sound-film microanalysis. This section will discuss the entertainment or synchronization of the *listener's* body motion organization to incoming speech. In this entrainment, the organizations of change, that is, process units, in the listener's movements are synchronized with the articulatory structure of the speaker's speech almost as well as the speaker's own body is synchronized with his speech. This often occurs in relation to sounds from inanimate objects as well. Entrainment occurs within a 42-msec latency following the sounds, like a car following a curving road. It implies that there is a basic short-latency auditory-motor linkage in which the motor processes reflect the structure of the incoming auditory signals, especially speech. The listener also tends to move faster at points of loudness in the speaker's speech. Entrainment is a complex phenomenon and is observable if the listener is moving while attending to the speaker. Obviously, if the listener is quite still, such entrainment cannot be easily detected.

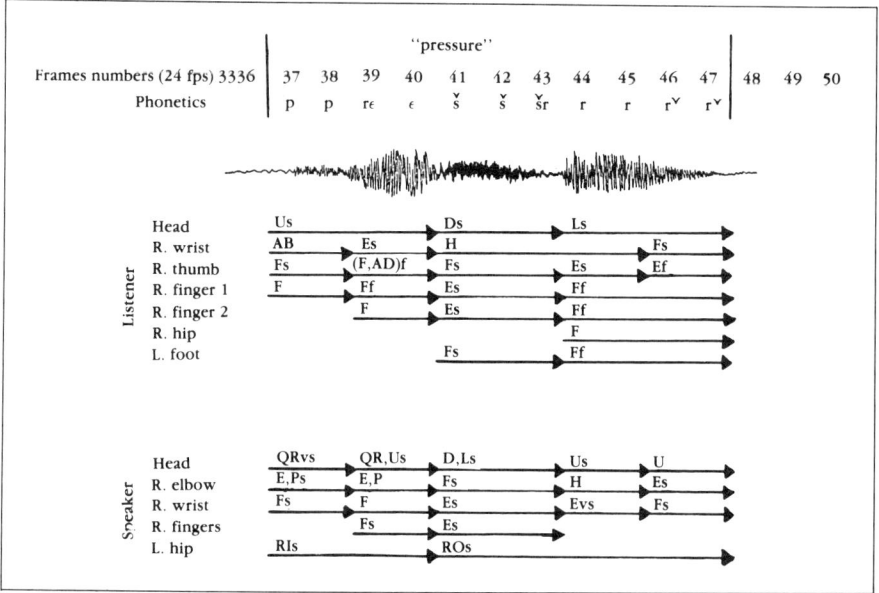

Fig. 8-4. Sound-film microanalysis of speaker and listener body motion during the word *pressure* shows interactional entrainment. The listener's process units and speed of movement entrain with the speaker's speech. (U = up; s = slow; D = down; L = left; R = right; AB = abduct; E = extend; H = hold or no movement; F = flex; AD = adduct; f = fast; Q = incline of head; v = very; P = pronate; RI = rotate in; RO = rotate out.)

Figure 8-4 illustrates the precision that is characteristic of entrainment. Two men who had never met before are seated and talking. A sound film was made at 24 fps. The speaker says, "Put the pressure on people on the job market." The word *pressure*, which will be used to illustrate entrainment, exhibits a constrasting sequence of voiced and unvoiced segments. An oscilloscopic display of the speech is presented to show that the sound pattern can be displayed visually. This is the same word shown in Figure 8-1. The voiced /ə/ sound terminating the word *the* is followed by the /p/ of *pressure*, which is unvoiced and lasts 2 frames. This is then followed by the voiced /rɛ/, which also lasts 2 frames. The /r/ flows smoothly into the /ɛ/, forming a unitary articulatory gesture. The unvoiced /s/ occurs next and lasts 3 frames. Finally, the terminal voiced /r/ occurs, lasting 4 frames. The total word covers 11 frames, or just slightly under ½ second. The body motion of the listener exhibits micromovement organizations, that is, process units, that occur isomorphically with the lengths of the units of the speaker's speech. This is seen particularly well in the listener's behavioral process unit that occurs with the 3 frames of /sss/ in *pressure*. The first and second fingers of the right hand had been flexing. They change direction and extend slightly across the 3-frame duration of /sss/ and then flex again at the end of the segment. The head also moves down slightly in contrast to a preceding upward movement and a following leftward movement.

The behavior of the listener in Figure 8-4 is not like that of a robot. The process units transform smoothly into each other and cannot be seen by the naked eye. They are part of the flow of ongoing behavior, but they are precisely synchronized with the articulatory structure of the speaker's speech. Such precise synchrony occurs constantly throughout this 12-minute film. This synchrony has been observed in all normal interactants studied thus far, including those in films of many different cultures. The form of organization of the listener's process units seems to be modulated by the structure of the speaker's speech. Whatever body parts the listener happens to be moving at that moment will follow the organization of the speaker's speech. Further, the listener's body often speeds up and slows down in relation to the softness or loudness of the speaker's speech. For example, in Figure 8-4, there is accelerated listener movement with the voiced /rɛ/ and with the voiced terminal /r/ in contrast to the unvoiced /p/ and /s/. This is seen in the lowercase *f*, which designates fast movement. There is a precise isomorphism between the flow of the speaker's behavior and that of the listener. Again, this occurs in all speaker/listener behaviors, and the illustration of it in Figure 8-4 is not an isolated instance.

The concept of *synchrony* is basic to the hypotheses of self-synchrony and entrainment. Both are organizational concepts. The units of speech and body motion are forms of organization or order in behavior. The structures that form the units of body motion, for example, are forms of organization and are identified by their order and not directly by the specific body parts that happen to be exemplifying that order at a given moment. In other words, no matter what body parts may be moving during speaking they tend to occur with characteristic forms of order that are synchronous with the co-occurring flow of speech. This is also true of listening behavior, but it is the phone types and word levels with which the listener's movements are primarily entrained, while entrainment with larger movements covering phrases is rarer. The precise organization and synchronization operating during normal speaking and listening behavior is a new dimension for exploration.

In another study, a normal infant as young as 20 minutes following birth was found to entrain with adult speech almost as well as an adult. This would suggest a basic biological preparedness for speech and human communication. Entrainment may occur in utero. Since it is not possible to show a motion picture of the phenomenon of entrainment to the reader, a series of still pictures taken from a 30-fps 16-mm sound film of a 2-day-old infant are presented in Figures 8-5 and 8-6. The infant is awake and alert. The male physician is standing to the infant's left out of view in Figure 8-6 and says, "Look over here . . . hum . . . not over there." The infant's organizations of movement during "not over there" were microanalyzed and are shown in Figure 8-5.

Figure 8-6 shows the actual series of still pictures of the movements taken from the film. Frame numbers can be seen at the bottom of the pictures. The first word, *not*, lasts for 7 frames, or approximately ⅕ second. What can be seen most clearly in the still pictures is the left arm sweeping up and out through frames 013208 through 013214. The baby had been still and begins to entrain at the onset of the word *not*. The second word, *over*, takes

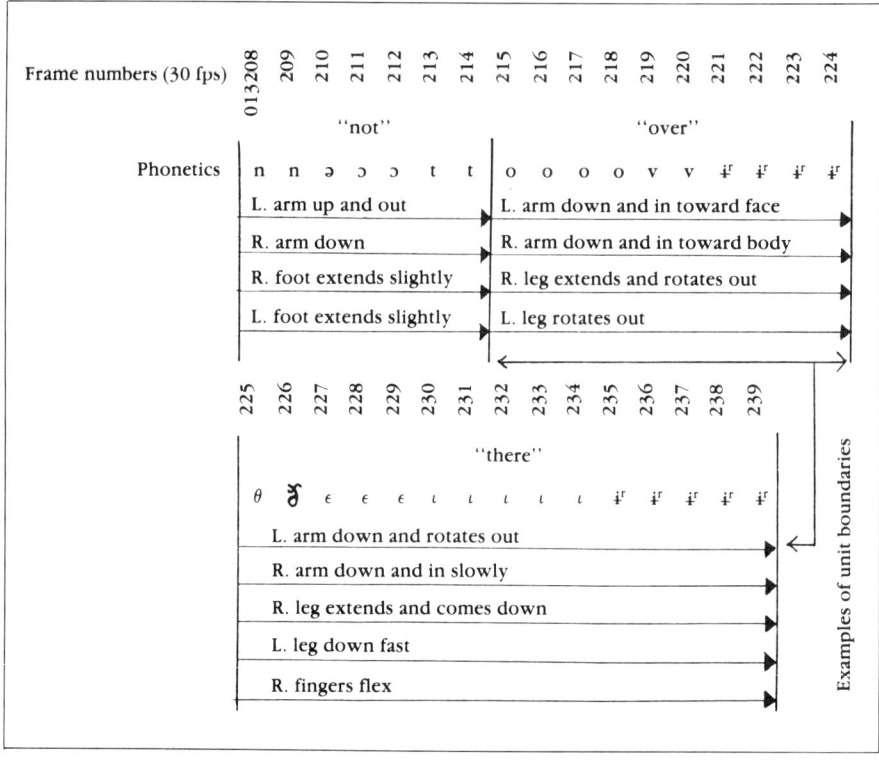

Fig. 8-5. Description of a 2-day-old infant's movements during the words *not over there* spoken by a male physician out of the infant's range of vision. Infants entrained equally well to tape-recorded human speech.

10 frames, from frame 013215 through 013224. The left arm now moves back in toward the face and across it. The arms cross each other over the baby's face. As this is occurring, the baby's left leg sweeps rapidly outward horizontally. During the word *there*, the left arm moves back to the left. This can be seen by the fingers of the left hand in relation to the white card on the back of the crib. The word *there* occurs across frames 013225 through 013239. The left leg comes down rapidly toward the mattress, and the fingers of the right hand flex.

The whole process lasts 32 frames or slightly over 1 second. It illustrates how much movement can occur in such a brief period, even in a 2-day-old infant. There are three clear process units that occur isomorphically with the three words uttered by the physician. This infant entrained in this same precise fashion across 89 consecutive words (in phrases) spoken by the physician. It is possible to analyze the film in reverse to provide additional evidence. This infant was among 16 normal 4-day-old infants who were studied for entrainment to adult speech [10]. All of the infants exhibited precise entrainment. A recent intensive analysis of a 48-fps high-speed film of a 2-day-old infant yielded marked entrainment to adult speech. There was precise entrainment of the organizations of change of the infant's body motion with both speech and tap sounds. The infant soon habituated to the tap sounds. It was as if the organization of the infant's body motion was being generated by the structure of the speech. The infant exhibited microstartle movements in response to the tap sounds within the first two frames following sound onset (i.e., within 42 msec). These were quite clear and convincing. The sustaining and changes of the articulatory units of the mother's speech were paralleled by almost simultaneous sustainings and changes in the organization of change of the infant's movements. The infant's movements would also accelerate in synchrony with louder sounds, especially the vowels. Speakers also characteristically accelerate movement with vowel sounds [9]. Such entrainment on the part of the infant would suggest a powerful and rapid linkage of the auditory and motor (striatal) systems, probably at the brainstem level.

Reliability studies have been conducted on entrainment. A judge segmented the speaker's speech without seeing a listener's body motion using a film with only numbers and a sound track. The same judge then segmented the listener's body motion using a different frame-numbered film and without sound. This blind analysis resulted in an agreement of 97 percent. This technique has obvious defects, but it is suggestive. In another, more rigorous study, 188 consecutive frames of a speaker's speech were segmented by one judge, and the body motion of the listener's behavior was segmented by another judge. These segmentations were in 87-percent agreement. In a third study, two independent judges analyzed the body motion of six normal children in response to 20 sounds for 10 frames of film following the onset of each sound. A significantly greater number of process-unit boundaries occurred in relation to the frame following sound onset for both judges for all six subjects. In another study [6], I found that listener eye blinks tended to occur at articulatory change points in a speaker's speech, supporting interactional entrainment.

There has been a series of recent studies concerned with the replication of interactional entrainment. McDowall [23] in Australia conducted the first study on adult entrainment. His study was defective in that he used the wrong analytical equipment, the wrong criteria for body motion change, and the wrong hypothesis. His study was criticized by Gatewood and Rosenwein [16] and Peery [27]. Austin and Peery [3] conducted an intensive study of infant entrainment with adult speech, spending at least one-half hour on each of 2,400 frames of mother-infant interaction. They state,

This research corroborates the Condon studies which showed synchrony or entrainment between neonates and adults in interactional situations. It is possible that McDowall did not find such levels of synchrony because, as indicated before, his use of an electronically operated projector did not allow observations meticulous enough to detect the phenomena.

Peery [27] has studied the facial approach and withdrawal between mother and infant and states,

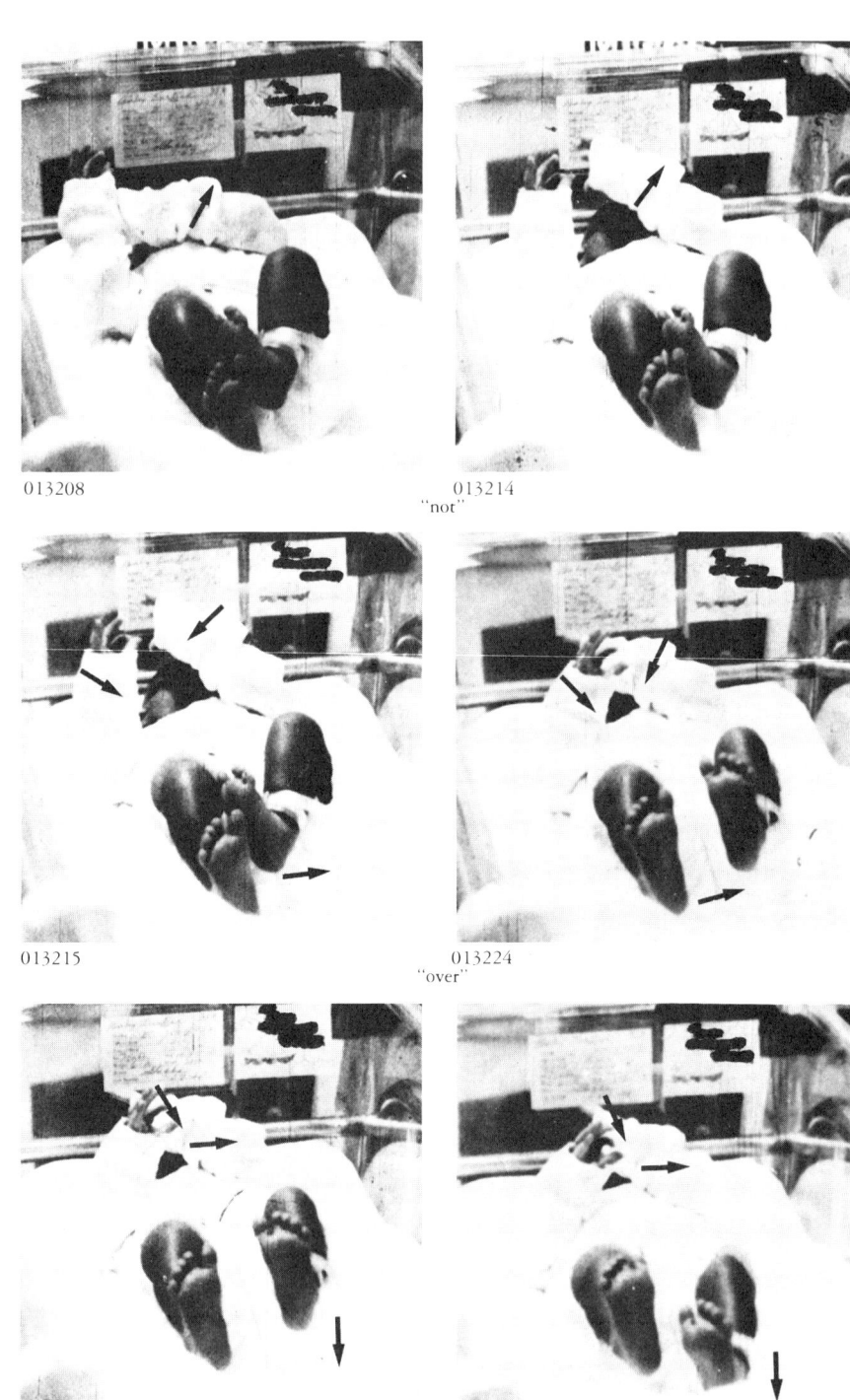

013208

013214
"not"

013215

013224
"over"

013225

013239
"there"

The most powerful relation is the simultaneous one. This simultaneity reflects the synchronous coordination of changes in direction of movement by the adult-infant dyad. . . . The same processes that produce interactional synchrony may be influencing the simultaneous regulation of the facial behavior we observed. In utero, the fetus has considerable experience with adult (mother's) rhythms of movement and with the relation between adult speech and movement. This experience may provide the base for the high degree of movement coordination required in both interactional synchrony and the simultaneous changes in facial behavior reported here.

In Japan, Kato et al. [20] have conducted the most intensive replication study thus far of infant entrainment to adult speech. They studied 32 full-term healthy infants. Each child's mother, a pediatrician, and a nurse were asked to talk to the infants, following a careful paradigm. The infants were videotaped and the results analyzed through linkage of a television with a computer. The neonates were found to synchronize with adult speech but not with white noise, tapping sounds, and nonpatterned sounds. The authors state,

Our work showed that the discrimination of voice was established within only the first week and that a neonate can correlate his movement with the voice not only from his mother but also from a doctor and nurse, who had been taking care of the neonates. . . . Our results suggest not only that the organization of the neonate's motor behavior reacts to and is synchronized with the organized speech behavior of adults in his environment, but that the neonate's movements influenced adult speech.

In a recent study of entrainment, Szajnberg and Hurt [30] state, "These data suggest that infant's movements show both quantitative (total movements/second) and qualitative (growing and unipolar movements/second) changes in response to mother's speech." Kendon [21] has studied human interaction intensively at the frame-by-frame level and states, "The phenomenon of synchrony has, in my view, been clearly demonstrated." Beebe, Stern, and Jaffe [4] have found that mothers and infants can follow the movements of each other at a mean rate of four film frames (100 msec). In some instances, this can occur as rapidly as one film frame. This seems to be visually mediated. Human infants seem to be able to entrain to different languages. For example, a 2-day-old American infant was able to entrain to Chinese speech [10].

Fig. 8-6. Pictures of infant's movements during the words *not over there*, taken from 16-mm sound film. Only the beginning and end pictures of each of the three body-motion process units are given because of space limitations. For example, frame number 013208 shows the body just as the movement sequence begins. Frame number 013214 shows the body at the end of the first sequence. The deleted pictures would show the smooth progression of movement between the first and last picture.

The preponderance of recent studies strongly supports the hypothesis of interactional entrainment. It appears that this hypothesis is going to be confirmed and will have to be evaluated for its implications for neurological speculation. The precision and speed with which the body motion organization of the listening organism follows or tracks the structure of incoming speech really needs to be seen on film to be fully appreciated. It can be considered to be a sort of involuntary, *organized* motor reflex to sound stimuli, especially to speech in humans. It has been observed in rhesus monkeys and may exist in all hearing creatures. Entrainment may have species-specific characteristics such that each species will entrain more readily to his own species' vocal patterns. The listening organism clearly reflects the minute patterns of change of the incoming signal in its own patterns of movement. There is some evidence that this may also be visually mediated. Indeed, it may be true to some degree for all sensory processes. Such a fundamental, entrained, organized response on the part of the motor system probably reflects aspects of the sensorimotor organization of the brain.

Sound-Film Microanalysis of Behavioral Disorders—Asynchrony

The existence of a basic auditory-motor reflex system that precisely, rapidly, and organizationally mirrors the structure of both spoken and heard speech would suggest that this system might become disordered or reflect disorder elsewhere. This appears to be the case. There are characteristic forms of organization in the disorganization. The disorganization itself is ordered. A major feature is an ordered desynchronization of both normal speaking and listening, auditory-motor synchrony. This is manifested as a sound-induced, asynchronous *multiple entrainment*. We have found that behavioral organization reflects brain organization, and disorders of brain organization appear in behavioral organization in subtle ways. This phenomenon can only be seen through frame-by-frame study of films. Analysis of behavior *as* organization provides a basis for correlating behavior and the brain. The intensive analysis and description of the microorganization of normal speaking and listening behavior also provide an essential framework for the comparative analysis of the organization of pathological behavior. Pathological, asynchronous multiple entrainment to sound was initially postulated as a result of the observation of "jumps" and "jerks" in the bodies of dysfunctional children following sound input. Normal speaker self-synchrony and listener entrainment appear to be functions of the same organizational processes. As there is normal synchrony, so there are forms of disorder of this synchrony. Asynchronous, multiple entrainment is postulated to be a major feature accompanying a variety of disorders. It is possible that the term *multiple entrainment* can be applied to both the speaking and listening behavior of the individual. When a dysfunctional person speaks, his body is out of phase with his own voice, in the same way it is when he is listening. Such multiple entrainment indirectly supports the hypothesis of entrainment.

An actual example of multiple entrainment will serve as an illustration. We analyzed one film in which a 4-year-old autistic girl is playing with blocks at a table with her mother. She sits back in her chair, remaining relatively still. Her mother drops a block on the table, which makes a loud sound. The child responds only minimally to this sound at the time it actually occurs, but approximately 1 second (23 frames) after the sound occurs, she jerks her head sharply as if slapped. No other sounds or events have occurred that might account for this sudden strange movement. It is certainly conceivable that she just randomly happens to move at this time. It was possible, however, to go through the film and locate the precise onset of many such sounds in relation to frame numbers. If there were a systematic relationship between the child's seemingly bizarre movements and the sounds that occurred earlier, then one should be able to predict, for this particular child, a marked movement organization change, a *process-unit boundary*, exactly 23 frames after the frame number of onset for most of the sounds occurring around her. This hypothesis proved to be true, thus enabling the investigator to count out to the twenty-third frame after the onset point of a given sound and find that the child jerked or moved at precisely that frame. Continued intensive analysis revealed that this child also exhibited not just one, but several systematic delayed entrainments, reinforcing the hypothesis of multiple entrainment to sound. Intensive analysis of the other frames after sound onset did not reveal this entrainment. There were few process-unit boundaries occurring at these other frames.

Studies of the Relationship Between Multiple Entrainment and Sound

A study [7] was conducted comparing the post–sound-stimulus behavior of six autistic children with that of six normal subjects, controlled for age and sex, by two independent judges. The subjects ranged in age from 5 to 14 years old. All subjects were presented with the same tape recording of random sounds while being sound-filmed. The sounds consisted of taps interspersed with short vowel-like sounds. It was determined at which frame numbers after each sound onset process-unit boundaries occurred. These were then summed across all sound onsets and a percentage obtained for each subject for each frame following sound onsets. The hypothesis examined was that, following sound stimuli, the autistic children would exhibit peaks or sums of process-unit boundaries that were significantly larger than those of the normal controls. This proved to be the case. Table 8-1 compares the post–sound-stimulus behavior of the autistic children with that of the normal controls.

The sum of process-unit boundaries occurring on the first frame following all sound onsets for each child was adopted as the measure of comparison for the sums of process units occurring for all onsets in the following frames 2 to 10 for that child. In essence, all autistic children had some later peaks (sums) of process-unit boundaries that exceeded the amount at their first frame, and all of the normals had peaks less than the amount at their first frame. This supported the hypothesis of marked points of delayed entrainment for

Table 8-1. Six autistic children compared by two independent judges to six normal controls for process-unit boundaries following sound onsets[a]

Judge	Subject Pairs	Autistic (X)	Normal (Y)	$X - Y$[b]
I	1	0	−1	−1
	2	+3	−8	−11
	3	+3	0	−3
	4	+1	−2	−3
	5	+8	−3	−11
	6	−3	−6	−3
II	1	+2	−8	−10
	2	+6	−17	−23
	3	0	−7	−7
	4	+7	−5	−12
	5	+14	−3	−17
	6	0	−17	−17

$p < .05$ by Signs test.
[a] Values represent a judged comparison between the sum of process units occurring in the largest peak for each subject subsequent to the first film frame after sound onset with the sum of process units occurring on the first frame.
[b] Difference between values for normal and autistic children. Normal children were found to have consistently lower values than autistic children.

the autistic group. Table 8-1 shows the difference between the largest later peak in frames 2 to 10 of the autistic subject compared to the largest later peak in frames 2 to 10 for the normal control subject. The normals' later peaks were always less than those of the autistics for both judges.

Dyslexic and autistic children continued to be sound-filmed and studied in the same intensive microanalytical way normal behavior had been studied. Marked differences were observed, and a basic pattern was detected. These children were both self-asynchronous and interactionally asynchronous. It was observed that their eyes might not track precisely together, one eyelid might be slightly out of phase with the other during an eye blink, or one side of the body might move before the other. As previously stated, in normal behavior, the total organism moves in bilateral synchrony with the incoming speech structure within 42 msec. The continued analysis of dyslexia, autism, and several other disorders led to the general hypothesis of an abnormal multiple entrainment to sound that has a characteristic pattern. A more specific hypothesis is that this pattern is bilaterally asynchronous. The left side tends to be delayed behind the right side in dyslexia, and the right side tends to be delayed behind the left in autism. There appear to be four multiple entrainments in the body within the first second following sounds in dyslexia, autism, and the other disorders. This occurs in relation to almost all the sounds and speech around them, including their own voice.

The following case illustrates the findings about sound-induced motor asynchrony in dyslexia. The subject was a 9-year-old boy. The family history indicated previous cases of dyslexia. A 10-minute, 30-fps sound film was made while he sat in a chair. He was able to move naturally. A recording of randomly spaced, short vowel-like sounds and tapping sounds was played. His teacher was with him, and they also talked together. Part of the film included a close-up of his face while he was talking and reading aloud. The dyslexic boy manifested an entrainment on the right side within 42 msec (by 1 film frame) following sound onset, which is when one should occur, but his entrainments were excessive. He oriented normally at 10 frames (333 msec) following the onset of the sound of his name when called. However, his left side entrained with the same sound, including speech, after a delay of 7 film frames (233 msec). The entrainment gave the appearance of flowing from the right side to the left side. Some aspect of the right side would move in response to sound and then, after a delay of 233 msec, the left side would move. The movements did not occur in the same body part(s). At one time the arm moved, at another time the head moved, or the eyes blinked. Several body parts often moved together. The boy also had jerks in his body at 10 film frames and 17 film frames. These were the four multiple entrainments per 1 second mentioned previously. We observed that the multiple entrainment pattern is the same for different dyslexic subjects, but the latency intervals may vary, that is, one child may have a pattern of 1, 4, 10, and 14 intervals, while another may have a pattern of 1, 6, 10, and 16. This characteristic pattern has also been observed in subjects with autism, Huntington's disease, Parkinson's disease, cerebral palsy, schizophrenia, and stuttering.

Entrainment 1 occurs within the first frame following sound onset. Entrainment 2 ranges between 3 frames (100 msec) and 8 frames (266 msec) following sound onset and is stable for a given child. Entrainment 3 tends to occur at 10 frames (333 msec) following sound onset. Entrainment 4 follows Entrainment 2 by 10 film frames. Speculatively, it appears as if there is a normal, bilaterally synchronized, 333-msec auditory input cycle. The precise *a*synchronous 333-msec pattern suggests this. When a normal person is called by name, the body begins to entrain to the sound within 42 msec, and then at about 10 film frames from the time of *onset* of the name, he or she will begin to turn toward the caller. In multiple entrainment, it looks as if this 333-msec cycle is out of phase, resulting in abnormal, multiple body motion entrainment at the out-of-phase points.

Figure 8-7 illustrates this hypothesized normal 333-msec cycle with the out-of-phase multiple entrainment pattern of the dyslexic boy shown in Figure 8-8. He exhibits marked peaks of process-unit boundaries at frames 1, 7, 10, and 17 following 47 sound onsets. At Entrainment 1, right-side movements predominate, and at Entrainment 2, left-side movements predominate. The sound on a copy of this subject's film was delayed for 7 frames, and in this altered film, the body parts on the left side of his body can be seen to move in precise synchrony with most of the sounds around him, including his own voice.

Table 8-2 shows the results of a study of six dyslexic children and six autistic children, controlled for age and sex. All 12 subjects exhibited the characteristic multiple entrainment pattern. Dyslexic child number 3 in the table is the boy described above. The left side of his face often pulls markedly

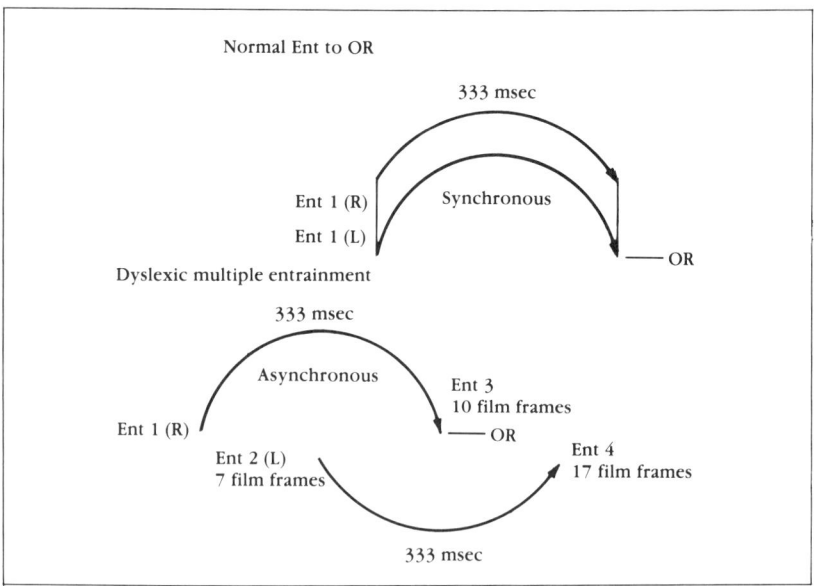

Fig. 8-7. Drawing of a suspected bilateral, 333-msec input cycle. The normal synchronized cycle is depicted at the top, and an out-of-phase cycle, postulated in a variety of disorders, is below. (*Ent L* = left-side entrainment; *Ent R* = right-side entrainment; *OR* = orienting response to the sound stimulus.)

Fig. 8-8. Close-up picture taken from 16-mm film showing delayed entrainment in a dyslexic boy to a marked sound change point (from /f/ to /l/ in the word *flying*, which he uttered 233 msec earlier). The left side of the face pulls up. The terminal frame of that movement is shown.

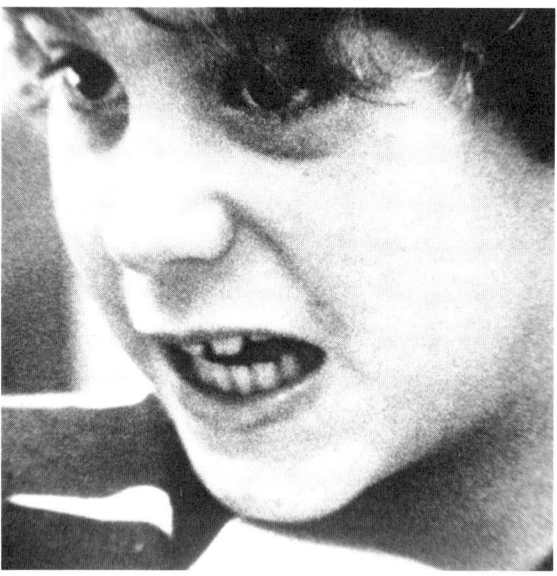

to the left at seven frames following louder units in his speech, particularly vowel onset points. Figure 8-8 shows his face pulled to the left seven frames following the initial voiced /l/ of the word *flying*. The left side of his body often moves in precise synchrony with speech that occurred seven frames earlier.

Plooij [28] in Amsterdam conducted a preliminary replication study of entrainment and multiple entrainment using two television cameras at different angles. Around the lenses of the cameras a ring of light sources emitted infrared light. Conically shaped reflectors were placed on the subject's body, reflecting the light straight back to the cameras. These reflectors appear as small, bright light-circles on the television monitor. The moving information from the two cameras on the television monitor was fed into a PDP-11/25 computer. Several years of prior work had been done to ensure the reliability of this process. Plooij studied an 11-year-old dyslexic child and a normal control in response to 58 sounds (the same sounds I used). At frame 1 following sound onset, in both the dyslexic and the normal child, there was a sharp increase or decrease of movement, which supports the hypothesis of normal entrainment within 42 msec. However, the graphs of the dyslexic were quite different from those of the normal control. There were several peaks centered around frames 1, 4, 9 to 10, and 14 to 15. Plooij states, "This is reminiscent of Condon's multiple entrainment." That a computer could pick up an almost identical delayed pattern as that predicted is most promising. Plooij is presently studying more subjects.

Oxman et al. [26] in Canada tried to replicate multiple entrainment in autistic children. They used only five sound stimuli and did not use process-unit boundaries as the criteria for co-occurring body motion changes. They did not observe multiple entrainment. They did, however, detect marked awkward movements in the behavior of the autistic subjects.

There appears to be two broad categories of autism: (1) the high-functioning autistic children, with speech and (2) the more severely autistic children, who tend to lack speech or who have very little speech. The high-functioning children are self-asynchronous and exhibit a clear multiple entrainment. One high-functioning man said that he heard sounds echo until he was 24 years old and that these echoes recurred at times in later years. Another had the following comment when asked how sounds were for him: "Like . . . sounds like . . . maybe the echoes for example. Like you repeat the same things over and over . . . six or eight times."

Severely autistic persons often seem withdrawn from the world. Sound-film microanalysis indicates that they exhibit a marked multiple entrainment *and* a multiple orienting response. They look around many times to the same sound as if it were repeating and coming from several different directions. They do not seem able to shut this off. It occurs even in relation to the sound of their own voice. We think the child is out of contact because he is not responding to *our* world. In fact, the child is not strange but may have a distorted world with which he is trying to cope.

The multiple orienting response appears to have some relationship to the multiple entrainment. Since the multiple orienting response tends to occur late, usually over a second later and may repeat two or three times, no one

Table 8-2. Percent of process-unit boundaries and their locations for 19 frames following sound onsets for six dyslexics, six autistics, and a Huntington's disease patient and for 11 frames following sound onset for six normals

Subject, Age (years)	Frame Number																			
	1	2	3	4	5	6	7	8	9	10	11	12	13	14	15	16	17	18	19
Dyslexic																			
1. Boy, 6	88	4	8	0	92	8	4	13	8	96	8	17	25	0	92	13	13	17	13
2. Boy, 8	96	0	25	21	92	0	38	33	8	92	0	29	17	17	92	4	17	21	21
3. Boy, 9	83	2	14	11	28	9	75	2	9	43	6	17	23	17	19	9	68	6	6
4. Boy, 10	93	0	7	7	86	3	17	17	30	63	13	10	27	10	56	0	13	17	23
5. Boy, 12	90	10	13	27	17	77	3	40	20	80	10	20	27	20	10	80	17	13	13
6. Girl, 12	92	8	88	4	20	32	29	20	8	65	8	4	84	4	8	25	25	20	20
Autistic																			
7. Boy, 6	78	12	6	84	4	10	18	20	14	36	20	12	4	62	4	8	12	12	12
8. Boy, 7	98	18	38	38	45	30	35	95	15	73	18	38	35	35	30	33	18	88	5
9. Boy, 7	83	10	13	15	75	10	17	31	13	71	8	17	37	21	69	2	13	19	23
10. Boy, 11	88	17	29	17	100	8	20	42	17	88	0	32	20	29	83	17	32	25	20
11. Boy, 12	100	0	8	32	24	4	84	20	4	88	8	12	36	12	36	4	80	8	8
12. Girl, 12	96	13	20	32	25	100	13	25	20	96	13	16	32	44	20	96	0	20	16

Normal

13. Boy[b]	75	12	21	42	40	20	45	21	40	35	25	
14. Boy	75	20	35	25	27	20	25	30	23	20	15	
15. Boy	75	20	35	30	30	50	30	32	35	30	25	
16. Boy	72	20	30	35	20	30	45	20	22	35	35	
17. Boy	65	27	27	35	32	35	55	22	25	35	32	
18. Boy	70	15	20	15	17	20	17	20	20	17	25	

Huntington's disease

19. Man, 40	88	0	25	22	93	9	28	28	9	88	6	19	38	9	88	9	10	25	15

[a] Some numbers are boxed to emphasize the high percentage of process-unit boundaries occurring at these particular frames following sound onsets for the subjects. The boxed numbers for the dyslexic, autistic, and Huntington's disease subjects follow the hypothesized pattern. For example, dyslexic boy 1 has marked peaks of process-unit boundaries at frames 1, 5, 10, and 15.

[b] The ages of the six normal boys, from another study, are approximately the same as those of the dyslexic and autistic subjects.

seems to have been aware of it. The multiple orienting response may be enslaved in some way to the multiple entrainment. The child does not seem to have any choice. He orients this way and that, two or three times, to almost every sound around him and seldom in the actual direction of the sound's source. A study was conducted [8] comparing the orienting responses of 8 autistic children with 8 normal children, controlled for age and sex. Each subject was filmed and presented with 26 tape-recorded, random sounds. All eye movements for all 16 subjects were noted for 30 frames following each of the 26 sounds by two independent judges. There was high reliability between the independent judges in detecting eye movements. The autistic children exhibited a significantly greater number of orienting responses ($p < .001$, Wilcoxon Rank Sum Test—two-tailed test). Table 8-3 presents the results.

The orienting responses (ORs) of seven autistic children were compared following sound onsets with silent epochs [8]. There were significantly more orienting responses following sound onsets, indicating that the multiple orienting response was related to sound onset. One minute (1,800 frames) was randomly selected from a sound film of an autistic boy and compared for orienting responses with a comparable minute from a normal control. There were 55 sounds for each subject in that minute. The autistic child exhibited 120 orienting responses (eye movements) during that minute, and the control exhibited 23. There does not seem to be any habituation in either multiple entrainment or multiple orienting response.

Figure 8-9 shows a histogram of the orienting responses following 87 sounds in a 15-year-old autistic girl. Her left side tended to move in synchrony with sound at the first frame (42 msec). There was a delayed response on her right side at 7 frames. The histogram begins with frame 7; there were no marked peaks of orienting response prior to this frame. The subject exhibited pronounced peaks of orienting at frames 27 and 47 following sound onsets. Each

Table 8-3. Comparison of eight autistic children with eight normal controls on the number of orienting responses (ORs) following 26 random sound onsets

Autistic subjects	Number of ORs	Rank*	Normal subjects	Number of ORs	Rank*
1	49	16	1	28	7
2	38	13	2	7	1
3	31	10	3	12	5.5
4	42	15	4	12	5.5
5	29	8	5	10	2
6	31	10	6	11	3.5
7	39	14	7	11	3.5
8	34	12	8	31	10
	Σ of Ranks = 98			Σ of Ranks = 38	

$p < .001$ (Wilcoxon Rank Sum Test—two-tailed). If the data were analyzed pairwise, the difference between autistic and normal subjects would still be highly significant.
* Rank: lowest number of responses yields rank of 1.

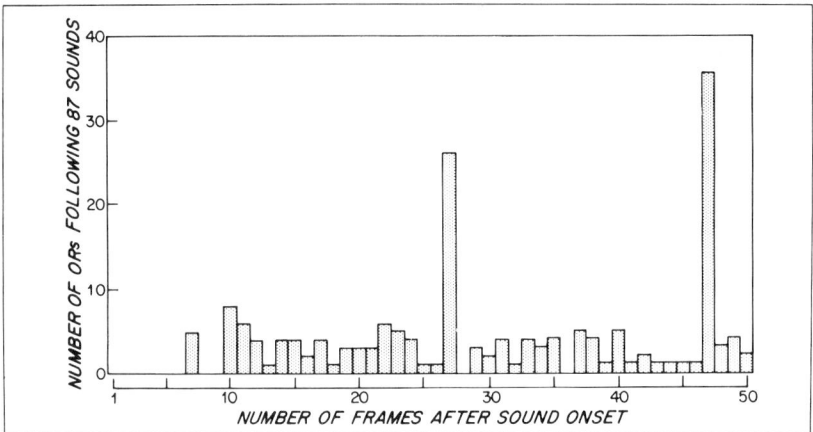

Fig. 8-9. Histogram of the number of orienting responses for 50 frames following each of 87 random sounds in a 15-year-old autistic girl. For example, there are 36 orienting responses at frame 47 following sound onsets.

of the 50 frames following each of the 87 sounds was examined for the occurrence of orienting responses. It is clear that there was a massing of orienting responses at frames 27 and 47. The very surprising thing is the precision. Figure 8-10 illustrates the delayed orienting at 47 frames (over 1.5 seconds after sound onset) with pictures taken from the subject's 16-mm film. In Figure 8-10A the subject is sitting quietly with her right hand up to her mouth and looking forward. A tap sound had occurred 46 frames earlier. This picture is from frame 46 following the onset of the tap sound. Beginning on frame 47, as if responding to the tap sound, she begins to orient up and to her left. Figure 8-10B shows the terminal position of that orienting response. The great majority of her orienting responses at the 47-frame delay point are toward the left.

In Figure 8-10C she is again sitting quietly with her head bent down looking into her hand. This is frame 46 following the onset of another tap sound. At frame 47 after the sound, her arm begins to go down to her lap and she orients up and to the left. Figure 8-10D shows the terminal position of the orienting response. This suggests that entrainment may also be involved, leading to the speculation that the delayed orienting responses may be enslaved to the multiple entrainment.

Figure 8-10E shows the girl looking forward toward the teacher at frame 46 following the onset of a short vowel sound uttered by the teacher. On frame 47 she begins an orienting response to the left and down. The termination of the orienting response is seen in Figure 8-10F. She looks away from the person making the sound. This may be part of the reason these persons are said to be withdrawn.

The soundtrack on a copy of her film was delayed 47 frames. One can go through this film and show her almost constantly orienting this way and that in precise entrainment with the systematically delayed sounds. The 36 orienting responses at frame 47 following the 87 sounds seen in Figure 8-9 are

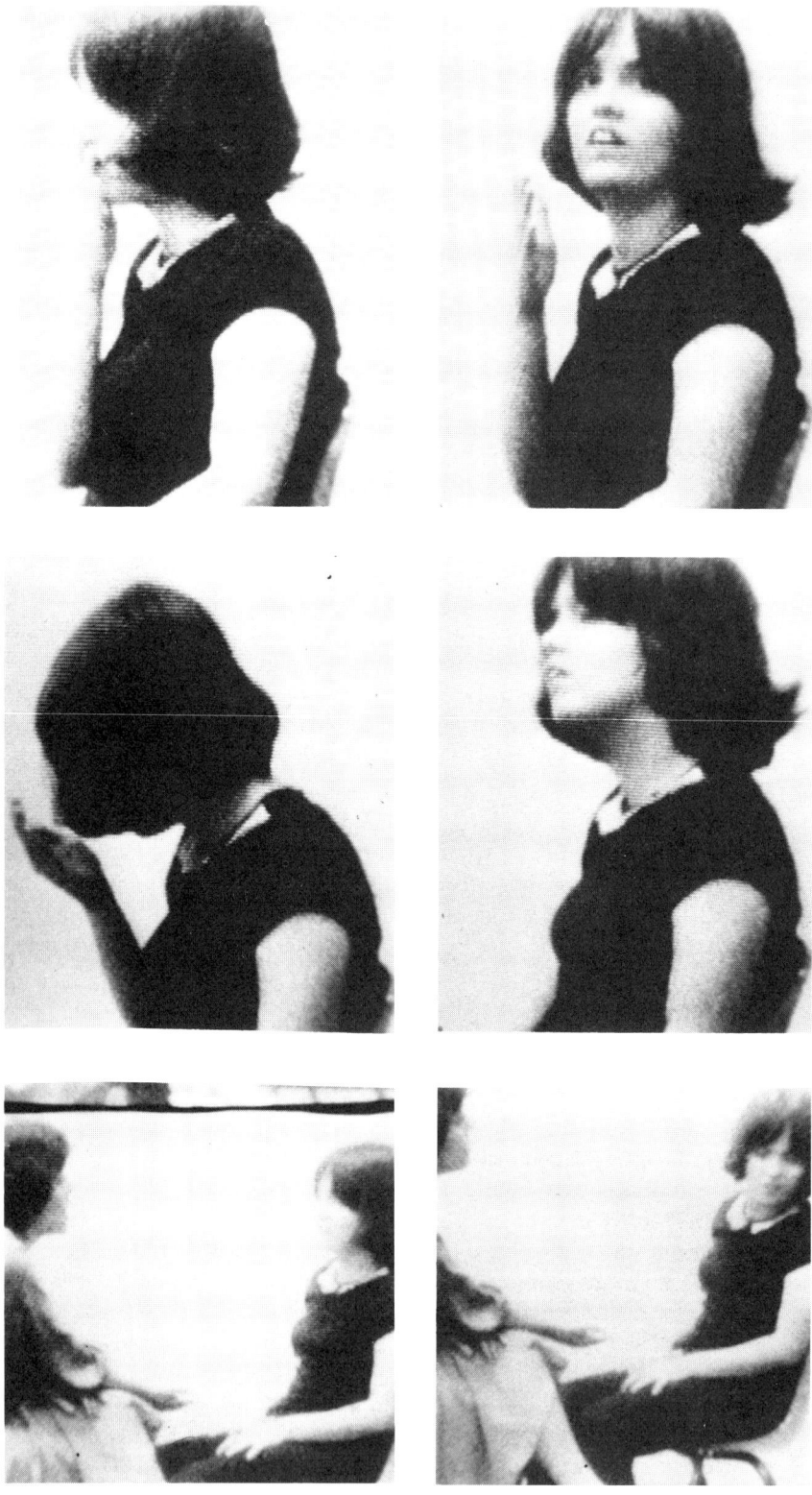

similar to those illustrated above. The occurrence of the orienting responses precisely at frame 47 implies a disturbed processing factor that is constant.

Sound-related self-asynchrony and multiple entrainment have been observed at the microlevel in a variety of other disorders, including schizophrenia, cerebral palsy, Huntington's disease, Parkinson's disease, hyperactivity, and stuttering. For example, two Huntington's disease patients were sound-film microanalyzed. The following points summarize the salient observations of the analysis.

1. Both patients exhibited a marked facial asymmetry, with the left side of the face pulled upward in contrast to the right. This was there most of the time.
2. Both patients manifested a multiple, asynchronous, sound-induced entrainment with a tendency for the delay to be on the right side. This would be compatible with facial asymmetry. The multiple entrainment resembles that seen in autistic subjects. However, the Huntington's disease patients can converse coherently. The latency of the delayed entrainment on the right is approximately the same in both patients at 167 msec.
3. The patients exhibited the characteristic four multiple entrainments within the first $2/3$ second, having the same 10-frame (333 msec) sequencing as the six dyslexic and six autistic subjects shown in Table 8-2.

Both patients manifested a noticeable amount of dysarthria. The multiple entrainment pattern in Huntington's disease is distinctly different from that of the other disorders and may be characteristic of Huntington's disease. The percentages of process-unit boundaries for one of the Huntington's disease subjects is provided in Table 8-2.

Brain Asymmetry and Sound-Induced Behavioral Asynchrony

Many students suggest that asymmetry is a concomitant feature of various forms of brain impairment. John [19] indicates that "most neurological diseases involve a unilateral disruption of the structure and/or function of the brain and might be expected to cause a concomitant decrease in electrical symmetry." After discussing many studies relating to aging, vascular accidents, and head traumas, John further states, "The reader may have noticed that amplitude decreases, frequency slowing, and asymmetry were abnormal signs found in a variety of different disorders." These appear to be analogous to the patterns observed in the overt behavior of many different disorders, suggesting that behavioral organization reflects brain organization in both normal *and* pathological conditions.

Fig. 8-10. Three of the orienting responses (taken from 16-mm film) beginning precisely 47 frames after sound onset and not in the direction of the actual sound are presented to illustrate multiple orienting response. These are characteristic of this 15-year-old autistic girl.

Duffy and associates [12], using brain electrical activity mapping (BEAM), studied the brain flow process in normal and dysfunctional subjects. He states, "Waveform components appearing at differing latencies at different scalp sites may, in fact, represent the same wave front slowly progressing across the scalp surface." Normal wave fronts were found to flow synchronously, and abnormal wave fronts were observed to flow asymmetrically. His analysis of tumor patients revealed an abnormal brain wave flow or processing pattern that bears a striking resemblance to the multiple entrainment pattern revealed by sound-film microanalysis. This suggests that as the synchronous order of normal behavior reflects normal symmetrical brain wave processing so asymmetrical brain wave processing may be reflected in asynchronous behavior. Duffy and colleagues [13] also observed increased slow activity and decreased fast activity overlaying tumor sites. A similar observation was made by Ahn and associates [1], who noted that the excess slow waves (delta and theta) in the parieto-occipital regions were much more frequent than any other frequency or regional abnormality in neurological subjects, learning-disabled children with generalized learning disabilities, and specific learning-disabled children. Duffy's group [13] also found differences in the left posterior quadrant between dyslexics and normals but observed the greatest difference anteriorly in the supplemental motor area bilaterally. Multiple entrainment may be related to such brain processing asymmetries, and it may occur in a variety of disorders. Duffy and colleagues [13] report on asynchronous repeating innervation: "Thus the process of first appearance in the right occipital region, spread forward on the right only, and late activation of the left occipital region from the right was repeated twice."

The various examples provided indicate that sound-film microanalysis reveals an asynchronous flow of innervation in overt behavior that appears to have a specific pattern in several disorders. Five stutterers were examined using sound-film microanalysis. All exhibited the multiple entrainment pattern like that shown in Table 8-2. The pattern was similar to that of dyslexics.

Mirsky and associates [25] studied the effects of total or partial asphyxia on auditory evoked potentials in rhesus monkeys. They indicated that many asphyxiates showed deviant latencies and grossly asynchronous responses from the two sides of the head. I filmed one of these monkeys (TZ) through the courtesy of Mirsky and observed a clear multiple entrainment and multiple orienting response. Gottschaldt and Vahle-Hinz [17] used an electron microscope and electrophysiology to investigate Merkel's cell mechanoreception. They found that these cells respond with very precise phase-locking to high-frequency vibratory stimuli. Diamond [11] reports that responses of the eye to flickering light is very precise. If every other flash in the flicker is displaced by as little as 30 μ, an associated and synchronized asymmetry appears in the brain's alternating voltage. Thompson and Masterson [31] studied the brainstem auditory pathways involved in reflexive head orientation to sound in the cat. Normal cats turn quickly toward a sound source, with a latency of 20 to 80 msec. They found that a subcortical unilateral lesion at various levels could affect the latency of the response contralaterally (out of phase), the appropriateness of the initial movement (in the wrong direction), and the accuracy of head orientation. Skoff [29] reports finding weak, delayed, and absent left brainstem auditory evoked potentials (BSAEP) in a series of autistic subjects. Arick [2] reports that six autistic subjects showed significantly longer latency in wave IV from the left ear. He suspects the presence of dysfunction in the brainstem of these children.

Efron [14] speaks of the possibility of a double input due to "timing asynchrony," especially with patients with lesions in the dominant hemisphere. Under normal conditions, the two hemispheres receive information at almost the same time. He feels that if the transmission from one hemisphere to the other is delayed by several hundred milliseconds, the person might infer that two different events had occurred. He suggests this may be part of the defect in aphasia, and I suspect it may be occurring in autism. Efron believes that the area of temporal discrimination lies in the temporal lobe and extends back to the angular gyrus.

Out-of-phase processing could result in perceptual difficulties, including distorted perception. The observations emerging from sound-film microanalysis suggest that such out-of-phase behavior, seen in self-asynchrony and multiple entrainment, is characteristic of several disorders. As a further example, a Parkinson's disease patient was sound-filmed at 30 fps, and his behavior in response to random sound stimuli was microanalyzed. At the time of filming, he was overmedicated with Sinemet, making him overactive. In this overmedicated condition, he manifested a multiple entrainment pattern very similar to that of a dyslexic subject. He had a very precise entrainment on the right at 42 msec, but a delayed entrainment on the left at seven frames. There was a marked pull to the right in his face at sound onset. Figure 8-11 shows this asynchrony.

As indicated, eye blinks tend to occur at prominent articulatory change points in normal speech behavior, especially at phone boundaries. In one of the Huntington's disease patients mentioned previously, the eye blinks tended to occur at Entrainment 1 and also at Entrainment 2. It was as if the blinks occurred where they should in relation to speech at Entrainment 1 but also

Fig. 8-11. Close-up of the face of Parkinson's disease patient taken from 16-mm film. He is overmedicated with Sinemet. His face pulls markedly to the right at the onset of sound. This response is very similar to that of stutterers and some dyslexics.

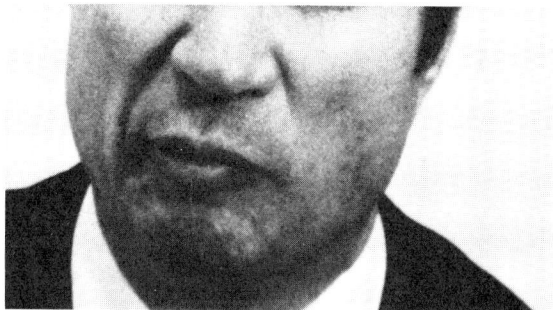

recurred in relation to speech at Entrainment 2 as if speech were also recurring, even though not heard by the subject. The sound track of the film was delayed to coincide with the Entrainment-2 point, and many of the eye blinks could be shown to be occurring in precise synchrony with speech units at that point.

Conclusions

The preceding observations on the organization of normal and disordered human speaker and listener behavior at the microlevel must be considered as tentative at the present time. Sound-film microanalysis is a recently emerging discipline, and only a few investigators are working at this level. Much further work needs to be done.

Sound-film microanalysis has revealed behavior to be fundamentally organized across many levels. As a result of repeated, intensive analyses, structures of organization "hidden" in the rapid, ongoing flow of behavior became a central focus. The "units" of behavior were seen to be forms of organization. This emerged through the analysis of how the parts of the body changed movement, sustained movement, and ceased movement in complex relationships with each other *and* with the units of speech. The body was discovered to move in terms of microforms of organization, which were called process units. The most minimal units of detectable body motion using frame-by-frame film analysis were *already* forms of organization and were not parts which were put together to form organization. Continued analysis indicated that the structures of the organization of speech and body motion were precisely synchronized across several levels at the same time. This was called self-synchrony and has been observed for many different cultures around the world. Animals also move in this self-synchronous manner. This pervasive self-synchrony implied integrated, multilevel neurological processes synchronizing speech and body motion across these multiple levels. Speech/body motions seem to be the unitary behavior of the organism. Speech/body motion behavior also exhibited characteristic periodicities across these several levels, leading to behavior being interpreted as wavelike. Thus, when a person speaks, his words and gestures can be considered as forms of behavioral waves integrated across several levels at the same time. The periodicities of these behavioral waves are similar to the delta, theta, alpha, and beta waves of the brain.

The body of the normal listener was discovered to move in precise synchrony with the articulatory units of the speaker's speech. A short-latency, synchronous entrainment to sound has been hypothesized to be a basic response characteristic of normal listening behavior. This normal entrainment was found to be disturbed in various disorders; including dyslexia, autism, hyperactivity, cerebral palsy, schizophrenia, Huntington's disease, Parkinson's disease, and stuttering. There is an *a*synchronous, or out-of-phase, entrainment to sound, which has a similar pattern in the various disorders.

The *and* in "behavior *and* the brain" does not signify a separation between two disconnected entities. Brain and behavior are profoundly unified organizationally so that the distinction of "inside of" and "outside of" the skull does not create a severance of their operational unity. That which they have in common is participation in shared order. Behavior is what the body does as a consequence of the kind of organization of its nervous system. Sound-film microanalysis reveals linkages of order between clinical behavior, as studied by Geschwind, Denckla, and Rudel, and brain electrical activity, as studied by Duffy and John.

References

1. Ahn, H., et al. Developmental equations reflect brain dysfunctions. *Science* 210:1259, 1980.
2. Arick, J. Auditory brainstem evoked response: Comparative analysis of autistic, mentally retarded and normal children and normal toddlers. Paper presented at NSAC Annual Meeting, Salt Lake City, Utah, July, 1983.
3. Austin, A. M., and Peery, J. C. Analysis of adult-neonate synchrony during speech and nonspeech. *Percept. Mot. Skills* 57:455, 1983.
4. Beebe, B., Stern, D., and Jaffe, J. The Kinesic Rhythm of Mother-Infant Interactions. In A. Siegman and S. Feldstein (Eds.), *Of Speech and Time*. Hillsdale, N.J.: Erlbaum, 1979. Pp. 23–24.
5. Condon, W. S. Synchrony units and the communicational hierarchy. Paper presented at Western Psychiatric Institute & Clinics, Pittsburgh, Penn. March, 1963.
6. Condon, W. S. Speech and Body Motion Synchrony of the Speaker-Hearer. In D. L. Horton and J. J. Jenkins (Eds.), *Perception of Language*. Columbus, Ohio: Merrill, 1971. Pp. 150–173.
7. Condon, W. S. Multiple response to sound in autistic-like children. *Proceedings of the National Society for Autistic Children Conference*, Washington, D.C., June, 1974.
8. Condon, W. S. Asynchrony and communication disorders. *Proceedings of Autism Research Symposium*, 2nd Annual Conference Canadian Society for Autistic Children, Vancouver, 1978.
9. Condon, W. S. Cultural Microrhythms. In M. Davis (Ed.), *Interaction Rhythms*. New York: Human Sciences, 1982.
10. Condon, W.S., and Sander, L. W. Neonate movement is synchronized with adult speech: Interactional participation and language acquisition. *Science* 183:99, 1974.
11. Diamond, A. Microsecond sensitivity of the human visual system to irregular flicker. *Science* 206 (4419):708, 1979.
12. Duffy, F., et al. Brain electrical activity mapping (BEAM): A method for extending the clinical utility of EEG and evoked potential data. *Ann. Neurol.* 5(4):309, 1979.
13. Duffy, F., et al. Dyslexia: Regional differences in brain electrical activity by topographic mapping. *Ann. Neurol.* 7(5):412, 1980.
14. Efron, R. Temporal perception, aphasia, and déjà vu. *Brain* 86:403-424, 1963.
15. Francis, N.W. *The Structure of American English*. New York: Ronald, 1958.
16. Gatewood, J., and Rosenwein, R. Interactional synchrony: Genuine or spurious? A critique of recent research. *J. Nonverbal Behav.* 6(1):12, 1981.

17. Gottschaldt, K., and Vahle-Hinz, C. Merkel cell receptors: Structure and transducer function. *Science* 214(4517):183, 1981.
18. Grobecker, D. B., and Pietsch, T. W. High-speed cinematographic evidence for ultrafast feeding in Antennariid Anglerfishes. *Science* 205(14):1161, 1979.
19. John, E. R. *Neurometrics: Clinical Applications of Quantitative Electrophysiology.* New York: Wiley, 1977.
20. Kato, T., et al. A computer analysis of infant movements synchronized with adult speech. *Pediatr. Res.* 17:625, 1983.
21. Kendon, A. Coordination of Action and Framing in Face-to-Face Interaction. In M. Davis (Ed.), *Interaction Rhythms*. New York: Human Services, 1982.
22. Matekundt and Groff, The men behind the work. A General Motors advertisement in *Science News* Vol. 118, No. 23, 1980.
23. McDowall, J. Interactional synchrony: A reappraisal. *J. Pers. Soc. Psychol.* 36(9):963, 1978.
24. Miller, J. A. Cell-e-vision. *Science News* 119:234, 1981.
25. Mirsky, A., et al. Auditory evoked potentials and auditory behavior following prenatal and perinatal asphyxia in rhesus monkeys. *Dev. Psychol.* 12(4):369, 1979.
26. Oxman, J., et al. Condon's multiple response phenomenon in severely dysfunctional children: An attempt at replication. *Proceedings of Autism Research Symposium*, 2nd Annual Conference, Canadian Society for Autistic Children, Vancouver, 1978.
27. Peery, J. C. Neonate-adult head movement: No and yes revisited. *Dev. Psychol.* 16(4):245, 1980.
28. Plooij, F. The relationship between ethology and paedology. *Neth. J. Zoo.* In press, 1983.
29. Skoff, B. Prolonged brainstem transmission time in autism. *Psychiatry Res.* 2(2):157, 1980.
30. Szajnberg, N., and Hurt, S. Infant cross-modal movement response to maternal speech. Paper presented at American Academy of Child Psychiatry, San Francisco, Calif., Fall 1983.
31. Thompson, G. C., and Masterson, B. Brainstem auditory pathways involved in reflexic head orientation to sound. *J. Neurophysiol.* 41(5):1183, 1978.

9 Neurometric Evaluation of Brain Electrical Activity in Children with Learning Disabilities

E. Roy John, Leslie S. Prichep, Jacob Fridman, Hansook Ahn, Herbert Kaye, and Henry Baird

There are many possible reasons for children's failure to learn basic skills in school. Two groups can be distinguished within the population of children with learning difficulties: *learning-disordered children*, whose problems are primarily due to social, motivational, psychological, or emotional factors, and *learning-disabled children*, whose problems are primarily due to brain dysfunctions. Estimates of the percentage of schoolchildren in the United States whose learning handicaps are due to brain dysfunction range widely, from 3 to 13 percent [4, 14, 25, 28, 35]. Thus, included among the 16 million U.S. children in the lowest quartile of academic performance, there are an uncertain number, between 2 and 8 million, with learning disabilities.

Logically, one of the essential prerequisites for effective individualized remediation for any learning-handicapped child must be the understanding of not only which tasks are difficult for the child to master but also the reasons for such difficulties. A particular behavioral symptom such as reading underachievement may be due to a wide variety of reasons. Treatment of the symptom without knowledge of its cause, by any standardized remedial procedure, must necessarily be ineffectual for a substantial proportion of the heterogeneous population of children who display that symptom. Haphazard, "shotgun" remedial procedures not only are costly and inefficient but also may be counterproductive, leading both the pupil and the teacher (and often the parent) to conclude that failure to learn is somehow the fault of the child rather than of an inappropriately chosen remedial procedure.

We believe that the first step toward helping a child with learning problems is to differentiate between learning disorder and learning disability, as defined above. Psychological and neurological examinations are widely used for this purpose. Psychometric tests evaluate behavioral products that are substantially dependent on skills acquired by prior learning and attempt to infer deficient processes from inadequate products. Aside from these inherent shortcomings, the results of psychometric tests are further questionable because of their cultural biases. Neurological examinations are primarily devised to detect structural lesions or relatively gross sensory or motor impairment. They provide sparse insights into information processing and cognitive functions. Neuropsychological evaluations, while superior in our opinion to conventional psychological and neurological assessments of the child with learning difficulties, are nonetheless limited in their ability to pinpoint deficient processes. A diagnostic method is needed that not only differentiates between learning disorder and disability but can also provide a differential diagnosis among the many types of brain dysfunction that may underlie any particular learning

---

The work reported in this chapter was supported in part by National Science Foundation grants DAR 78-18772 and APR 76-24662 and by grant G00604516 from the Office of Education, Bureau of Education for the Handicapped. All data analysis was performed by Neurometrics, Inc., 17 John Street, New York, New York 10038.

disability. (Admittedly, the practical utility of such differential diagnosis for facilitation of remediation cannot be demonstrated, since the corresponding differential remedial procedures do not exist. Yet, it seems reasonable to suggest that differential remedial procedures, at least for some causes of learning disability, will inevitably be forthcoming once adequate differential diagnosis can be precisely achieved.)

However, even if current psychometric, neurological, and neuropsychological methods were to possess the necessary precision and sensitivity, the number and geographical distribution of qualified specialists in these various disciplines seems quite insufficient to evaluate the huge numbers of children with learning problems, to distinguish between those whose problems are probably attributable to learning disorders and those with learning disabilities, and to provide the desirable differential diagnoses. For example, there are less than 500 pediatric neurologists in the United States, and most of these work in a relatively small number of metropolitan areas.

This chapter describes our attempts to provide a *practical* and precise computer method for the differential diagnosis of children with learning difficulties. This method, called neurometrics, is based on the statistical evaluation of quantitative features of brain electrical activity, objectively extracted by automatic computer analysis of the electroencephalogram (EEG) and sensory evoked or "event-related" potentials (EPs). Neurometrics is intended to supplement the existing methods of the psychologist or neurologist for examination of children with learning problems, revealing abnormal features of brain electrical activity in children with learning disabilities and providing an objective basis for differential diagnosis of various brain dysfunctions that may underlie the same behavioral symptoms. It is our hope that these computer methods, applied by personnel without specialized training in statistics, psychology, or neurology, will also serve a useful preliminary diagnostic function in those numerous regions where the appropriate specialists are insufficient in number to meet practical demands of the school system.

Undoubtedly, some of the more subtle signs of brain dysfunction that can be detected by the experienced EEG analyst will be overlooked by relatively simple computer algorithms. However, many important diagnostic features can be reliably detected by computer algorithms with extremely high precision and sensitivity. We believe that loss of the subtle sensitivity of the experienced clinician is offset by the facts that not all clinicians are equally skillful, that even skillful clinicians show inconsistencies, which are often exacerbated by a uniformly heavy case load, and most decisively, that there are simply not enough trained EEG analysts to evaluate all the children at risk for brain dysfunction, especially in smaller communities and in developing countries. In contrast, computer feature extraction remains consistently accurate no matter what the workload, is completely independent of the skill of the examiner, and can be made generally available because of the increasingly powerful capability and steadily decreasing cost of microprocessor systems.

This chapter presents the principles of neurometric analysis of EEG activity. *Quantitative EEG features will be described that are replicable and fall within a predictable range for most normally functioning individuals but lie outside this range for a high proportion of persons with cognitive dysfunctions, as well as those with a variety of neurological disorders*. The principles of neurometric analysis of EP activity are essentially identical with those for the EEG, but they will not be discussed in this chapter. All computational details will be published elsewhere, but will be provided upon request to the authors.

Background

Abundant evidence suggests that observations of brain electrical activity may be of great utility for differentiating between learning-disordered and learning-disabled children and for development of individualized prescriptive remediation. In spite of the pressing needs that have been discussed in the preceding section, electrophysiological methods have not been widely adopted for such purposes. Actually, many workers in the field of special education have come to regard such methods as being of little or no use for their purposes. Several reasons exist for this negative response. For many years, EEG evaluation of learning-handicapped children relied on the subjective judgments of electroencephalographers, based on visual examination of paper records of the EEG. Except with severe neurological disorders such as epilepsy, this visual pattern recognition usually yielded negative findings. Although a consensus gradually emerged among electroencephalographers that certain patterns were often found among learning-handicapped children, such patterns could frequently be observed in normally functioning children as well and so had no specific implications. Further, repeated studies revealed poor concordance between different clinicians examining the same records, even in cases with neurological disorders less subtle than those that can disrupt learning. The same clinician might even reach different conclusions when evaluating the same record on different occasions.

The qualitative nature of visual EEG interpretations, together with the failure of the conventional neurological examination to yield positive findings in the great majority of learning-handicapped children, contributed to the concept of minimal brain dysfunction (MBD), in vogue during the 1970s. Minimal brain dysfunction was often reminiscent of "Catch-22"; MBD was a brain dysfunction so slight that one could not prove its presence. Understandably, the vague nature of this diagnosis, the fact that its description included a wide diversity of symptoms commonly displayed by children with neither behavioral nor learning problems, and the absence of any unequivocal or unique symptoms, as well as the absence of individualized prescriptive remediation other than medication with stimulant or sedative drugs, caused many parents and educators to suspect the validity of conclusions derived from the EEG or the convential neurological examination.

Quantitative Electrophysiological Evaluation of Brain Dysfunction

In spite of the inherent limitations of visual EEG interpretation and the conventional neurological examination, we believe that qualitative analysis of the electrical activity of the brain can be the basis for differential diagnosis of the learning-handicapped population. Spontaneous fluctuations of minute electrical voltages, on the order of 50-millionths of a volt (50 μv), can be recorded using sensitive amplifiers connected to electrodes affixed to the scalp with a conductive paste. Certain aspects of these rhythmic electrical oscillations, referred to as the EEG, have long been known to reflect the anatomical integrity, functional status, and maturational level of the brain.

With the advent of powerful and economic minicomputers, many investigators who were convinced that the electrical activity of the brain contained much more subtle and diagnostically useful information than was accessible by visual inspection of the conventional EEG turned their attention to the problem of quantitative analysis of electrophysiological data. Their goal was to devise objective methods for extracting features of diagnostic value in numerical form. A brief overview of some representative EEG findings that are most relevant to evaluation of learning-disabled children is presented in the following section. Greater detail can be found in numerous review articles and books [2, 3, 5, 6, 12, 20, 23, 30, 33].

Relevant Electroencephalographic Studies

Normative data for the mean amplitude of the wide frequency bands of the EEG from various regions of the scalp for a large sample of healthy Swedish children across the age range from birth to maturity have recently been published [11, 26]. These norms reveal a systemic change in these features with maturation. In general, there is a steady decrease in the amount of slow waves in each region with maturation.

Many studies have revealed a high incidence of abnormal EEG activity in children who were "underachievers" or who had speech problems, dyslexia, or other learning or behavioral difficulties. Usually, the neurological examination of such children has been within normal limits and their intelligence was average [16, 18, 36]. Excessive slow-wave activity is seen in 14 percent of unselected pediatric neurological referrals and is commonly associated with learning or behavioral difficulties [24, 37]. Some workers have asserted that the most common EEG abnormality found in learning-disabled or "hyperactive" children is excessive slow waves [15, 34]. Kinsbourne [24] proposed that excessive slow-wave activity represents a "maturational lag" in brain development, characteristic of a substantial subgroup of learning-disabled children.

There is general agreement that the EEG recorded from bilaterally symmetrical, or homologous, regions of the scalp in normal healthy persons is extremely symmetrical with respect to both amplitude and waveshape, whether analyzed qualitatively [10] or quantitatively [13, 26]. Some investigators have reported a high incidence of asymmetry in the resting EEG of dyslexic children or underachievers [9, 29] and in a wide variety of neurological disorders [12].

This review, representative rather than exhaustive, indicates the major kinds of EEG observations that support the belief that quantitative analyses of the EEG might usefully contribute to the diagnosis of learning disabilities in children.

Neurometrics

If measurements of brain electrical activity are to become of practical utility for routine evaluation, differential diagnosis, and eventual guidance in the treatment of children with learning difficulties, methods have to be devised to circumvent the complexity of the measurement techniques, the subjective nature of qualitative data evaluation by experienced specialists, and the paucity of specialists, however well qualified. These considerations define a set of requirements that neurometric methods are intended to fulfill:

1. Electrophysiological data of acceptable quality should be gathered in a standardized way, using automated microprocessor-controlled equipment requiring minimum expertise.
2. Univariate diagnostic features should be extracted from the raw data in an objective manner, using quantitative computer analysis.
3. Each quantitative feature should be subject to those transformations required to achieve Gaussian (or "normal") distributions in the healthy population. Such "Gaussianity" would have to be confirmed if parametric statistical inferences are to be applied validly.
4. Age-regression equations should be derived, if possible, that describe the progressive alterations of the mean value and the standard deviation of each defined feature across the age range of interest for a data base of healthy, normally functioning subjects.
5. Every quantitative univariate feature extracted from the raw electrophysiological data of each subject should be referred to the normative data base, with appropriate regression for the age of the subject, to assess its *relative probability* (using the Z-transformation; see p. 164).
6. Combinatorial methods should be devised to compress different univariate features within an anatomical region or similar univariate features across diverse regions into multivariate composites that could be scaled on a comparable metric of relative probability.
7. The neurometric examination of each subject should be represented as a Z-matrix, with columns corresponding to univariate anatomical derivations or multivariate composites and rows corresponding to quantitative extracted univariate or multivariate features. This Z-matrix would constitute a profile of those features in the subject's EEG that were *improbable in the healthy population*, or *"abnormal."*

The intent of these procedures is to replace the subjective judgment of the skilled EEG clinician by routine statistical evaluation by a computer. *Abnormal* becomes redefined as "improbable in a healthy person." Disrespectful of human expertise though this strategy may appear, its credibility ultimately depends not on possibly emotional reactions to the suggestion that evaluation of complex diagnostic data can be performed better by computers, but on the legitimacy of the statistical procedures and assumptions and the reproducibility of the results. Since neurometric assessment is based on well-known and acceptable parametric statistical procedures, straightforward methods exist to test or demonstrate their validity. First, neurometric procedures must be described. The next section of this chapter is devoted to various demonstrations of validity of neurometric measures. The last section presents evidence that these valid measures are in fact sensitive and useful for "automatic" and reproducible detection of brain dysfunction and for differential diagnosis of persons with cognitive dysfunctions.

Neurometric Procedures

Data Acquisition

Neurometric analysis of the EEG begins by obtaining a sample of 60 seconds of artifact-free, eyes-closed, resting EEG. Since we want to be able to compare similar data from different people or repeated measures from the same person, precautions are necessary to reduce or eliminate sources of variability in these measures. Test conditions must be carefully standardized. The subject is seated in a comfortable chair in a dimly lit, quiet test chamber. Silver disk electrodes are pasted on the scalp at measured positions defined by the International 10-20 Electrode Placement System [21], as shown in Figure 9-1. Care is also taken to ensure that the subject is comfortable, relaxed, and not apprehensive, and the whole procedure is described in simple language beforehand. To reassure young children, a familiar adult should sit in an adjacent chair, making soothing remarks and reminding the child to remain with eyes closed, if this is necessary. Older subjects are continuously observed by means of closed-circuit television, while a two-way intercom permits verbal interactions between the subject and the examiner.

Uniform quality of electrical recordings is achieved by placing data acquisition fully under control of a microprocessor. The microprocessor automatically tests electrode impedances, calibrates the amplifiers, and most importantly, uses artifact rejection algorithms (computational procedures) to

Fig. 9-1. Electrode placements according to the International 10-20 System.

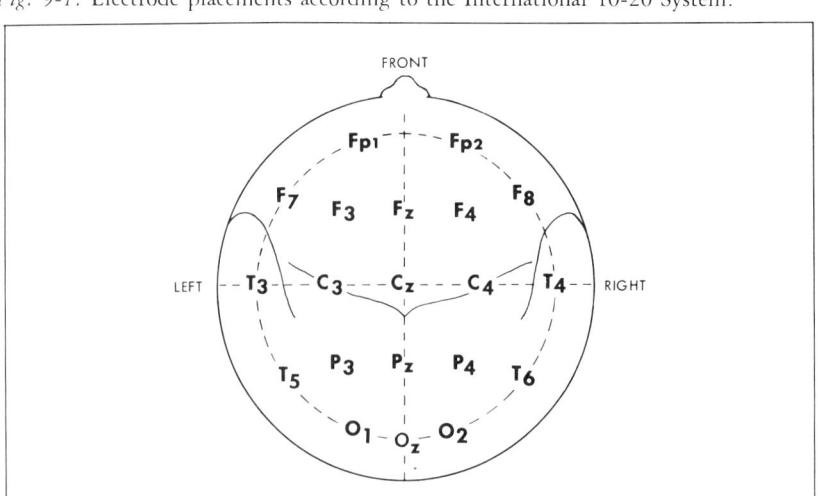

monitor the recordings. The complex algorithms use a variety of criteria to reject all data contaminated by voltages that do not come from brain electrical activity, including artifacts caused by eye movements, blinks, changes in body position or muscle tension, and sources of electrical noise in the environment. All data accepted as artifact-free by these computer programs are recorded in digital format on magnetic disks. *All data are reconstructed and graphically displayed for visual inspection.* Invalid data that may have eluded the computer artifact rejection procedures are then edited out of the record, prior to qualitative analysis.

Objective Extraction of Quantitative Univariate Features
To eliminate subjective evaluation of the electrophysiological data, analytical programs were written to extract many quantitative features of the EEG that had been reported to be of diagnostic utility in the prior literature. These individual, or *univariate*, features were extracted from eight bipolar electrode combinations, or *derivations*: bilateral frontotemporal (F_7T_3/F_8T_4), temporal (T_3T_5/T_4T_6), central (C_3C_z/C_4C_z), and parieto-occipital (P_3O_1/P_4O_2). The letters and subscripts in parentheses refer to electrode positions in the International 10-20 System (Fig. 9-1). The basic univariate features consisted of the *total absolute power* in the frequency range 0.5 to 25.0 Hz; the *relative (%) power* in the delta (1.5–3.5Hz), theta (3.5–7.5 Hz), alpha (7.5–12.5 Hz), and beta (12.5–25.0 Hz) frequency bands; the average *coherence* (% phase-locked power) within each of these four frequency bands between each of the four pairs of symmetrically placed electrodes; and the *power asymmetry* within each of the four frequency bands between each symmetrical pair.

Transforms to Achieve Gaussian Feature Distributions
Under standardization conditions, EEG and EP samples designed to comprise a normative data base have been gathered from a large representative sample of healthy, normally functioning children across the age range from 6 to 16 years. Parenthetically, this normative data base is currently being expanded to encompass most of the human life span, 2 to 90 years. School records, health records, and parent questionnaires were used to exclude all children from this normative sample if they had a history of neurological disorders, school failure, or any event that might have caused brain damage. The Wechsler's Intelligence Scale for Children–Revised (WISC-R) or the Peabody Picture Vocabulary Test was administered to provide reassurance that each child was within the normal intelligence range, and the Wide Range Achievement Test was administered to confirm that each child was functioning at appropriate grade level with respect to reading and arithmetic skills.

Each of the univariate features defined previously was extracted from the EEG sample recorded from every child in the normative sample ($n = 306$). We examined distributions of each feature as a function of age. For every feature, transforms were sought to convert the observed initial distribution into one with known statistical properties, such as the Gaussian distribution. Generally, when a transform has been found that establishes a well-understood distribution, it becomes legitimate to apply a variety of powerful statistical procedures to determine the probability that any feature obtained from an individual subject might have been obtained from a person in the normally functioning population.

The following transformations were found to achieve acceptable Gaussian distributions, where X stands for the initial value of each feature; absolute power $= \log X$; relative power and coherence $= \log (X/100 - X)$; and power asymmetry $= \log (X_{LEFT}/X_{RIGHT})$. The results of statistical tests that were carried out to confirm the adequacy of these transformations will be discussed in a later section.

Age-Regression Equations

All of the EEG features that we have studied show systematic changes with age. To evaluate the probability that the observed value of some feature extracted from a particular subject might be obtained by chance in a member of the healthy population, it is first necessary to take these systematic age effects into account. Values within the normal range at one age might be outside the normal range at some different age. Accordingly, age-regression equations were computed for the mean values and the standard deviations of the distributions of each feature after all data have been subjected to the transforms required to achieve Gaussiantity. For every feature i, the changes in mean values and standard deviations as a function of age could be satisfactorily described by simple polynomial functions of the form

$$\bar{V}_i(t) = C_0 + C_1 t + C_2 t^2 + \ldots C_n t^n$$

where $\bar{V}_i(t)$ denotes the predicted mean value or standard deviation of the distribution of the relevant transformed feature i in the normal population and C_i denotes the values of constant coefficients for each term in the corresponding polynomial. The actual values of C_i change from feature to feature and derivation to derivation. The only variable in any of these polynomials is t, the chronological age of the subject. Obviously, separate equations are used to obtain the expected mean values and the standard deviations.

At present, age-regression equations for the mean values and standard deviations of 286 univariate and multivariate features have been derived from our normative EEG data base. (See the discussion Multivariate Features). Although polynomials of the fourth order or higher are required to describe the evolution of these EEG features across the age range from 1 to 90 years old, changes across the restricted school age of 6 to 16 years can be well described by first-order linear equation of the form $C_0 + C_1 t$. Some of those equations have already been published [20, 21].

Z-Transformation

The statistical properties of the Gaussian distribution, also referred to as the bell-shaped curve, are very familiar. Among these properties are symmetry about the mean value and the fact that if the total area under the curve is understood to include 100 percent of the population, then the mean ± 1 standard deviation (SD) subsumes 65 percent of the population, the mean

±2 SD subsumes 95 percent, the mean ±2.5 SD subsumes 99 percent, and so on. Given any observed value of some variable *i* known to be distributed in a Gaussian manner among the healthy normal population, the *probability* that a value that large might be obtained by chance in a member of the normal population can be precisely estimated. This estimate is obtained by subtracting the value $V_i(t)$ observed in an individual subject of age *t*, from the mean value of that variable in the normal population of age *t*, $\bar{V}_i(t)$, and dividing by the standard deviation of the distribution of the variable *i* at that age, $S_i(t)$. Thus,

$$Z_i = \frac{\bar{V}_i(t) - V_i(t)}{S_i(t)}$$

It should be clear that the values of $\bar{V}_i(t)$ and $S_i(t)$ are calculated by inserting the age *t* of the subject into the regressional equations for the mean value and standard deviation of variable *i*, while the value of $V_i(t)$ is obtained by performing the appropriate transformation for Gaussianity on the extracted feature *i*. A value of Z_i can be thus calculated for every quantitative feature *i* extracted from the EEG sample recorded from each subject.

The Z-transformation rescales the distance between the observed value and the expected mean value of any feature into multiples of the standard deviation. *The Z-value is proportional to the relative probability of abnormality,* since the probability of obtaining a value as large or larger than the observed value in a normal person is the percentage of the area under the bell-shaped curve that lies equal to, or farther from, the mean than the observed value. This probability can be looked up in any book of statistical tables.

Multivariate Features

An important consequence of Z-transformation is that all extracted EEG features are reduced to the common metric of relative probability even though their initial physical dimensions (e.g., μv^2, % power in a given frequency range, % phase-locked power at a specified frequency) were not readily comparable. Not only does Z-transformation facilitate ready interpretation of the diagnostic significance of any quantitative feature extracted from an individual EEG, it is now possible to combine subjects of disparate univariate features into composite multivariate features without any serious problems of scaling.

The potential utility of multivariate composite features should be obvious. If many different univariate features can be Z-transformed and combined, it becomes possible to construct operational definitions for such notions as "the overall abnormality (improbability) of a given brain region across all EEG features," "the overall abnormality of a particular EEG feature across all brain regions," or "the overall abnormality of the EEG examinations across all brain regions and across all measured features."

In spite of the common metric provided by the Z-transform for all features, a major obstacle to the computation of such multivariate indices arises from the fact that many of the measure features are correlated, or nonindependent. This redundancy precludes simple combinations such as computing the square root of the sum of squares of a set of Z-transformed features (the Euclidean distance). Principle component factor analysis is one way to compensate for the presence of intercorrelated measures. Another way, called the Mahalanobis distance, uses the matrix of covariance between measures to define a complex correlation for the intercorrelations within any set of features.

We have determined the distribution of the Mahalanobis distances for a variety of multivariate combinations of univariate neurometric EEG features. Appropriate transforms, usually of the form log X, have been found to make these distributions of multivariate features Gaussian, and age-regression equations for the mean values and standard deviations of these distributions have been derived. Accordingly, it is now possible to calculate the probability of obtaining any observed *combination of univariate EEG features* in a member of the normal population by Z-transformation of the corresponding Mahalanobis distance, exactly as for any univariate feature. The Z-transformation of the Mahalanobis distance across any set of univariate features i is denoted in what follows by the symbol $\bar{Z}_i$.

Mahalanobis distance age-regression equations are now available for the following composites of univariate EEG features:

Combinations of Univariate Features Within any Region. These composites include slow-wave excess within any region (delta + theta), total relative power abnormality within any region (delta + theta + alpha + beta), total coherence abnormality across all four frequency bands between two asymmetrical derivations, total power asymmetry across all four frequency bands between two symmetrical derivations, and total regional abnormality across all measures obtained from the regions (absolute power, relative power, coherence, symmetry).

Combinations of Univariate or Multivariate Features Across Regions. These composites include total abnormality for the specified combination of features in the whole left hemisphere, the whole right hemisphere, the anterior half of the head, the posterior half of the head, or the total head (all measures in all regions).

The Z-transform of each of these multivariate features, relative to the age-regression equation derived from the normative data base, provides the same metric of *relative probability* for all multivariate $\bar{Z}_i$ as for the univariate Z_i. Thus, both univariate and multivariate features can be included in such computations, for example, as stepwise discriminant functions.

Special Multivariate Features: Maturational Lag and Developmental Deviation

Two multivariate features are of special interest because of the prognostic implication that they suggest on purely intuitional grounds: maturational lag and developmental deviation. If we examine the age-regression equation for any single univariate feature, it is a curve that ascends or descends rather smoothly over a substantial age range. Within reasonable limits, any plausible value of a single univariate feature obtained from a particular subject can be found someplace on that curve, even if it is not found at the point that corresponds to the age of the subject. No objective criterion comes to mind that might aid the distinction between an improbable single feature value

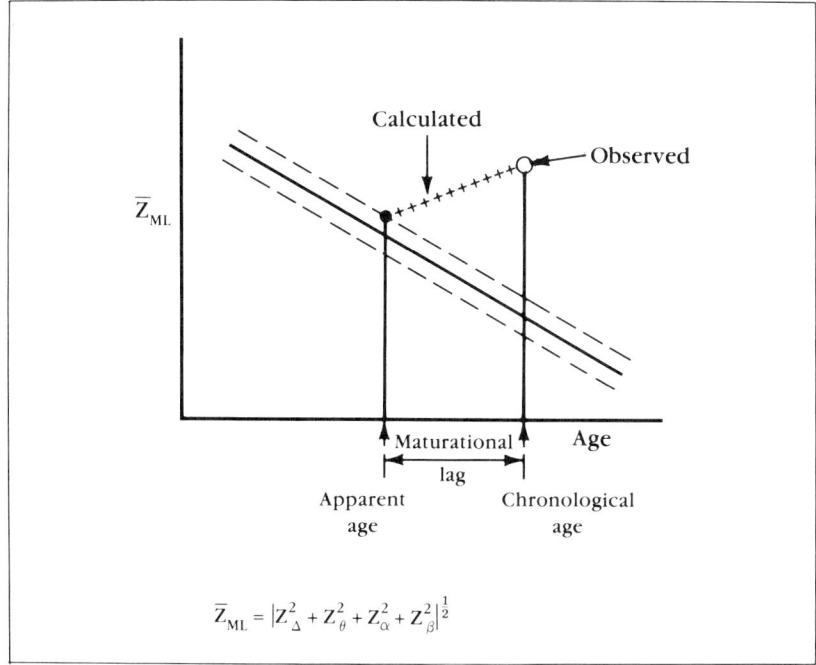

Fig. 9-2. The straight line from upper left to lower right is an idealized representation of the power in the four-dimensional delta, theta, alpha, beta frequency band "space" predicted by the normative age regression equations for a particular derivation. The dotted lines represent the confidence intervals. The open circle represents, in that space, the Z-transformed EEG spectral values actually observed in a patient with the indicated chronological age. If values of age different from this actual age are inserted in the age regression equations, the consequent changes in Z-values move the patient closer to the normative region. The age for which the distance between the observed and predicted spectrum is *minimum* is the apparent EEG age. At this age, the observed value may no longer be significantly different from the predicated value. The discrepancy between actual and apparent age is the maturational lag.

that could reasonably be interpreted as unusually *slow* (or fast) maturation versus *abnormal* development.

However, the situation is somewhat different when we consider "natural" combinations of univariate features. For example, the multivariate feature $\bar{Z}_{FREQ}$ represents the $\bar{Z}$-transform of the Mahalanobis distance across the full set of four frequency bands in all eight derivations. $\bar{Z}_{FREQ}$ thus quantifies the overall abnormality in the power spectrum of the total EEG record, subsuming 32 measurements. The age-regression equation for the mean value of $\bar{Z}_{FREQ}$ defines a multidimensional trajectory, and the age-regression equation for the standard deviation defines a region around that trajectory. One can visualize this as akin to a "developmental tunnel," with a slope defined by the mean value and a diameter proportional to the standard deviation of $\bar{Z}_{FREQ}$ at any age (Fig. 9-2).

Now imagine an individual whose $\bar{Z}_{FREQ}$ value lies significantly further from the point, in this multidimensional "frequency composition of the EEG in all brain regions" space, expected for a healthy person at that age than would be probable if one considers the standard deviation at that age. In such an instance, one possibility is that the overall discrepancy in the EEG spectra of the various regions systematically decreases as ages other than the chronological age of the subjects are inserted into the 32 age-regression equations used to compute the univariate Z-transforms on which $\bar{Z}_{FREQ}$ is based. Further, at some age different from that of the subject, $\bar{Z}_{FREQ}$ falls inside the developmental tunnel; that is, the overall frequency profile of the brain, considering all eight regions analyzed, looks like that which would be expected from a normal person younger (or older) than the subject. The apparent abnormality in the frequency composition of the EEG can be considered as a *maturational lag* quantified by the interval between the "apparent EEG age" and the actual chronological age of the subject [7]. Such a case is illustrated in the example presented in Figure 9-2.

In such a case, it would seem especially important to perform a second neurometric evaluation after a reasonably long time, say 6 months to 1 year later. If the value of $\bar{Z}_{FREQ}$ and the length of the maturational lag *have not increased* (i.e., the apparent physiological age has shifted), then maturation is progressing but with a constant developmental gap between the subject and his age peers. Intuitively, one might predict that this subject will follow a normal sequence of development, although milestones will be reached later than is usual. While there might be concern about social and psychological consequences of this delay, it seems reasonable to expect that this subject will eventually reach the same educational goals as his peers. On the other hand, if the apparent physiological age remains the same after passage of time, then maturation would appear to have reached an asymptote. The intuitive prognosis in such a case would appear less reassuring, suggesting that there may be some constraint that will prevent the subject from developing beyond a certain level. One might speculate that certain kinds of mental retardation might have such an effect.

A second possibility exists if $\bar{Z}_{FREQ}$ exceeds the probable confidence limits. That is, no matter what ages are inserted into the age-regression equations from which the univariate Z-values are computed, the value of $\bar{Z}_{FREQ}$ cannot be made acceptably small (Fig. 9-3). Stated another way, there is no age at which a healthy normal person might be expected to display the overall EEG frequency profile found in this subject. Such a profile is defined as a *developmental deviation*, since the EEG of this subject lies outside the developmental tunnel for any hypothetical age. Intuitively, one has no basis for a prognosis of eventual normal development in such a case, especially if the deviational classification remains unaltered at a second neurometric examination after a reasonable time interval. Developmental deviations would seem likely to reflect serious disturbances of brain state, such as might be caused by drugs, systemic disorders, or neurological diseases. In such cases, it would seem worthwhile to seek further for the cause of the abnormal brain state and to consider carefully the possibility of pharmacological or other intervention.

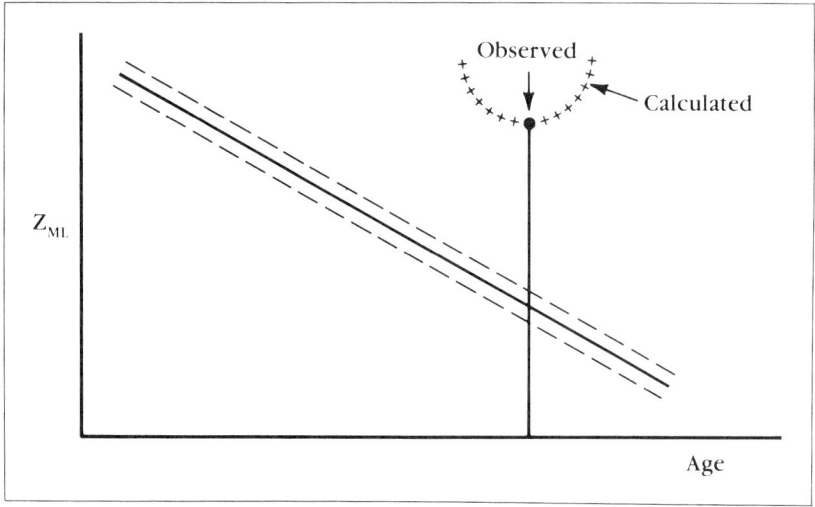

Fig. 9-3. At the age where the discrepancy between the observed and predicted spectrum is minimized, substitution of larger or smaller age in the regression equations will increase this discrepancy. To the extent that the *minimum* discrepancy is significant, this EEG would not lie within normal limits in a subject of *any* age. This residual represents functional deviation, or developmental deviation.

As with other multivariate measures, the size and distribution of maturational lags and developmental deviations in our normal data base have been analyzed and age-regression equations computed so that the probability of observed values of these multivariate features can be estimated. Perhaps we should emphasize that throughout our discussion of maturational lag and developmental deviation, we have consistently inserted the qualification "intuitively" prefatory to our speculations about the possible prognostic value of these new multivariate descriptors of the EEG. At present, the only information available about these features is their relative incidence in populations of children with various types of problems. No follow-up nor correlative data have been obtained to provide any support for our conjectures. Nonetheless, we feel that the potential utility of these features for patient management and remedial treatment justifies this detailed discussion.

The Abnormality or Z-Matrix
The quantitative results of a neurometric evaluation of the EEG are presented as an "abnormality matrix," or "Z-matrix." Every entry in this matrix represents a Z-transformation computed from age-regression equations defining the mean value and standard deviation of the distribution of the corresponding univariate or multivariate feature, derived from a healthy, normally functioning population. The EEG abnormality matrix consists of 13 columns: four symmetrical pairs of bipolar derivations *plus* two composite left and right hemispheric measures *plus* two composite anterior and posterior measures *plus* one total head measure. This matrix contains 22 rows consisting of univariate

Table 9-1. EEG abnormality matrix

Electrophysiological Features	Regions											
	Frontotemporal		Temporal		Central		Parieto-occipital		Z_L	Z_R	Z_A^a	Z_P^b	Z_{Row}^c
	L(1)	R(2)	L(3)	R(4)	L(5)	R(6)	L(7)	R(8)					
Relative Power													
1. % delta	Z_{11}	Z_{12}	Z_{13}	Z_{14}	Z_{15}	Z_{16}	Z_{17}	Z_{18}	Z_{1L}	Z_{1R}	Z_{1A}	Z_{1P}	Z_{1Row}
2. % theta	Z_{21}	Z_{22}	Z_{23}	Z_{24}	•	•	•	•	•	•	•	•	•
3. % alpha	Z_{31}												
4. % beta	Z_{41}												
5. % delta + theta	Z_{51}												
Frequency Composites													
6. Z_f spectrum	Z_{61}												
7. Z_m best fit	•												
8. Maturational lag	•												
9. Developmental deviation	•												
Absolute Power													
10. Absolute power	•												
11. Power asymmetry	•												

Z-Matrix = region (columns) × feature (rows)

Coherence
12. delta
13. theta
14. alpha
15. beta

Coherence composite
16. Z_c coherence

Power asymmetry
17. delta
18. theta
19. alpha
20. beta

Asymmetry composite
21. Z_a amplitude asymmetry

Overall regional dysfunction
22. Z_{R1}

Z_{HEAD} [c]

[a] Composite of frontotemporal and temporal regions (anterior).
[b] Composite of central and parieto-occipital regions (posterior).
[c] Overall abnormality for feature across regions.
[d] Overall abnormality for region across feature.
[e] Overall abnormality across features across regions.

features quantifying absolute power, absolute power asymmetry, the relative power, coherence and asymmetry in four frequency bands, and multivariate features quantifying combinations of relative power, coherence, and symmetry across all frequency bands with each column, as well as the composite of all available measures. This matrix, which is constructed from evaluation of the EEG record of each individual subject, is illustrated in Table 9-1.

Validation of Neurometric Procedures

Before presentation of the currently available evidence about the diagnostic utility of neurometric evaluation of the EEG, it is desirable to provide some concise documentation that the basic requirements on which the complex statistical procedures described above depend have indeed been satisfied and that the quantitative data contained in a Z-matrix are stable and consistent within an individual, and to provide a meaningful framework within which to evaluate some aspects of brain function as reflected in the EEG. Complete documentation will be provided in more extensive publications currently in preparation.

Validation of Automatic Artifact Rejection Method
Careful examination of EEG records reconstructed from our digital records showed that most records contained segments accepted by the computer artifact rejection algorithm that an experienced EEG technician would have rejected. Accordingly, such reconstructed records from 20 children were subjected to subsequent human editing. Quantitative analyses were carried out on the records as initially edited by the computer and as finally edited by skilled personnel. Cross-correlations were computed for each measure between the analytical results with and without human editing.

Correlations for relative power features ranged from .99 to .83, for coherence features from .99 to .75, and for power asymmetry features from .99 to .89. Less than 20 percent of all features showed correlations below .9. These results indicate that the majority of artifacts that elude the computer rejection algorithm lie above or below the frequency band of 1.5 to 25.0 Hz, from which these neurometric features are extracted. This is in agreement with reports that eye movements and muscle contractions produce artifacts that are outside this frequency band. Although these results suggest that automatic computer artifact rejection provides valid estimates of neurometric EEG features, all data presented in this chapter were derived from recordings that had been visually edited prior to quantitative analyses.

Validation of Sample Length
Some workers have suggested that EEG segments as short as 8 to 10 seconds will provide accurate estimates of spectral features. We examined cross-correlations between features extracted from successively longer segments within the same individual recordings. The results indicate that estimates based on 20 seconds of computer-artifacted EEG recording were in good agreement with those obtained from records 60 seconds long. Accordingly, data were

considered adequate for inclusion in the studies reported here if 30 seconds or more of EEG record were considered artifact-free after visual editing.

Test-Retest Reliability

From each subject, two 60-second artifact-free samples of eyes-open and eyes-closed EEG were recorded, one of each at the beginning and end of an evoked potential testing session about 1 hour long. After visual editing, spectral analyses were carried out on each sample from every subject. The absolute power and relative (%) power in each frequency band were computed for every derivation in each sample. Test-retest correlations were then computed to compare, across subjects, the values of each feature between the beginning and end of session samples.

Data obtained in the eyes-closed condition were significantly more reliable than in the eyes-open condition. Absolute power measures were far less reliable than relative power measures. The average overall reliability of relative power estimates from eyes-closed EEG records, based on 32 values (four frequency bands in eight derivations), was .83 after 1 hour. With an intertest interval of 1 week, the average correlation remained at .83. For a group of 30 children with an average test-retest interval of 0.62 years, the average correlation was .73, and when the two tests were separated by an average of 2.46 years, the average correlation was .68.

These results, based on age-regression Z-transforms or relative power in the delta, theta, alpha, and beta bands, demonstrate that these neurometric features are reasonably stable and replicable characteristics of the individual. The data presented in this chapter focus on relative power features extracted from the eyes-closed EEG, on the associated coherence and power asymmetry features that could be extracted from these stable spectra, and on multivariate features compressing these univariate features.

Tests of Gaussianity of Univariate and Multivariate Features

The distributions of all univariate and multivariate features, defined previously and included in the Z-matrix, were studied in the large sample of normal children (n = 306) described in the subsequent section Diagnostic Utility of Neurometric Procedures. For this purpose, this sample was divided into two "split-half" groups using a randomization procedure that balanced the age distribution in the two groups (normal groups N-I and N-II). Age-regression equations were first constructed for the mean value and standard deviation of each univariate and multivariate feature using group N-I. Each feature extracted from every member of group N-II was then Z-transformed relative to the appropriate age-regression equation from N-I. Conversely, a corresponding set of age-regression equations for all neurometric EEG features was constructed from the data of N-II. Features from N-I were then Z-transformed relative to the normative functions derived from N-II. This procedure permitted us to use each subject in our normal sample twice, once as a member of a group to construct "split-half norms" and once as a member of a group providing an independent "split-half test" of the validity of the norms derived from the other group.

The age-regression equations derived from both groups were examined, as were the distributions of Z-transformed values resulting from this "crossover norming," for every univariate and multivariate feature tested in both split-half normal groups. The coefficients of the age-regression equations for corresponding features were closely similar in the two split-half samples. *All Z-distributions were found to have a mean value very close to 0 and a standard deviation very close to 1.00*. The incidence of false-positives (Z-transforms with a probability beyond a specified confidence level) was acceptably close to 5 percent at the 0.05 level and 1 percent at the 0.01 level. Only a few features showed an incidence of false-positives more than 2 to 3 percent above the level that might be expected by chance.

These results, which were published in detail elsewhere [21], demonstrated that the two split-half normal groups showed homogeneity of variance and *the various transforms*, applied to the univariate raw feature values extracted from the EEG and to the multivariate features constructed from combinations of those univariate features, *yielded Gaussian distributions in our normal population. Therefore, the use of conventional parametric statistical procedures to assess such features must be considered legitimate and can be expected to yield replicable results.*

Age-Regression Equations

The tests described demonstrated that the neurometric feature extraction and transformation procedures that we had devised yielded measures that should be statistically "well behaved" and that displayed homogeneity of variance in the two split-half normal groups N-I and N-II. Accordingly, the two split-half normal groups were combined to maximize the final sample size to obtain the most accurate descriptors, and age-regression equations were computed for every univariate and multivariate neurometric EEG feature using the full sample of 306 healthy, normally functioning children. The values of the coefficients of some of these age-regression equations for the range 6 to 16 years of age, for the means and standard deviations of 32 relative power features (four frequency bands × eight bipolar derivations), have been published previously [20]. We have since extended the age range of our normative sample up to 90 years of age, and the full set of polynomial functions defining the age-regression equations for all univariate and multivariate neurometric EEG features contained in the Z-matrix presented in Table 9-1 has been published elsewhere [21].

Culture-Fair Nature of Neurometric EEG Features

Age-regression equations for the mean values and standard deviations of 16 relative power features (four frequency bands × four averaged left-and-right bipolar derivations) were also computed using absolute power data published by Matoušek and Petersén [27], which we converted to relative power. Across the age range 6 to 16 years, the equations that we derived from our sample of healthy U.S. children and computed from the published normative values of healthy Swedish children were in close correspondence. These findings are graphically depicted in Figure 9-4 [20].

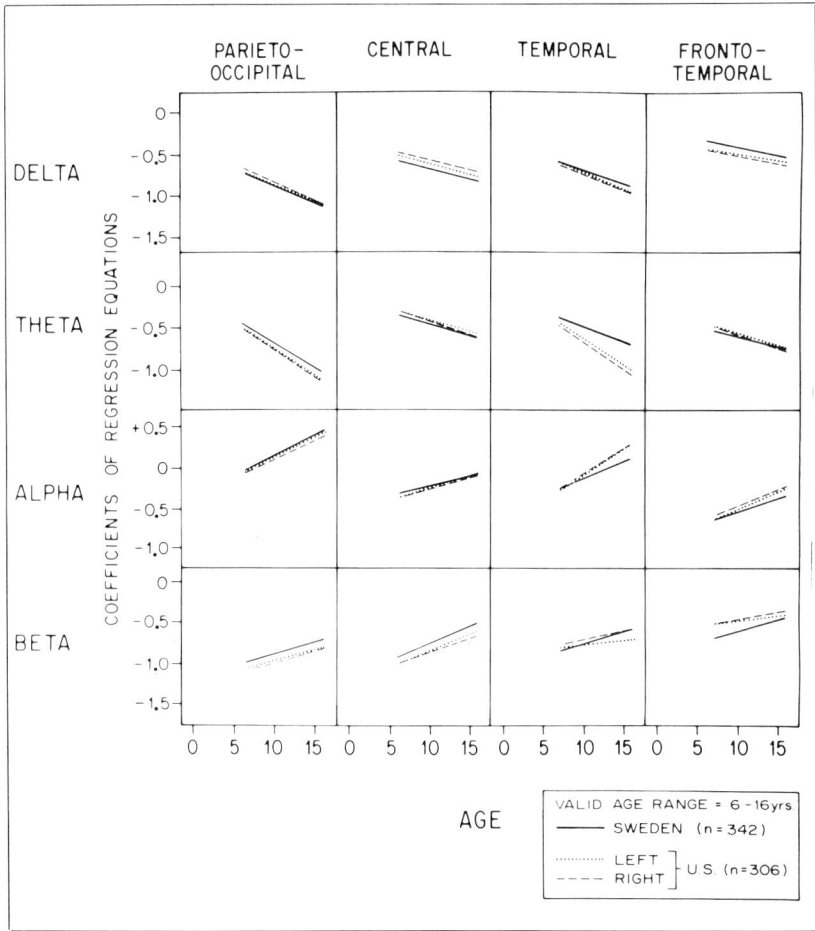

Fig. 9-4. Regression equations for data from U.S. children (n = 306) and Swedish children (n = 342) for each frequency band and derivation. (From E. R. John et al., Developmental equations for the electroencephalogram. *Science* 210:1255, 1980. Copyright 1980 by the American Association for the Advancement of Science.)

These equations were used to Z-transform relative power features extracted from EEG recordings obtained from groups of urban, suburban, rural, black, white, male, and female normal U.S. children (n = 25 for each group) and from a group of normal children from Barbados (n = 91). The incidence of false-positives was at the chance level for each of these groups, and no group differed significantly from any other group on any of these measures [1, 20]. Preliminary results from other laboratories [8] have confirmed that our published transforms and age-regression equations for these EEG features well describe the distribution of such measures in children from diverse cultural and ethnic backgrounds. *This evidence suggests that the univariate and multivariate neurometric EEG features defined previously and described in these age-regression equa-*

tions may provide quantitive indices of the development of the healthy, normal human brain that are independent of socioeconomic, cultural, and ethnic factors.

Diagnostic Utility of Neurometric Procedures

Deviations from the distributions of univariate and multivariate EEG features apparently well described for diverse populations of healthy children by the age-regression equations were studied in large populations of children with learning disabilities, children with a wide variety of neurological disorders, and normal children. The results, which indicate that these valid, replicable measures of brain activity are sensitive to brain dysfunctions that are highly correlated with cognitive problems as well as neurological diseases, are presented in this section.

Subjects

"Normal" U.S. Children. A sample of "normal" U.S. children was gathered by using newspaper ads and notices in local schools to inform the metropolitan New York area that healthy, normally functioning children were needed to serve as control subjects in a research project intended to develop quantitative measures of brain dysfunctions related to learning disabilities. In addition, parents of learning-disabled children who wanted to serve as subjects on this project were asked to use their personal contacts to recruit a normally functioning child who would serve as a matched control. In an initial screening telephone interview, parents were informed that to be accepted as normal subjects for this study, children must have been born after an uneventful full-term pregnancy with no peri- or postnatal complications, should never have suffered head injury or high-febrile illness resulting in loss of consciousness, should have no history of convulsions or neurological disease, should be of normal intelligence, and should currently be at age-appropriate grade level in school with no history of failure at any prior level, as confirmed by school report cards. Parents of children who met these criteria received $10 for permitting their child to undergo several hours of behavioral testing and a painless and harmless recording of spontaneous and evoked brain electrical activity. The electrophysiological testing procedure was described in easily understood language.

Further evaluation consisted of a detailed interview and questionnaire completed by the parent who accompanied the child to the testing session, administration of the Peabody Picture Vocabulary Test (PPVT) to provide an estimate of intelligence, and administration of the Wide Range Achievement Test (WRAT) to provide an estimate of the child's actual scholastic achievement level. The final sample considered admissible to a normative population contained 306 children. All of these children had uneventful histories, scores of 90 or higher on the PPVT, and standard scores of 90 or higher on all sections of the WRAT. In subsequent discussion, this group is divided into N-I and N-II, each with 153 patients.

A Word of Caution About Norms. A fundamental issue cannot be evaded in the construction of developmental "norms": Should children who seem to have compensated for events that obviously place them at risk be included in a normative sample, and should children who fail to meet criteria defined by laboratory measures for normality be excluded even though they have not *as yet* displayed inability to meet the demands of daily life and are not obviously at risk by historical criteria? Exclusion of all subjects from the control population who might conceivably be at risk for any reason minimizes the standard deviation of normative data and can be expected to maximize the subsequent incidence of false-positives, that is, individuals who lie outside the normative range even though they are asymptomatic. Conversely, inclusion of subjects obviously at risk although currently asymptomatic maximizes the standard deviation of the normative data and can be expected to minimize the subsequent incidence of false-positives while decreasing detection of true abnormalities.

It must be emphasized that the definition of a normative reference is not absolute but relative and involves a value judgment about the respective risk-benefit ratio of the false-positive and false-negative errors that will result from that definition. The consequences of failure to detect the presence of neurological disease are obviously different from failure to detect possible brain dysfunction related to a learning disability. Neurometric assessments should only serve as one input to a multidisciplinary evaluation of any patient. While neurometric findings may serve to "raise a flag" to indicate that a patient is at risk for brain dysfunction, careful replication of abnormal neurometric findings and confirmatory evidence from other modes of assessment are required to minimize the chance of a false-positive finding. Conversely, the absence of neurometric findings cannot be considered as definitive evidence of the absence of any brain dysfunction. No technology relieves the user of that responsibility to evaluate critically the results that it provides.

In our decisions about the composition of a normative sample, we endeavor to tread a conservative path, constructing relatively "tight" reference data and relying on stringent statistical criteria and the expected strong effects of true brain dysfunction to discriminate between false-positives and true abnormalities.

Normal Barbados Children. A sample of 129 normally functioning children from rural communities in Barbados was gathered, using well-documented developmental data.* These children all had uneventful histories, had full scale scores of 85 or above on the Wechsler's Intelligence Scale for Children–Revised (WISC-R), and were at appropriate grade level for their age. The WISC-R had been modified by Galler to make it culturally relevant for Barbados children. The recording of deficiencies and gross abnormalities discerned by visual examination of the EEG and EP records reduced this sample of normal children to 91.

Learning-Disabled Children. A group of 139 learning-disabled children were recruited from a special education facility, the James E. Allen Learning Center, Board of Cooperative Educational Services (BOCES), District #3, Dix Hills,

---

*The study was conducted in collaboration with F. Ramsey, J. Galler, and G. Solimano and was supported by the Ford Foundation, grant 770-0471.

New York. These children had no known neurological diseases but had IQ scores between 65 and 84 on the WISC-R and standard scores below 90 in language and/or arithmetic skills on the WRAT. In subsequent discussion, this group is divided into LD_1 (n = 89) and LD_2 (n = 50).

Specifically Learning-Disabled Children. A group of 159 children with "specific learning disabilities" were recruited from local schools (or the James E. Allen Learning Center). These children had no known neurological diseases but had IQ scores above 85 on the WISC-R and WRAT standard scores below 90 in language and/or arithmetic skills. In the subsequent discussion, this group will sometimes be referred to as SLD.

Neurologically "At Risk" Children. The last group consists of 533 patients 6 to 16 years of age who were referred to a pediatric neurology service because they were considered at risk for neurological disorders.* This group included children diagnosed as having a variety of disorders, including cerebral palsy, severe mental retardation, phenylketonuria, renal disease, epilepsy, emotional disturbances, and learning disabilities.

The learning-disabled children contained in this heterogeneous group were removed to constitute a separate subgroup, referred to as LD_3 (n = 71). In addition, 85 epileptic children were removed and combined into another subgroup, EPILEPTIC. NEURO (Table 9-2) refers to the 462 children who remained in that group after removal of LD_3. NEUROLOGICAL (Table 9-3) refers to 377 children who remained after the removal of epileptic patients (n = 85).

Sensitivity of Univariate Neurometric EEG Features to Brain Dysfunction

The results presented earlier in this chapter demonstrated that Z-transforms of quantitative EEG features provided replicable and culture-fair predictors of the frequency composition of the EEG recorded from various electrode locations on the scalp of healthy, normally functioning children. The incidence of Z-values significant at the .05 and .01 levels of probability was studied for these EEG features in the various populations of normal, specifically learning-disabled (SLD), learning-disabled (LD), and neurologically at risk (NEURO) children already defined [1]. The results are shown in Figure 9-5.

Inspection of the histogram in Figure 9-5 shows that the proportion of Z-values significant at the .05 level (white band) and .01 level (shaded bars) was at or below the incidence expected by chance for the distributions of most of these features in the samples of normal U.S. (N-I) and Barbados (N-II) children. However, in the SLD, LD, and NEURO groups, the proportion of Z-values at or above the .01 (as well as the .05) level was much greater than expected by chance. It is noteworthy that the incidence of significant findings in the NEURO group, at risk for a variety of neurological disorders, is not qualitatively greater than in the SLD and LD groups, who display learning disabilities in the absence of known neurological disorders.

*Subjects were patients of Pediatric Neurology Service, Handicapped Children's Unit, St. Christopher's Hospital for Children, Philadelphia. The study was supported in part by NIH general CRC grant RR-75. Disks from the neurometric examinations of 533 neurological patients were sent to New York University for analysis with no information other than the age of the patient.

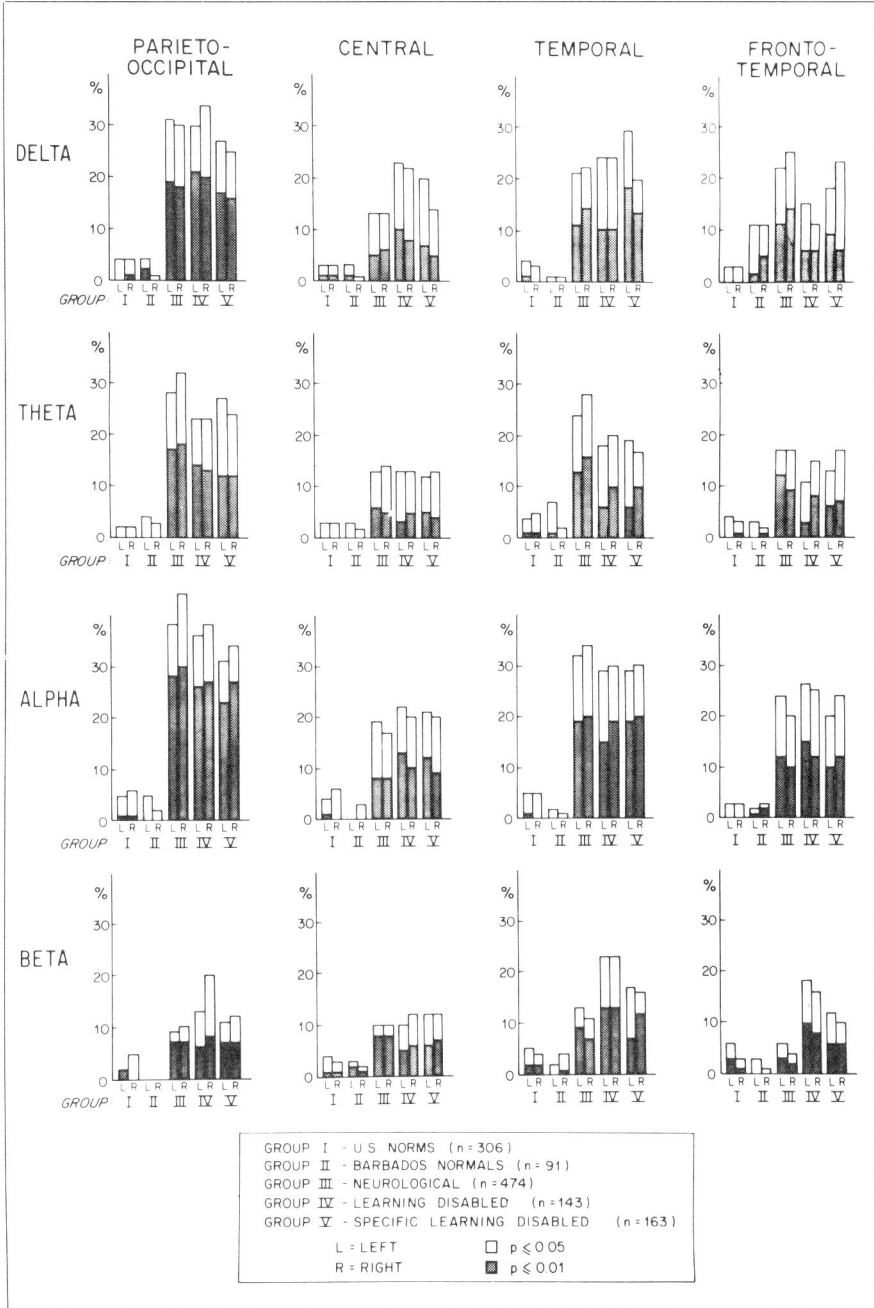

Fig. 9-5. Percentage distribution of hits for five groups of children. Height of bars corresponds to hits at the p ≤ .05 level; shaded portion corresponds to hits at the p ≤ .01 level. (From H. Ahn et al., Developmental equations reflect brain dysfunctions. *Science* 210:1259, 1980. Copyright 1980 by the American Association for the Advancement of Science.)

Table 9-2. Classification of normal and dysfunctional children by stepwise discriminant function

	Group	Sample Size	% Classified as	
			Normal	Abnormal
Original discriminant function	N-I	n = 153	86.3	13.7
	LD_1	n = 89	33.7	66.3
Independent replication				
	N-II	n = 153	78.4	21.6
	SLD	n = 159	53.5	46.5
	LD_2	n = 50	24.0	76.0
	LD_3	n = 71	21.1	79.9
	NEURO	n = 462	11.1	88.9

Note: LD_1 and LD_2 were selected only on the basis of academic performance. LD_3 had been referred to a pediatric neurologist because they were considered at risk for brain dysfunction by the referring physician.

Classification of Normal and Dysfunctional Children by Stepwise Discriminant Functions

Using only the univariate and multivariate neurometric features based on the relative power of the EEG in the four frequency bands, an optimized stepwise discriminant function was computed using one split-half of the U.S. normal group (N-I) and one learning-disabled group (LD_1). The classification accuracy achieved with this mixed "training set" of normal and dysfunctional children is shown in Table 9-2.

Table 9-2 shows the classification accuracy achieved by this stepwise discriminant in the two groups that composed the training set and in five additional groups that composed the "test set" used to provide independent replications of the training set results. For each group, Table 9-2 presents the percentage classified as "normal" and the percentage classified as "abnormal." Inspection of the results on the training set (split-half N-I and group LD_1) show that 86.3 percent of the normal children in the training set were correctly classified as normal, while 66.3 percent of the LD children in the training set were correctly classified as abnormal.

Table 9-2 shows that 78.4 percent of the normal children in the independent test set were correctly classified, using the discriminant function derived from the training set. Approximately 47 percent of the SLD group, 76 percent of the LD_2, 80 percent of the LD_3, and 89 percent of the NEURO group were classified as abnormal. These results constitute independent replications of the classification accuracy of the discriminant function and demonstrate that reliable differences in patterns of abnormal neurometric EEG features exist between groups of normal children and dysfunctional children.

Preliminary results show that different behavior deficits seem to be associated with different profiles of neurometric abnormality [21, 22, 32]. These differential behavioral correlates of particular profiles of neurometric abnormality cannot be presented in the limited space available for this chapter.

Sensitivity of Multivariate Neurometric Features to Brain Dysfunction
The results of classification using stepwise discriminant functions, presented in the previous section, demonstrate that the neurometric measures contained in the abnormality matrix are not highly redundant. While the incidence of significantly abnormal univariate neurometric features in dysfunctional children ranges from 10 to 40 percent, the stepwise discriminant function that utilizes multiple features achieves 80 to 90 percent classification accuracy. This finding justifies the expectation that multivariate Mahalanobis distance features, which combine multiple univariate neurometric measures while correcting for their intercorrelations, should display an even higher incidence of abnormal findings by concatenation of weak effects.

Table 9-3 shows the incidence of positive findings significant at the .05 level for several "whole head" neurometric features: $\bar{Z}_{FREQ}$, maturational lag, developmental deviation, $\bar{Z}_{COH}$, $\bar{Z}_{ASYM}$, $\bar{Z}_{HEAD}$, $\bar{Z}_{ABS\ POW}$ and $\bar{Z}_{TOTAL\ POW\ ASYM}$. These data are tallied separately for eight groups: split-half N-I used for development of initial normative values (n = 153), split-half N-II used for independent replication of the norms developed from N-I (n = 153), the "clinical norm" group constructed by subsequent combination of N-I and N-II (n = 306), the SLD group (n = 159), group LD_1 and LD_2 (n = 139) and LD_3 (n = 71), and the NEUROLOGICAL group (n = 377) minus its epileptic subgroup (n = 85).

Inspection of Table 9-3 shows that the incidence of false-positives at the .05 level is no more than 5.9 percent in N-I and no more than 7.8 percent in N-II. This was considered an acceptable independent replication of our estimates of the distribution of these various multivariate features in the normal population. Accordingly, N-I and N-II were combined (Clinical Norms). In this combined normal group, no multivariate feature displayed an incidence of false-positives greater than 5.0 percent at the .05 confidence level.

The neurometric feature $\bar{Z}_{FREQ}$ showed an increase in significant (positive) findings that ranges from 30.2 to 52.9 percent in the five dysfunctional groups. Maturational lag showed an incidence of false-positives of 4.9 percent in the clinical norms group and fluctuated between 26.4 and 35.3 percent in the dysfunctional groups. Developmental deviation showed no incidence of false-positives in the normal groups and ranged from 3.8 to 17.7 percent in the dysfunctional groups. Absolute power abnormalities ranged from 10.0 to 49.1 percent in the dysfunctional groups. $\bar{Z}_{COH}$ ranged from 10.7 to 38.8 percent, $\bar{Z}_{ASYM}$ from 9.4 to 27.1 percent, and $\bar{Z}_{HEAD}$, which combines overall frequency, coherence, and asymmetry features, from 30.8 to 60.0 percent. Total power asymmetry ranged from 5.0 to 18.8 percent. These data illustrate that the reliability and sensitivity of whole head Mahalanobis distance multivariate composites of neurometric EEG features substantially exceeds that of the constituent univariate features. At the time that this chapter was written, we had not yet incorporated these powerful new multivariate features into a step-

Table 9-3. Percent incidence of positive findings at .05 (.01) level[a] in multivariate features[b]

Group	$\bar{Z}_{FREQ}$	ML	DD	$\bar{Z}_{COH}$	$\bar{Z}_{ASYM}$	$\bar{Z}_{HEAD}$	$\bar{Z}_{ABS\ POW}$	$\bar{Z}_{TOTAL\ POW\ ASYM}$
Split-half N-I (n = 153)	5.2 (1.3)	5.2 (1.3)	0.0 (0.0)	5.2 (1.3)	5.2 (1.3)	5.2 (1.3)	5.2 (1.3)	5.9 (1.3)
Split-half N-II (n = 153)	3.3 (2.0)	4.5 (3.3)	0.0 (0.0)	5.9 (3.9)	7.8 (0.7)	6.5 (2.0)	6.5 (2.0)	4.6 (0.0)
Clinical norms (n = 306)	4.9 (1.0)	4.9 (1.0)	0.0 (0.0)	4.9 (1.0)	4.9 (1.0)	4.9 (1.0)	5.0 (1.0)	4.9 (1.0)
SLD (n = 159)	30.2 (20.1)	26.4 (22.0)	3.8 (0.0)	10.7 (6.9)	9.4 (3.1)	30.8 (19.5)	10.0 (6.3)	5.0 (0.6)
LD$_1$ + LD$_2$ (n = 139)	39.6 (25.9)	26.6 (20.1)	13.0 (5.8)	23.0 (13.7)	14.4 (7.9)	33.9 (28.1)	19.4 (15.1)	7.2 (4.3)
LD$_3$ (n = 71)	33.8 (28.2)	33.8 (22.5)	0.0 (5.7)	33.8 (23.9)	19.7 (14.1)	43.7 (35.2)	43.7 (40.8)	12.7 (4.2)
NEUROLOGICAL (n = 377)	45.4 (32.1)	35.3 (25.9)	10.1 (6.3)	31.6 (21.4)	27.1 (13.8)	54.6 (38.2)	49.1 (44.3)	14.1 (4.2)
Epileptic (n = 85)	52.9 (38.8)	35.2 (30.6)	17.7 (6.2)	38.8 (25.9)	24.7 (11.8)	60.0 (43.5)	34.1 (28.2)	18.8 (7.1)

[a]In each cell of this table, the percentage without parentheses refers to positive findings at the .05 level, and the percentage within parentheses refers to findings at the .01 level.
[b]In computing Mahalanobis distances, all terms in the covariance matrix referring to correlations between features in different anatomical regions were set to 0.

$\bar{Z}_{FREQ}$ = Mahalanobis distance across all relative power features across the whole head; ML = maturational lag across the whole head; DD = developmental deviation across the whole head; Z_{COH} = Mahalanobis distance across all coherence features across the whole head; Z_{ASYM} = Mahalanobis distance across all asymmetry features across the whole head; Z_{HEAD} = Mahalanobis distance across all relative power, coherence, and symmetry features across the whole head; $Z_{ABS\ POW}$ = Mahalanobis distance across absolute power features across the whole head; $Z_{TOTAL\ POW\ ASYM}$ = Mahalanobis distance across total power asymmetry across the whole head.

wise discriminant function; however, subsequent articles provide a detailed description of this method [21, 31]. Even if the classification accuracy of such a function were not significantly improved over one based on primarily univariate features, these multivariate compressions have one strong advantage. Recall the empirical "rule of thumb" that the ratio of subjects to variables should be at least 5:1 and preferably 10:1 if the structure of cluster analyses is to be expected to be replicable. Obviously, use of these multivariate compressed features should theoretically permit the definition of replicable clusters using a substantially smaller sample of subjects.

Extensions to Dysfunction in Adults: Preliminary Results

In an earlier section, we indicated that our normative age-regression equations had been extended to cover the age range from 6 to 90 years. Currently, we have accumulated reasonably substantial neurometric data on a variety of adult groups who have been evaluated as behaviorally normal or abnormal by clinical or behavioral criteria. The groups that have been thus studied include normal elderly subjects, elderly subjects with signs of cognitive impairment, normal mature adults who have been diagnosed as chronic alcoholics, manic-depressives, and victims of mild head injuries. Stepwise and multiple discriminant functions have been computed using neurometric EEG data from these various groups. Results [32] indicate that the same neurometric EEG features that permit accurate discrimination between normal and cognitively impaired children also permit accurate discrimination between normal and cognitively dysfunctional adults. Stepwise discriminant functions have been constructed that separate normal from cognitively impaired elderly subjects with no false-positives and 98-percent correct classification of patients with mild to moderate senile dementia. Further, these features appear to permit differential diagnosis of adult groups who display similar behavioral impairments attributable to different causal factors. Multiple discriminant functions have been constructed that separate normal adults, chronic alcoholics, manic-depressives, mild head-injury patients, and mildly and moderately impaired senile dementia patients (Alzheimer's disease) with 64- to 85-percent correct classification [31].

Electroencephalographic features not only may provide the basis for identification of individuals whose cognitive dysfunctions can be attributed to abnormal brain activity, but may also permit the subdivision of cognitively impaired adults with similar behavioral deficits into relatively homogeneous subgroups, each of which shares a common etiology and each of which may respond preferentially to a differentiated prescriptive intervention.

The optimal application of this new methodology requires systematic correlation of the outcome of different modes of treatment with different patterns of neurometric abnormality.

References

1. Ahn, H., et al. Developmental equations reflect brain dysfunctions. *Science* 210:1259, 1980.

2. Begleiter, H. (Ed.). *Evoked Brain Potentials and Behavior*. New York: Plenum, 1979.
3. Callaway, E., Tueting, P., and Koslow, S. (Eds.). *Event Related Potentials in Man*. New York: Academic, 1978.
4. Conely, R. *The Economics of Mental Retardation*. Springfield, Ill.: Thomas, 1973.
5. Desmedt, J. (Ed.). *Visual Evoked Potentials in Man*. Oxford: Clarendon, 1977.
6. Dolce, G., and Kunkel, H. (Eds.). *CEAN Computerized EEG Analysis*. Stuttgart: Fischer Verlag, 1975.
7. Fridman, J., et al. Quantification of maturational lag and functional deviation by neurometric evaluation of the EEG. In preparation.
8. Gasser, T., Bacher, P., and Mochs, J. Transformation towards the normal distribution of broad band spectrum parameters of the EEG. *Electroencephalogr. Clin. Neurophysiol.* 53:119, 1982.
9. Gergen, J., et al. Personal communication, 1965.
10. Gibbs, F. A., and Gibbs, E. L. *Atlas of Electroencephalography*, Vol. III. Cambridge, Mass.: Addison-Wesley, 1964.
11. Hagne, I., et al. Spectral Analysis Via Fast Fourier Transform of Waking EEG in Normal Infants. In P. Kellaway and I. Petersén (Eds.), *Automation of Clinical Electroencephalography*. New York: Raven, 1973.
12. Harmony, T. *Functional Neuroscience*, Vol. III: *Neurometric Assessment of Brain Dysfunction in Neurological Patients*. Hillsdale, N.J.: Erlbaum, 1984.
13. Harmony, T., et al. Polarity coincidence correlation coefficient and signal energy ratio of the ongoing EEG activity: I. Normative data. *Brain Res.* 61:133, 1973.
14. Health, Education and Welfare National Advisory Committee on Dyslexia and Related Reading Disorders. *Reading Disorders in the United States*. Washington, D.C.: Department of Health, Education and Welfare, 1969.
15. Hughes, J. R. Electroencephalography and Learning. In H. R. Myklebust (Ed.), *Progress in Learning Disabilities*, Vol. I. New York: Grune & Stratton, 1968.
16. Hughes, J. R., and Denckla, M. G. Outline of a Pilot Study of Electroencephalographic Correlates of Dyslexia. In A. L. Benton and D. Pearl (Eds.), *Dyslexia—An Appraisal of Current Knowledge*. New York: Oxford University Press, 1978.
17. Jasper, H. H. The ten-twenty electrode system of the International Federation. *Electroencephalogr. Clin. Neurophysiol.* 10:371, 1958.
18. John, E. R. *Functional Neuroscience*, Vol. II: *Neurometrics: Clinical Applications of Quantitative Electrophysiology*. Hillsdale, N.J.: Erlbaum, 1977.
19. John, E. R., Herrington, R. N., and Sutton, S. Effects of visual form on the evoked response. *Science* 155:1439, 1967.
20. John, E. R., et al. Developmental equations for the electrocephalogram. *Science* 210:1255, 1980.
21. John, E. R., et al. Neurometric evaluation of cognitive dysfunctions and neurological disorders in children. *Progr. Neurobiol.* 21:239, 1983.
22. Kaye, H., et al. Neurometric evaluation of learning disabled children. *Int. J. Neurosci.* 13:15, 1981.
23. Kellaway, P., and Petersén, I. (Eds.). *Automation of Clinical Electroencephalography*. New York: Raven, 1973.
24. Kinsbourne, M. Minimal Brain Dysfunction as a Neurodevelopmental Lag. In F. de la Cruz, B. H. Fox, and R. H. Roberts (Eds.), *Minimal Brain Dysfunction*. New York: New York Academy of Sciences, 1973. Pp. 268–273.
25. Kratoville, B. L. *Youth in Trouble*. San Rafael, Calif.: Academic Therapy Publications, 1974.

26. Matoušek, M., and Petersén, I. Frequency Analysis of the EEG in Normal Children and Adolescents. In P. Kellaway and I. Petersén (Eds.), *Automation of Clinical Electroencephalography*. New York: Raven, 1973.
27. Matoušek, M., and Petersén, I. Automatic evaluation of EEG background activity by means of age-dependent EEG quotients. *Electroencephalogr. Clin. Neurophysiol.* 35:603, 1973.
28. Menkes, M., Rowe, J. S., and Menkes, J. H. A twenty-four year follow-up study on hyperkinetic child with minimal brain dysfunction. *Pediatrics* 39:393, 1967.
29. Muehl, S., Knott, J., and Benton, A. EEG abnormality and psychological test performance in reading disability. *Cortex* 1:434, 1965.
30. Otto, D. (Ed.). *Multidisciplinary Perspectives in Event-Related Brain Potential Research*, EPA 600/9-77-043. Washington, D.C.: U.S. Government Printing Office, 1978.
31. Prichep, L., et al. Neurometric Electroencephalographic Characteristics of Dementia. In B. Reisberg (Ed.), *Alzheimer's Disease: The Standard Reference*. New York: The Free Press, 1983.
32. Prichep, L., et al. Neurometrics: Quantitative Evaluation of Brain Dysfunction in Children. In M. Rutter (Ed.), *Developmental Neuropsychiatry*. London: Guilford, 1983.
33. Regan, D. *Evoked Potentials in Psychology, Sensory Physiology and Clinical Medicine*. London: Wiley-Interscience, 1972.
34. Satterfield, J. H., et al. Physiological studies of the hyperkinetic child. *Am. J. Psychiatry* 128:1418, 1972.
35. U.S. Bureau of the Census. *Statistical Abstract of the U.S., 1971 Census*. Washington, D.C.: U.S. Government Printing Office, 1971.
36. Wender, P. H. *Minimal Brain Dysfunction in Children*. New York: Wiley-Interscience, 1971.
37. Wikler, A., Dixon, J. F., and Parker, J. B. Brain function in problem children and controls: Psychometric, neurological, and electroencephalographic comparisons. *Am. J. Psychiatry* 127:634, 1970.

10 Motor Coordination in Dyslexic Children: Theoretical and Clinical Implications

Martha Bridge Denckla

Since the publications of Samuel Torrey Orton, developmentally dyslexic children have been described as frequently exhibiting the pattern of hand and eye preference known as mixed dominance. This, along with other minor but repeatedly observable motor characteristics, has long been noted by educators and clinicians who deal with many dyslexic children. For example, Critchley [4] and Benton and Pearl [2] cited reports of fine motor coordination problems and "perceptual-motor" difficulties (known to educators as "eye-hand" problems) among developmentally dyslexic children. In this chapter, I will explore the specific characteristics of the skill and preference patterns of dyslexic children, as contrasted with those of other types of learning-disabled children (e.g., the attention deficit disorder/hyperactive group or the nondyslexic, otherwise learning-disabled group).

Since Chapter 3 addresses the development of an inclusionary set of biological characteristics for the definition of dyslexia, I will limit myself to drawing an enclusionary circle around the term *dyslexia,* to distinguish it especially from "dyslexia-plus," which includes a very large group of children who have elements of both dyslexia and attention deficit disorder. In other words, when I use the word *dyslexia* in the pages that follow, I am subscribing to the usual exclusion of motor handicaps in the sense of cerebral palsy, of classic or traditional neurological impairment, and of visual, auditory, other sensory, major psychiatric, and intellectual deficits. Roughly speaking, I am therefore subscribing to the World Federation of Neurology definition of dyslexia with the further particular refinement of the exclusion of children with elements of attention deficit disorder. The present criteria for considering a child free of dyslexia-plus attentional characteristics are the following: below-threshold scores on the teacher and parent rating scales of Connors [3]; normal scores on observational tests of impulsivity, vigilance, and continuance performance; and in the clinical interview with parents and other referring personnel, absence of anecdotal history of problems with attention or conformity behavior.

Both practical and theoretical implications follow from a careful description of the coordination deficits of dyslexic children. There is, for example, a common tendency among some clinicians to use the word *dyspraxia* rather liberally, even in reference to disorders that these clinicians regard as coordination deficits, related to brainstem or vestibular connections. This leads to considerable confusion, since parents are exposed to the same term used in quite diverse ways, with disparate implications by different professionals who also make quite different recommendations based on their understanding of the motor descriptor terminology. Furthermore, it has recently been stressed that even within the medical profession there is considerable misunderstanding of the nonspecific developmental awkwardness often seen as a correlate of dyslexia, which some may attribute to "cerebellar" dysfunction. Far from being harmless, the utilization of such terminology, which inevitably leads to many different interpretations, has been one of the factors leading to pharmacological therapies directed toward parts of the nervous system that appear to have little direct relevance to the acquisition of reading skills. One such example is afforded by theories of dyslexia based on defects in cerebellar or the oculomotor tracking performance, which have in turn led to particular forms of pharmacological intervention.

Motor Characteristics of Learning-Disabled Children

Let us return to previous descriptions of children designated as dyslexic. One excellent epidemiological study that addressed these issues did not use the term *dyslexia;* instead it investigated the children who met the criterion of reading underachievement in the entire population of one California town. The underachieving readers were matched not only with same-sex siblings who had scored normally in reading, but also with the remainder of the control population. This study, which is liberally quoted and reviewed in Benton and Pearl [2], found that poor rapid alternating finger movements in the classic neurological examination were the sole finding distinguishing the developmentally reading-disabled group from the control group. In addition, eye-hand impairment was documented by means of performance on the task of design-copying in the Bender-Gestalt test, widely used by school psychologists in the diagnosis of neurologically based learning disabilities. These elementary-school-age poor readers in Palo Alto did indeed copy the Bender-Gestalt designs poorly compared to their own normally achieving siblings and peers. However, the use of a clever maneuver helped to avoid "ego assault" and at the same time get at the issue of separating "perception" from "motor function." The researchers in this study gave each of the dyslexic children a paper of another child to score. The researchers then evaluated the *judgment* of reproductive accuracy on the part of every child participating in this study. It was determined that the poor copiers were better judges of accuracy of others. The judgmental level of accuracy of the reading-disabled children was closer to that of professional psychologists than was that of their siblings or peers who were reading normally! This study, the largest survey of an entire population done in the United States, indicates that there are perceptual-motor and fine motor impairments in a large group of dyslexic children (not pure in the sense of having been separated out neurologically or by questionnaire, but homogeneous in the sense that all were attending normal public schools). There are strong suggestions that the "perceptual" part of the perceptual-motor is not the important locus of the problem.

Careful observation has often confirmed that the elementary-school-age child referred for a reading problem often also performs below age level on copy-forms tests. Further, the child appears to have some knowledge of his own poor performance, but he is unable to make the pencil do his bidding! Whether it be the Bender-Gestalt or the Beery-Buktenica visual-motor integration test (VMI), difficulties are often observed in executing the angles in the designs, completing the contact at the corners, and generally achieving precision. At the Boston Children's Hospital Learning Disabilities Clinic, we also noticed that many times the best design completed on the VMI was surprisingly more difficult than the simpler designs, where errors were made and formal scores were given for precision of copying. Another remarkable clinical observation is that although poor copying was a pretty reliable correlate of reading retardation in most cases before the age of 11 years, in longitudinally followed cases this particular correlate seemed to have disappeared by junior high school. A problem that may arise in the school system when this occurs is that the child is often classified as "an emotional problem," since school psychologists have relied very heavily on the poor eye-hand coordination or copying tasks as an indicator or marker of physical or biological dysfunction as opposed to environmental-emotional dysfunction. The controversy, Is it neurological or is it emotional?, emerged regularly as longitudinally followed dyslexic children passed over the pubertal line and rapidly became excellent copiers of whatever materials were placed before them.

Performance on the Rey-Osterreith Complex Figure, a critical tool with which I also became familiar through my colleagues at the Boston Children's Hospital Learning Disabilities Clinic, gave further evidence of the nature of the early problems of dyslexics. There were difficulties with internal detail, with mutual articulation of lines, and more generally, with the precise characteristics of the figure to be copied. It was dramatic to find that these disorders were often coupled with an extraordinarily good spontaneous memory for the general configuration (with a tendency toward rotation of the figures by 90% and toward "emptiness" of the insides of the configuration). As these children are followed into adolescence, we see the same change described on the performance of copy-forms tests, that is, the subjects frequently become excellent copiers of this complex design, even with respect to the inner details. In general, however, the rotation problem and the tendency to *recall* more of the configurational and relational aspects than the details persist.

Another remarkable clinical observation is that of a visible shift in pencil grasp, depending on the task, in this reading-disabled population. When the subject shifts from a precision-oriented copying task or, even more spectacularly, from a writing to a drawing task, one observes a change in the pencil grasp from a cramped grasp with distally collapsed fingers to a grasp in which the pencil is more loosely held with several fingers, much in the manner of a paintbrush or a large piece of chalk to be used on a chalkboard. Broad, free, flowing lines emerge. As the figure being drawn becomes less constrained and less detail-oriented, the grasp and line quality become freer and more flowing.

Another interesting clinical observation is the fact that the examination of motor coordination in the office seems to have minimal correlation with the individual history of athletic ability. On the other hand, I have recently found in an analytical review of my records that tests of spatial ability correlate highly with a history of athletic ability. There is a particularly strong positive correlation between spatial scores and success in sports, especially in team sports requiring awareness of placement of other players. Thus, again, one has to be careful about the word *coordination* and its implications, even when one is not using neurological terminology such as *apraxic* or *cerebellar* to arrive at therapeutic implications. Coordination, however tested in the office, appears to have a kind of "hothouse" specificity, which, related to certain subsystems of the "motor analyzer" [11] and office findings, should not be used by the clinician to extrapolate to real-life skills across the board. It is particularly ironic that what most of us think of immediately when the word *coordination* is mentioned, namely athletic skills, is very poorly correlated with the motor coordination testing we do in our standard neurological examination of repetitive and alternating movements.

Another observation that illustrates changes over time and the different definitions of coordination comes from the studies of Denckla, Rudel, and Broman [9] on map-walking. We used the test first developed by Semmes and associates [15] in studying head injury cases from World War II and Korean War veterans' groups. Dots are placed on the floor, and the subject is required to follow a path given on a piece of cardboard on which a route is outlined in ink, connecting ink dots that correspond to those on the floor. We studied dyslexic, otherwise learning-disabled, and normal control children. The younger dyslexic children, that is, children below the age of 10 years (and therefore prepubertal) had the worst performance of the three groups, as measured by walking these routes correctly. A startling "late blooming" effect, however, shone forth in the data on children over 10 years old. The teenaged dyslexic group, and in particular the familial dyslexic adolescents, demonstrated superior performance on this test, averaging better scores than the nondyslexic, otherwise learning-disabled and the normal groups.

Possible Interpretations of Clinical Data

What could these results possibly mean, and what do they have to do with the history of good athletic ability, which is so startlingly disassociated from the office coordination studies? In addition, what do they have to do with the "outgrowing" poor Bender-Gestalt copying? After discussing this for many years, Dr. Rudel and I have come to the conclusion that the most parsimonious explanation is as follows: the part of the "motor analyzer" that is dependent on the left hemisphere and has been found to be important for timed, sequential, detailed movements is deficient in the first decade of life in this group of children whom we call dyslexic. We have proposed a maturational lag in this system. Thus, even if there is an inefficient or deficient substrate on the left side of the brain, this motor system, whatever its nomenclature may be, can mature so as to reach an adequate level at or around the time of puberty; previously "locked-in" abilities of a spatial and visual-perceptual nature now become available to the child. In other words, even when there is lifelong deficiency of certain left hemisphere–subserved capabilities, those that are part of the motor analyzer system in the left hemisphere may improve sufficiently to act as a means of expression for the adequate or even above-average functioning of a presumably right hemisphere–subserved set of capabilities, such as athletics and perception of spatial relationships and visual design.

Recent Investigations of Motor Development

Let us turn now to some limited studies that we have carried out on a particular aspect of motor behavior, rapid repetitive and alternating movements. In the early 1970s, I performed a survey of large populations in the normal school system [5, 6]. I obtained normative data on toe taps, heel-toe alternations, hand pats, hand pronation-supination alternations, and finger repetitive and successive opposition to thumb alternating sequences. (In addition, recent data have been collected on tongue wiggles! These are not included in the results given below.) In 1978, Denckla and Rudel [8] described the anomalies of motor coordination in a carefully defined group of attention deficit disorder children, then still referred to as hyperactive. The children were selected for freedom from traditional neurological findings, however subtle. In addition, they were performing normally in school such that they were not learning disabled, even in the educational or legal sense. They were found by linear discriminant function analysis to be readily distinguished by the motor examination. The following features were particularly useful: (1) total body overflow movements, that is, synkinetic movements in the hands on moving the feet and mirror movements occurring extraneously during motor performances of the rapid repetitive and alternating types, and (2) very slow performance with the feet. This latter point appeared to be a confirmation of immaturity, since it is well-known to child neurologists that the development of motor control proceeds from head to feet (cephalocaudad). The excess overflow also appears to reflect "motor immaturity."

More recently, we have completed a study of a group of purely dyslexic children, defined on the basis of poor reading performance but completely free of questionnaire, historical, or examinational evidence of attention deficit characteristics. We were able to obtain a test group of 40 children who met these stringent criteria. When the same analysis of motor behavior was applied to them as had been applied to their peers diagnosed as having hyperactivity or attention deficit disorder, it was found that a quite different motoric picture emerged. First, they were not characterized by excessive overflow, so that age-specific lack of inhibition of the motor system was not characteristic of the pure dyslexic population. Second, they were not particularly slow and in fact were faster than the control group on several of the motor tasks. Only at ages 7 and 8 years were the dyslexic children slower than controls on the toe taps, and only at age 8 were they slower on the sequence of successive opposition of fingers and thumbs. On formal examination the sequencing often appeared awkward and effortful; it had to be rehearsed to be gotten in the correct sequence. This kind of "dyspraxic" learning of finger sequencing was not, however, reflected in the speed of execution once the sequence had been mastered. The other overall characteristic of the dyslexic group was a tendency toward large right-left differences, that is, a tendency for the left side, normally somewhat slower in a right-preferring population such as this one, to be even more so, excessively slow.

The last finding, really the only one of theoretical interest in the study of the motor behavior of the pure dyslexic group, reminded us of the findings of Badian and Wolff [1], who have found that dyslexic boys did more poorly with their left hands than did controls in performing a task of alternative rhythmic tapping entrained to a metronome. These boys were not inferior to controls when tapping with the right hand alone or the left hand alone, nor was their right-hand performance during the alternative rhythmic tapping inferior to that of controls. The performance of the left hand was inferior in the dyslexics only when entrained to a rhythm that had to alternate with the right hand. Badian and Wolff suggested that this might indicate a "significant delay in interhemisphere cooperation" as one of the mechanisms underlying dyslexia.

It is a frequent clinical observation that young children referred for poor progress in reading, particularly at the ages of 7 and 8 years, show large right-left differences such that they are frequently unable even to perform pantomimes of common daily activities with the left hand in response to verbal command. This observation is the more spectacular in referrals from among 6-year-olds because these children are considered to be at risk at the end of the kindergarten year. In addition, although there is no excessive overflow in these young predyslexic or dyslexic children, there is often observed a left-to-right (i.e., asymmetrical) elicitation of mirror movements during the pattern portion of the motor coordination battery, namely, with hand pronation-supination and successive finger-thumb opposition and to a lesser extent with heel-toe alternation.

What Does "Mixed Dominance" Mean?

Let us now return to the original observation of Orton on the motor characteristics of dyslexic populations and their mixed dominance. Mixed dominance in dyslexics refers in the great majority of cases to preference for the right *hand* but the left *eye*. Left-handedness per se has not been found to be more common among the dyslexic population than among the normal population, although this may be due to inadequate assessment of handedness. There is some suggestion that familial non-right-handedness is more common among dyslexics despite personal right-handedness. Perinatal research project data of the early 1970s document the fact that right-handed, left-eyed children constitute about 30 percent of the normal population. (It should be noted that one must rule out strabismus, ocular anomalies, and anisocoria or unequal visual acuity before one may conclude that the eyedness of any individual gives any information about the inferred "brainedness.") Over many years of observations of the preference patterns of a population referred for study of possible learning disabilities, it has been found that 60 percent of this clinical population demonstrates a right-handed, left-eyed pattern. In so overwhelming a majority that it does not even require statistical methodology to validate, these same persons have a first-degree left-handed relative [7]. During each year 1980 through 1983, the "reading referral" group in my practice was 70-percent right-handed and left-eyed.

In follow-up analysis, there does not appear to be any shift in preference patterns after the age of 6 years. Children who are right-handed and left-eyed who are performing tasks such as drawing a design that has no "conventional" directionality in ordinary linguistic usage very frequently draw from right to left. Yet, they will revert to the left-to-right direction when dealing with the learned convention of the English language. Furthermore, when asked to count a randomly assorted group of items scattered on a table in a nonlinear fashion, these same children will often use the right index finger to point to the items in a counterclockwise pattern. A study is now being planned that will further investigate this phenomenon and will also investigate the drawing of circles by nursery school children who have not yet had extensive instruction in the left-to-right direction of the reading or writing of English text. We will be recording whether the drawing of a circle is performed in the clockwise or counterclockwise direction. In addition, pennies will be spread randomly on a table for counting. Preliminary investigations indicate that a preference for proceeding from right to left or counterclockwise dominates the behavior of the preschool right-handed, left-eyed person.

What could be the theoretical significance of mixed dominance? In terms of practical implications, it is clearly not a cause in and of itself of failure to acquire skills of reading, but it does appear to be a factor requiring an additional level of conscious activity in the reading process in the early years. Mixed dominance, when occurring simultaneously with linguistic inefficiencies (see Chap. 3, for example), may be a risk factor because it is another thing with which the child must consciously deal. One first-grader explained to me that each time he wants to write a number, "I think of the way I like to see the numbers go and then write it in the opposite direction!" This clearly requires an added level of effort in the act of writing, which is stressful for a child who has other linguistic inefficiencies with which to cope. In a multifactorial within-brain model of the inefficiencies that underlie dyslexia, mixed dominance may be an early but relevant component.

Neurologically, mixed dominance may indicate that although handedness is dependent on a certain motor analyzer superiority when the hand is programmed on the left side of the brain, the oculomotor system, or the gaze system, may have its preponderant programming in the right hemisphere. Elsewhere, I have discussed the underlying relationship of eye preference to gaze rather than to visual field [8], referring to the work of a Canadian psychologist who demonstrated that only in the scanning condition is eye preference manifest in terms of skill.

Thus, Orton's concept of mixed dominance may be important not in terms of "competing engrams" in the visual field but rather in terms of competing motor coordination systems in the anterior portions of the brain. Rather than emphasizing a mirroring of the incoming information on the two sides, this model emphasizes the fact that the way in which a child actively gathers and reproduces information may be at conflict if he has oculomotor activity controlled predominantly by the right hemisphere and the motor control over the pencil used for copying controlled predominantly by the left hemisphere.

What theoretical possibilities exist to explain the findings about large left-right differences? Of relevance are several electroencephalographic studies (e.g., [10], [16]) showing lesser interhemispheric coherence function in dyslexics. The large left-right difference may indeed reflect "deficient interhemispheric cooperation" in the elementary-school-age group, arising out of the delayed development of some neural system. This may be the callosal system. Using the term *callosal* does not imply that a defect need be present in the fibers of the callosum; collosal transmission can be impaired by lesions in the cells of origin of the callosal fibers in the cortex or in the cortical cells on which the callosal fibers synapse. This is a point that has been repeatedly emphasized by Geschwind in his teaching. Thus, the large left-right difference with its implication of faulty hemispheric integration or cooperation does not necessarily differ in its implication from the evidence that suggests an inefficient, deficient, or maturationally delayed left hemisphere in the population of dyslexics [13, 14]. In fact, some of the previously presented data in this chapter on the shift during the second decade of life from poor map-walking to good map-walking and from poor copying of design to adequate copying of design, as well as the anecdotal accounts of late blooming in dyslexics, may be related to maturation to some adequate threshold level by some critical system within the left hemisphere. Such a maturation would then allow the superior capabilities of the right side of the brain to be allied with the now-adequate motor analyzer or motor programmer within the left hemisphere. (This type of motor maturation does not necessarily imply a parallel maturation of linguistic capabilities.) Thus, what has been "money in the bank" can now be usefully withdrawn and displayed.

Conclusions

Let me close with some clinical considerations. Consider the young dyslexic children who have poor control over a pencil in writing but can use that pencil in a broader, more brush-stroke-like fashion. Since we are concerned with providing kinesthetic experience to the central nervous system on the shapes of letters, let us use the blackboard, where the broad strokes of the upper arm using the chalk can be more comfortable for the child. In addition, since we are cognizant of the eventual improvement in the ability to copy designs, let us refrain from wasting the child's time with so-called prerequisite training that will make him the proud copier of designs but will probably not carry over into writing behavior. Let us also be constantly aware of the probability that our evaluations will show certain strengths. These strengths should be reported both to the parents and to other professionals so that they can search out activities that will bolster the total self-esteem and the "social currency" of the adjustment of the child. Such activities might include early involvement in music, art, athletics, crafts, or any other nonacademic skills that will give him the strength to carry on in his struggle to reach a "good enough" level in the academic ("three Rs") areas. In short, let us carefully follow the rule of prima non nocere, including the avoidance of unproved and time-wasting therapies; let us select our remedial procedures with a better knowledge of the natural history of the condition, and let us act as advocates for the child's talents.

References

1. Badian, N., and Wolff, P. Manual asymmetries of motor sequencing in boys with reading disability. *Cortex* 13:343, 1977.
2. Benton, A. L., and Pearl, D. (Eds.). *Dyslexia: An Appraisal of Current Knowledge*. New York: Oxford University Press, 1978.
3. Connors, C. K. Rating scales for use in drug studies with children. *Psychopharmacol. Bull.* special issue:24, 1973.
4. Critchley, M. *The Dyslexic Child*. Springfield, Ill.: Thomas, 1970.
5. Denckla, M. B. Development of speed in repetitive and successive finger movements in normal children. *Dev. Med. Child Neurol.* 15:635, 1973.
6. Denckla, M. B. Development of motor coordination in normal children. *Dev. Med. Child Neurol.* 16:729, 1974.
7. Denckla, M. B. Childhood Language and Learning Disabilities. In K. Heilman and E. Valenstein (Eds.), *Clinical Neuropsychology*. New York: Oxford University Press, 1979.
8. Denckla, M. B., and Rudel, R. G. Anomalies of motor development in hyperactive boys. *Ann. Neurol.* 3:231, 1978.
9. Denckla, M. B., Rudel, R. G., and Broman, M. The Development of a Spatial Orientation Skill in Normal, Learning-Disabled, and Neurologically Impaired Children. In D. Caplan (Ed.), *Biological Studies of Mental Processes*. Cambridge, Mass.: MIT Press, 1980.
10. Leisman, G., and Ashkenazi, M. Aetiological factors in dyslexia: IV. Cerebral hemispheres are functionally equivalent. *Neuroscience* 11:157, 1980.
11. Luria, A. R. Investigations of Motor Functions. In *Higher Cortical Functions in Man*. New York: Basic Books, 1966.
12. Owen, F. W., et al. Learning Disorders in Children: Sibling Studies, Serial #133. *Monogr. Soc. Res. Child Dev.* 1971.
13. Rourke, B. P. Reading Retardation in Children: Developmental Lag or Deficit? In R. M. Knights and D. J. Bakker (Eds.), *The Neuropsychology of Learning Disorders*. Baltimore: University Park Press, 1976.
14. Satz, P. Cerebral Dominance and Reading Disability: An Old Problem Revisited. In R. M. Knights and D. J. Bakker (Eds.), *The Neuropsychology of Learning Disorders*. Baltimore: University Park Press, 1976.
15. Semmes, J., et al. Correlates of impaired orientation in personal and extrapersonal space. *Brain* 86:747, 1963.
16. Sklar, B., Hanley, J., and Simmons, W. W. A computer analysis of EEG spectral signatures from normal and dyslexic children. *I.E.E.E. Trans. Biomed. Eng.* WME-20 (1):20, 1973.

11 Biological Foundations of Reading
Norman Geschwind

The Origins of Written Language

Reflecting on the biology of reading brings to mind a statement created for a different purpose but readily adaptable to my topic. The original version stated that there were more scientists living at this moment than in all past ages combined. It probably takes little calculation to come to the conclusion that the same is true for those who are literate, that is, there are probably more literate people now living than in all past periods combined. This is an important fact in any discussion of the biological basis of the capacity to read. While spoken language is the almost universal endowment of humans, it is likely that 100 years ago there was not one country in the world in which the majority of the population was literate. Even in the 1870s, Carl Wernicke, discussing the anatomical foundations of language, pointed out that the average patient seen by the neurologist was not endowed with the capacity to understand written language, a statement that achieves its full significance only when one realizes that Wernicke was talking about one of the most advanced societies in the world. Furthermore, written language, in the sense in which we use the term, is of remarkably recent origin. The usual estimates place the beginnings of written language no more than 10,000 years ago. It is possible that the real origins of written language lie in some more remote period of time, since our judgment must rely on the existence of documents on which writing appears. The dramatic recent investigations of Alexander Marshack on the cultural development of early human beings raise the possibility that written language existed earlier than is conventionally thought. Marshack has pointed out that as long ago as 30,000 years humans were already creating elaborate designs on pieces of bone. It was thought in the last century, and even well into this one, that these carvings simply represented decorations until Marshack showed quite clearly that those ancient humans who had scored the surface of those ancient bones were, in fact, producing methodical sets of marks. One is tempted to wonder as to whether some of the markings on these early artifacts were already early forms of writing, but for the moment this is purely speculative.

One may well ask why in a discussion of the biological foundations of reading so much time should be spent on the question of the first development of written language. The answer is that although we may never be able to ascertain the truth, it is of great theoretical importance whether written lan-

---

Supported in part by grants from the National Science Foundation (BNS 7823610), the National Institutes of Health (NS 14018-03 and NS 06209), the Orton Research Fund, and the Essel Foundation.

guage has a very long human history or a very short one. Let me clarify the reasons for this statement.

If written language appeared in some form a very long time ago, one could conjecture that even if the capacity for comprehending written language was present at that period in only a few humans, the processes of natural selection might lead to a spread of this capacity to the entire population. It should be pointed out, however, that even if written language were of very ancient origin, the fact that the majority of humans over most of history would not have had the opportunity to learn to read still makes it questionable that evolutionary selection would have played a role in ensuring the spread of this capacity throughout the population.

If, on the other hand, writing is a human invention, then one can argue that the capacity for reading must have a neurological basis that appeared because of its importance for some function other than reading itself; 5,000 years would not have been long enough for a widespread evolutionary change to take place in the human brain in all societies. Furthermore, we know that reading can be learned by most members of any society even when no ancestor of any member of that population was ever exposed to the written word.

The Acquisition of Reading

We must therefore account for the fact that most humans can learn to read, even in cases where they have had no literate ancestors. How can we account for this talent for reading, which appears to be latent in every population, despite the lack of contact with reading at any point in the evolution of that society? There are a couple of possibilities that might account for this. One might simply argue that the capacity to read is really not a *special* talent of humans and is rather like the capacity to learn to repair engines, which presumably depends on several of the inherited specializations of the brain. This type of explanation would also help to account for the fact that learning to read is usually a very slow process when compared to the capacity to acquire spoken language. A capacity that depends on a particular special innate brain system is usually very rapidly acquired, while one that depends on learning new linkages between many such systems is usually learned slowly. Spoken language comes quickly without special instruction, while, by contrast, even simple but not innately programmed acts such as tying one's shoelaces may require a remarkably long learning period. The years required in school for an adequate mastery of reading suggest that reading is in the latter class of skill acquisition.

There is, however, at least one piece of evidence that suggests this interpretation may be incorrect. That is, there appear to be some circumstances in which reading is acquired very rapidly. Before presenting this example, it is necessary to consider briefly exactly what is meant by *reading*. This may appear to be a simple question, since most people would assume that it means something like the ability to extract meaning from arbitrary visual linguistic symbols on paper or stone or some other such substance. I would argue, however, that this definition is too narrow. It is probably more reasonable to define *reading* as the ability to extract meaning from *any* type of visual representation of language. I would thus include in *reading* not merely the comprehension of the written language systems of the West, the hieroglyphics of ancient Egypt, and the ideographic languages of the Far East, but also the sign languages of the deaf. We are accustomed, as I have noted, to thinking that reading is a difficult task, since children almost universally acquire the comprehension of written language at a far slower pace than that of auditory language. Ursula Bellugi of the Salk Institute has, however, brought forth evidence that the congenitally deaf child born into a deaf family, and therefore exposed only to the sign language of the deaf, acquires it at high speed; in fact, she believes that the rate of acquisition of sign language by such children is comparable to that of the acquisition of spoken language by the hearing child. This finding therefore suggests that the brain does indeed contain a system that makes it possible to acquire linguistic symbol systems rapidly, regardless of the primary modality.

The Need to Communicate with Conspecifics

We are thus faced with an apparent paradox. There appears to be considerable evidence that reading is difficult for most children. Another measure of this difficulty is perhaps indicated by the fact that the number of people who are dyslexic, and thus have special difficulty in acquiring reading, is much higher than the number of children who have difficulty in acquiring spoken language. Yet we are also told that the congenitally deaf learn to "read" manual sign language very rapidly. We must therefore draw one of two conclusions. Either learning sign language is not equivalent to learning written language, or there is another factor at play that has not yet been considered. I will now argue that the latter may well be the case. Another important set of data casts light on a rather neglected aspect of language learning. When a child of, let us say, 5 years of age is moved from his own linguistic community to another one, he rapidly acquires the second language, and it is indeed not rare to find children who, in the course of movements among different countries in childhood, have acquired superb command of several languages—each spoken without an accent. Yet, when a child who has acquired his first language with great ease studies a second language *in school* he typically acquires only a mediocre knowledge, even if the teaching is begun at a very early age. The expectation that early teaching of foreign languages in school would make this type of learning easy has not been fulfilled. Let me advance the speculation that in order to acquire a language well *two* necessary conditions must be fulfilled. The first of these is the appropriate neurological substrate for language, and the second is the condition of being placed in an environment in which communication with one's peers is impossible unless one acquires the language.

This speculation, if correct, might have implications not only for the neurology of language acquisition, but perhaps even for the practical teaching of such skills as reading and foreign languages. In addition, it might have certain implications for the capacities of the dyslexic child. We know that, in general, dyslexic children have much more difficulty than the average child in learning foreign languages. It is reasonable, therefore, to ask about what happens to the dyslexic child whose parents move to another language community. I would predict that he would acquire the new language quite easily. It would not be surprising if he acquired it more slowly than the nondyslexic child, but the learning would probably still take place at a high rate. There is evidence suggesting that dyslexic children tend to acquire their first language more slowly than do nondyslexics, but it is clear that in most cases the first language is fairly readily mastered. In other words, the dyslexic may differ from the normal child in his neurological substrate, but under certain conditions of motivation, that is, the need to communicate with others, he will still acquire language quite readily. In contrast to the normal child, however, he has much more difficulty when the motivation for acquisition of a new language is relatively weak, that is, when this learning is not essential for communication with his peers. Thus, one might predict that if a child who would have been dyslexic were born deaf or became deaf at a very early age, he would still acquire sign language, that is, a visual language, quite well. Furthermore, if he became deaf *after* his acquisition of spoken language, he would also acquire sign language rapidly, although his capacity to learn written language of the usual form remained poor. He would thus acquire a particular type of visual language because it was essential to master it in order to communicate with others. This suggests that a dyslexic with adequate verbal communication skills who decided to learn sign language out of interest would find it far more difficult than would a nondyslexic.

The influence on the acquisition of language systems of the desire for communication with another member of the same species is thus probably extremely important. The motivation involved may well be a highly specific one, since it is quite likely that built into the nervous system of almost every species is a strong tendency to observe and learn from conspecifics. The biological importance of this inborn tendency is easy to understand. It makes sense that animals should be so designed that they learn most readily from observation of members of their own species, who are far more likely to have those stores of knowledge necessary for their survival than are members of other species. E. Roy John showed some years ago that a kitten can learn to perform certain tasks by observing another cat carrying them out. The kitten is furthermore more likely to learn these tasks if the mother is performing them than if the other cat is simply a random member of the species. It would be important to find out whether the kitten observing not another cat, but, for example, a dog or a monkey learning the same task, would learn less effectively or conceivably not at all.

These speculations may appear to be remote from our central concern of the neurology of reading, but I would argue that they are not. We must perhaps reformulate our notions concerning the learning of language in the following fashion: Language learning proceeds most rapidly when the child acquires a system of communication that is absolutely necessary for communication with peers. The neurological basis of language learning will therefore consist not only of the neurological substrate for language itself, but also of that remarkably powerful biological system that creates a necessity for interaction with other members of the same species. Let me recall the remarkable experiments that Harry Harlow carried out in Wisconsin some years ago. Infant monkeys were raised under unusual conditions, including that of contact with a nonliving "mother" who might supply food and warmth but did not move. The animal raised under these conditions was distinctly abnormal in adult life. Perhaps the most surprising finding was, however, that adult abnormalities were most striking when monkeys were raised without contact with others of the same age group. The permanent severe social impairment of these animals, which included not only isolation from the simian community but also failure to acquire normal sexual activity, reveals how powerful neurologically is the contact with conspecifics, especially those of the same age group.

It is conceivable that it is the lack of the neurological substrate for the motivation to communicate with conspecifics that may underlie certain dramatic developmental disorders that are often described as failures to acquire language. Thus, the autistic child is typically nonverbal. Yet he is likely to be far more impaired overall than is the child who cannot communicate because of more delimited neurological disorders. The autistic child is isolated, fails to form the powerful affectional ties that normally bind children to others, and shows a lack of interest in many forms of social interaction that are normally regarded as extremely powerful. Thus, many autistic children lack normal sexual interest, a feature in which they are very similar to the animals studied by Harlow who were raised without contact with conspecifics. It is also conceivable that a disturbance of this type on an acquired basis may underlie some of the most dramatic clinical features of schizophrenia, a disorder in which one typically finds a deterioration in the communicative aspects of language, a lack of contact with others, and a frequent loss of normal sexual interest.

Furthermore, there are some experiments that might give a clue as to the neurological basis for this normal motivated interaction with others of the same species. Let us consider the effect in rats of lesions of the septal nuclei and the amygdala. Rats who have lesions in the septum will tend to run closer together than do normal rats, a phenomenon known as the *septal cohesion effect*. By contrast, rats with lesions in the amygdala will tend to run more widely separated than do normal rats. As Kling showed some years ago, adult monkeys with lesions in the amygdala who are returned to a monkey colony will tend to be isolated from the remainder of the population and will often disappear in the jungle, presumably to die in isolation from their society. It is of interest, by contrast, that in some patients with limbic epilepsy, in which abnormally increased electrical activity in the amygdala often occurs, one may observe the opposite phenomenon, that is, a heightened tendency toward contact and communication with others. Thus, the temporal lobe epileptic often shows, in contrast to the schizophrenic, the quality of stickiness or viscosity, that is, a heightened tendency to remain in contact with someone with whom the patient is speaking. Furthermore, patients with temporal lobe epilepsy often show a remarkably increased drive to write extensively, so that their letters often extend to many pages, while other patients with this disorder tend to write sermons, essays, and poetry. It is conceivable that in this condition there is an intensification of the normal human instinct to associate and communicate with others. By contrast, some autistic children, despite their overall poor communicative ability, may become fascinated with language activities that can be carried on in isolation and without any communicative content. I can recall one autistic child who had as a hobby the finding of all the different words that could be formed with the letters contained in one long word in a text.

The Neurological Substrate of Reading

The preceding discussion tells us that we must make distinctions between different causes of failure to learn to read. Some children may have difficulty in acquisition of language because they lack the drive to communicate, while others may fail because of some deficit in what we might call the language instrumentalities themselves. It is also easy to conceive of children with defects in both of these abilities, for example, dyslexia associated with a distinct withdrawal from normal human contact. By contrast, however, the majority of dyslexic patients show quite normal capacity for communication and normal desire for human contact, and so it is important to examine in detail the instrumental abilities that underlie the capacity to learn to read.

Neurological Lesions that Impair Reading

We will now consider lesions of the nervous system that produce impairment in the capacity to read. An analysis of these syndromes may help in the formulation of theories concerning the structures essential for this process [1]. I shall present these syndromes in an unusual order in order to emphasize certain points.

Hemialexia
Hemialexia was first described by Trescher and Ford [17] of the Johns Hopkins Hospital and later by Paolo Maspes of Milan. The affected patient has normal vision in both halves of space but can understand written language *only in the right half of space* and not the left. There is destruction of a particular portion of the corpus callosum, the posterior end (splenium) of this great commissure. The mechanism is as follows: When a word is presented only to the left visual field of such a patient, it reaches his right visual cortex. In order to be understood as language, however, it must be transferred to the left hemisphere; this transfer is not possible because of the destruction of the fiber pathway that normally carries the visual stimulus from one side to the other. This syndrome, while fascinating, clearly does *not* involve the essential

neurological substrate of reading, since the patient is able to read quite normally in the right visual field. It tells us that the essential neural substrate for reading probably lies in the left hemisphere.

Alexia Without Agraphia

Alexia without agraphia is the most common of the isolated syndromes of reading deficit. The affected patient typically has a right visual field defect and, in addition, a lesion in the splenium, the posterior end of the corpus callosum. This syndrome occurs most commonly as a result of occlusion of the left posterior cerebral artery, which leads to destruction of the left visual cortex and the splenium [4, 11]. The patients are typically unable to comprehend written language, although they can copy correctly the words that they are unable to read. The mechanism of this syndrome is also easy to understand. The patient cannot read words in the right visual field because of the hemianopia. A word can therefore be seen only if it is located in the left visual field so that its image can reach the intact right visual cortex. The word must, however, be relayed to the left hemisphere to be understood as language; this transfer does not take place because of the lesion in the posterior corpus callosum.

The evidence is clear that in this syndrome the neural substrate of reading is intact. Thus, although these patients typically cannot read aloud or comprehend the printed word, they can "read" correctly letters traced on the hands or anagram letters that they hold while blindfolded. The reason for the success of these maneuvers is that the tactile information concerning the form of the word can reach the left hemisphere. Thus, when the letters are traced on or palpated with the right hand, they are conveyed directly to the left hemisphere. When they are palpated by the left hand, they reach the right hemisphere. Since the part of the callosum carrying somesthetic information between the hemispheres is intact, the tactile information can be transferred from the right to the left hemisphere. Similarly, these patients can comprehend words that are spelled aloud to them by the examiner, since the words reach the intact auditory language regions in the left hemisphere. In addition, these patients can write normally, thus indicating again that the systems for written language in the left hemisphere are intact. A little reflection will make clear that these patients are, to a great extent, similar to normals with their eyes closed: Although they are unable to read aloud or comprehend written language, they will still be able to write, to "read" palpated letters, and to comprehend words spelled aloud to them. Thus, this interesting syndrome involves a disconnection between the area in which the visual image of the word is perceived and the area in which the processing of the written word as language must take place.

Alexia With Agraphia

Alexia with agraphia, although rarer than alexia without agraphia, is critical to an understanding of the reading process. The affected patients usually have lesions in the cortex of the left hemisphere in the angular gyrus [3], that is, in the large association area that lies at the junction of the temporal, parietal, and occipital lobes. In many cases there is no visual field deficit. This is a point of considerable importance, since it shows that this syndrome is not the result of simply adding another lesion to the one that produces alexia *without* agraphia. The absence of a hemianopia in many cases of alexia *with* agraphia clearly shows that the lesion must be different from that of alexia *without* agraphia.

One might expect that patients with the syndrome of alexia *with* agraphia would show the same types of *reading* disturbances as patients with alexia *without* agraphia; they would then differ only in the fact that patients with alexia *with* agraphia also write incorrectly, either spontaneously or when copying. Careful observation, however, reveals that the reading disorder in the two syndromes is distinctly different in a way that casts very important light on the localization of structures essential for the reading process. As I have pointed out, the patient with alexia *without* agraphia can usually write correctly, either spontaneously on dictation or in copying (although the actual process of copying may be quite clumsy). In addition, he can correctly spell aloud words spoken to him by the examiner, can recognize words spelled aloud to him by the examiner, can correctly "read" palpated anagram letters or letters traced in his hand by the examiner, and can read large letters that he traces with his finger. As already stated, this patient is in many ways like a normal person with his eyes closed, who can correctly show his knowledge of reading by all of the processes just described (except, of course, copying of written words).

By contrast, the patient with alexia *with* agraphia differs markedly in all of these tasks. He writes incorrectly, either spontaneously or on dictation, and has much more difficulty in copying than does a patient from the first group. He cannot spell aloud words spoken to him by the examiner, and he usually does not recognize words spelled aloud to him, although he repeats correctly the uttered letter names. He fails to "read" correctly palpated anagram letters or letters traced on his hand and is usually not helped by tracing large letters with his finger. A little reflection will show that this patient is like an illiterate, who cannot read, write, spell, recognize spelled words, nor "read" through his hand or his ear, unlike the normal literate person.

It thus seems likely that in alexia *with* agraphia there is selective involvement of some system that is essential for reading, that is, for the processing of language in visual form so that it can arouse either the meaning or the sound. Some portion of the angular gyrus therefore appears to be more clearly related directly to the reading process than any other area of which we know. Chiarello, Knight, and Mandel [2] described a congenitally deaf patient who became aphasic after a lesion of the left angular gyrus. Although they describe this as a case of Wernicke's aphasia, the clinical picture was clearly that of alexia *with* agraphia, since the patient could neither "read" (comprehend) nor "write" (make the appropriate manual gestures) sign language. This is further support for the belief that the learning of manual sign language is essentially equivalent to learning how to read.

Wernicke's Aphasia

In Wernicke's aphasia, a lesion destroys a major speech area in the upper and posterior portion of the temporal lobe [9, 10]. These patients cannot understand the written word, but their language disability extends well beyond this level, since they also do not understand spoken language, produce incorrect spoken as well as written language, and repeat spoken words incorrectly. Obviously, damage to Wernicke's area leads to destruction of some neuronal processing system that seems to be involved in all aspects of language and not reading alone. Wernicke's area thus seems to be involved in widespread deficits of language.

Broca's Aphasia

In Broca's aphasia, the lesion involves the lower portion of the frontal lobe lying anterior to the face area of the classical motor cortex. A patient with Broca's aphasia produces aphasic spoken language, writes abnormally, and repeats incorrectly. He is quite likely, however, to show good comprehension of the written word, although in some instances he shows the rather curious inability to name letters. He may also suffer from difficulties in the processing of grammar, whether this be in spoken or written form. One might therefore suspect that this region is involved in at least some aspects of the reading process.

Possible Abnormalities in the Brain of the Dyslexic

As we review these syndromes for their relevance to the neurological substrate of reading, we can exclude the first two, hemialexia and alexia without agraphia, since these clearly involve disconnections from regions that are involved in the processing of written material. Let us ask where the other findings we have described lead us in terms of possible abnormalities in the brain of the childhood dyslexic. One would expect that some part of the angular gyrus would be an essential region for the acquisition of reading. It is a little more difficult to be certain of the status of early lesions of either Wernicke's area or Broca's area, since Wernicke's area produces a language disorder that goes well beyond written language, while in Broca's aphasia only certain aspects of written language are impaired. It is not clear, however, just what would be the effects of congenital abnormality of these regions. It is conceivable that the functions they support might at least be essential components in the initial acquisition of reading.

One first asks whether our knowledge of any of these regions really does cast light on failures to acquire reading. It has usually been taught that a lesion in the language areas of the left hemisphere in childhood produces an aphasia that usually recovers to a very considerable extent. It might therefore be argued that no unilateral disturbance occurring early in life could lead to a difficulty in learning to read, because the right side would presumably be able to take over. On the other hand, most would agree that a *bilateral* abnormality in the angular gyrus region might lead to a severe defect in the acquisition of reading. We must still ask whether any type of *unilateral* abnormality might produce this disability. As I will suggest, this is probably the case.

Comparison of Childhood and Fetal Lesions

The existence of good recovery from aphasia following unilateral lesions in *early childhood* has led to the following extrapolation: There must be even better preservation of function after a unilateral disturbance in *fetal life,* since this takes place even earlier. This extrapolation is almost certainly incorrect.

When a cortical region is damaged or malformed in fetal life, the response is quite different from that which occurs to trauma after birth. Damage to the left-sided speech regions in childhood appears to lead to a diminution of some of the usual right-hemispheric capacities, that is, in order for the right hemisphere to acquire language it must apparently give up space that would have been allocated to other activities. On the other hand, damage to language regions in the fetus may have quite different effects. In fact, it appears that what occurs after intrauterine damage is almost the reverse of what is seen in the postnatal period. Goldman [13] has shown that when a cortical region of the fetus is damaged, the corresponding region on the opposite side turns out to have a more extensive pattern of connections than normal. It sends many connections to regions to which the *damaged* area would have normally projected. The implication of this is that damage in the developing speech region on the left side may lead to an increase in right-hemispheric functions, while left-hemispheric functions are permanently diminished. Damage to a brain region in adult life might be thought of as removing some particular talent, while other abilities remain more or less intact. Damage in childhood results in a compensatory mechanism by which there is recovery, but at the expense of diminution of other abilities, so that overall performance is mediocre. Damage or maldevelopment in the fetus may lead to diminution of one particular talent, while talents subserved by other brain regions may achieve higher levels. Thus, impaired development of the cortex or a cortical lesion in intrauterine life may lead to poor development of the functions of the region involved, even when the abnormality is unilateral.

Structural Asymmetry of the Brain

It is useful to look at the pattern of asymmetries of the brain in relation to the structures that are essential for reading. The angular gyrus, which plays a special role in reading, is a large region, an area that has very likely expanded more in the human brain than any region in the brains of other primates [8]. It lies at the junction of the temporal, parietal, and occipital lobes. Let us consider the asymmetries in the neighborhood of the angular gyrus.

The cortical asymmetry described by Geschwind and Levitsky [12] is found on the upper surface of the temporal lobe, a region containing part of the classical speech area of Wernicke. A particular area, called the *planum temporale,* is visibly larger on the left side in most brains. As Galaburda [6] has shown, this gross anatomical asymmetry reflects the fact that an area of defined cellular structure is of greater extent on the left than the similar structure on the right side.

The Sylvian fissure, separating the temporal lobe below from the parietal lobe above, contains asymmetries. In the first place, the left Sylvian fissure is normally longer than the right. In addition, as LeMay and Culebras [16] showed, the right Sylvian fissure is angled up more at its end than is the left (which therefore runs more horizontally). Another asymmetry in this neighborhood is that of the posterior horn of the lateral ventricle, which is typically longer on the left side than on the right. A fourth asymmetry in this region was described by LeMay [15] on the basis of studies of computed tomographic (CT) scans. The left posterior region of the hemisphere is typically wider than the right posterior region. Thus, there are multiple asymmetries in the vicinity of the angular gyrus, reflecting the greater growth both of the angular gyrus itself and of regions of specified cellular architecture that border on it [7].

Accompaniments of Dyslexia

We might expect the anomalies in the brain accompanying developmental dyslexia to involve parts of the angular gyrus itself or lie along its borders. It is therefore illuminating to consider the kind of functional disabilities that may accompany dyslexia. In a certain number of dyslexic patients one finds the components of the Gerstmann syndrome. In the adult, this syndrome results from damage to a portion of the left angular gyrus and consists of difficulties in calculation, right-left orientation, identification and recognition of the fingers, and writing. Disturbances in writing are, of course, a universal characteristic of the dyslexic patient. As is well known from the literature, a certain number of dyslexic patients also suffer from the other components of the Gerstmann syndrome, but this is not seen in all dyslexics. This suggests, therefore, that those dyslexics with the Gerstmann components might have a somewhat different pattern of maldevelopment or damage from others. An anomaly of the angular gyrus might also extend into Wernicke's area, very likely with a somewhat different set of accompanying difficulties. A large number of dyslexics have difficulties not only in reading but also in other aspects of language, such as discrimination of phonemes. Finally, the type of mechanism previously mentioned, in which an intrauterine disturbance on the left side might lead to hypertrophy of right-hemispheric functions, appears also to be operative, since it is increasingly becoming clear that in many dyslexics the language-related difficulties are associated with preserved and, in many instances, clearly superior right-hemispheric talents, so that superior artistic, athletic, and spatial abilities are quite frequently seen in this population.

Lesions of the Dyslexic Brain

There is distinct evidence of malformation in the neighborhood of Wernicke's area in the dyslexic brain. In the case of Galaburda and Kemper [5], one found a set of anomalies in the pattern of cellular architecture in Wernicke's area, as well as islands of nerve cells that had failed to reach the cortex. Similar anomalies have further been found in three brains of dyslexics, and no negative cases have yet been found.

The dyslexic patient described by Galaburda and Kemper [5] had a series of disorders that are very concordant with our earlier discussion. In this patient, there was a failure of normal migration of nerve cells to the cortex, found only on the left side, with special involvement of one of the major language areas. As a result of this disordered pattern of neuronal migration, at least one of the areas involved in language, Wernicke's area, was probably much smaller than it would have been normally. In addition, the pattern of cellular architecture within Wernicke's area was quite abnormal. This whole pattern of anomalies suggests that the brain in this region was improperly wired and therefore did not function correctly. It should be noted that this patient was left-handed and was a highly talented metalsmith, characteristics that fit with the earlier suggestion that intrauterine maldevelopment of the brain occurring on the left side may lead to greater development of right-sided functions.

Many authors have assumed that any impairment in the functioning of the brain must result either from chemical abnormalities or the presence of cells of abnormal structure. On the other hand, this case illustrates the important possibility that even if every individual cell were normal, there might be grossly abnormal functioning because of miswiring, that is, abnormal patterns of the connections of certain brain regions. Secondly, some brain regions that are made up of quite normal cells may function poorly simply because they have not achieved their usual size and are therefore inadequate for the information or memory load placed on them.

It has also been suggested by Hier and associates [14] that in dyslexics with delayed speech, the usual pattern seen on the CT scan in which the left posterior brain region is wider may be changed so that there is an increased number of cases with a wider right posterior region. These results are still, however, controversial since, while all observers seem to agree that the left posterior region is usually the wider, there is considerable uncertainty about the exact proportion of cases in the general population in which the right posterior region may be the wider one.

Hyperlexia

A brief comment is appropriate on what, in some ways, appears to be the opposite syndrome, which is called *hyperlexia*. Hyperlexic patients show very rapid and early acquisition of the capacity to read in the sense that they learn to read aloud correctly, including even the many irregular words in English. Despite this apparent precocity in reading aloud, however, the patients continue to show poor reading comprehension. In these cases, one might postulate that the area involved in acquisition of grapheme-phoneme conversion rules is well developed while the pattern of connections from it to other brain regions is defective.

Certain defects that are commonly associated with difficulty in the comprehension of the written word may occur independently of it. The dyslexic typically has difficulty in acquiring writing and, in particular, spelling skills. There are, however, a certain number of cases in which writing and spelling capacities are impaired in the face of even quite superior abilities for comprehension of written language. Many students of this problem have taken the stand that these agraphic patients were really all dyslexic at one time. This need not necessarily be the case, since some of the patients with disorders in writing appear to have acquired the capacity to comprehend written material very early and very well. It is possible that in these cases there is a much more delimited involvement of those systems that control writing, while reading itself may be unimpaired.

Implications for Future Research

Why should we place so much emphasis on the neurological substrate of reading? There is a common belief that the finding of anomalies in the dyslexic brain would simply encourage therapeutic nihilism, but I believe that this is quite incorrect. In the first place, the presence of some failure of full development of the system involved in reading should in no way lead to the conclusion that educational measures would be useless. When the system is in its full normal state, only a minimum of teaching is needed and reading will be acquired quite easily and with a minimum of direction. Educational measures are most necessary in those cases in which the system is in some way deficient. In such a circumstance, well-designed teaching may enable the most efficient use of the limited neuronal substratum of reading and may furthermore enable the person to use strategies other than those employed by the majority of people.

Secondly, the notion that structural neurological abnormality implies that the system cannot be altered is, of course, also incorrect. It has been a repeated experience throughout the history of medicine that the finding of structural abnormality has led to the development of highly effective treatments. One need only recall the discovery that the pancreas and indeed particular portions of the pancreas were involved in secretion of some substance that controlled the blood sugar level, which led to the discovery of insulin and the beginnings of modern effective therapy for diabetes. Furthermore, the fact that a particular brain region is not wired correctly as a result of events that occur during intrauterine life clearly raises the possibility that one may be able to prevent the occurrence of such anomalous developments by appropriate chemical manipulations during pregnancy.

Animal Models of the Dyslexic Brain

There is another very important reason for the stress on the study of the neurological substrate of dyslexia. It has invariably been the case in the history of medicine that whenever an animal model becomes available for the study of any type of disorder, there is a rapid advance in research on mechanisms and on the possibilities of prevention and therapy. The availability of a nonhuman animal model makes possible a whole array of experiments that could not possibly be carried out in humans, especially when one is dealing with a disorder that is not fatal and is compatible in most cases with reasonable, even if not always fully effective, functioning. Until recently, it was commonly accepted that no animal model could possibly be available for the study of dominance and its disorders, and it was therefore always assumed that research in this area would inevitably be subject to major limitations. It is now, however, clear that the pathway is open for research on the influences in intrauterine life that might lead to similar anomalies in the brains of other species and on methods for preventing the occurrence of these anomalies or diminishing their severity.

References

1. Benson, D. F., and Geschwind, N. The Alexias. In P. J. Vinken and G. W. Bruyn (Eds.), *Handbook of Clinical Neurology*, Vol. 4. Amsterdam: Elsevier North-Holland, 1969. Pp. 112–140.
2. Chiarello, C., Knight, R., and Mandel, M. Aphasia in a prelingually deaf woman. *Brain* 105:29, 1982.
3. Dejerine, J. Sur un cas de cécité verbale avec agraphie, suivi d'autopsie. *Mém. Soc. Biol.* 3:197, 1891.
4. Dejerine, J. Contribution à l'étude anatomopathologique et clinique des différentes variétés de cécité verbale. *Mém. Soc. Biol.* 4:61, 1892.
5. Galaburda, A. M., and Kemper, T. L. Cytoarchitectonic abnormalities in developmental dyslexia: A case study. *Ann. Neurol.* 6:94, 1979.
6. Galaburda, A. M., Sanides, F., and Geschwind, N. Human brain: Cytoarchitectonic left-right asymmetries in the temporal speech region. *Arch. Neurol.* 35:812, 1978.
7. Galaburda, A. M., et al. Right-left asymmetries in the brain. *Science* 199:852, 1978.

8. Geschwind, N. The development of the brain and the evolution of language. *Monogr. Ser. Lang. Linguist.* 17:155, 1964.
9. Geschwind, N. Disconnexion syndromes in animals and man. *Brain* 88:237, 1965.
10. Geschwind, N. The organization of language and the brain. *Science* 170:940, 1970.
11. Geschwind, N., and Fusillo, M. Color-naming defects in association with alexia. *Arch. Neurol.* 15:137, 1966.
12. Geschwind, N., and Levitsky, W. Human brain: Left-right asymmetries in temporal speech regions. *Science* 161:186, 1968.
13. Goldman, P. S. Neuronal plasticity in primate telencephalon: Anomalous crossed cortico-caudate connections induced by prenatal removal of frontal association cortex. *Science* 202:768, 1978.
14. Hier, D. B., et al. Developmental dyslexia. *Arch. Neurol.* 35:90, 1978.
15. LeMay, M. Morphological Cerebral Asymmetries of Modern Man, Fossil Man, and Non-human Primates. In S. R. Harnad, H. D. Steklis, and J. Lancaster (Eds.), *Origins and Evolution of Language and Speech.* New York: New York Academy of Sciences, 1976.
16. LeMay, M., and Culebras, A. Human brain: Morphological differences in the hemispheres demonstrable by carotid arteriography. *N. Engl. J. Med.* 287:168, 1972.
17. Trescher, J. H., and Ford, F. R. Colloid cyst of the third ventricle. *Arch. Neurol. Psychiatry* 37:959, 1937.

Index

Page numbers followed by *t* indicate tables; those followed by *f* indicate figures.

Acquired dyslexia
  phonological, 62–64
  Reading by lexical route, 62–64
  relationship to developmental dyslexia
    classification by association, 55–57
    routes to reading, 57–64
    symptoms, 56
    taxonomy, 56
Adult(s)
  accompaniments of dyslexia, 207
  neurometric evaluation, 183
  with probable constitutional dyslexia, 23–24
Age, 38*t*, 40
  Correlation with motor coordination, 44, 45*t*
  for dyslexia classification, 26
  effect on reading latency, 48
Age-regression equations, 161, 164, 167, 173–176
Agraphia, with alexia, 1, 203–204
Alcoholism, 183
Alexia, 47
  with agraphia, 1, 203–204
  without agraphia, 203, 205
Alphabetic system, 100–101
Alzheimer's disease, 183
American Speech, Language, and Hearing Association, 9
Angular gyrus, 119, 153
  asymmetries near, 206–207
  bilateral abnormality, 206
  damage, 207
  left, 55
  unilateral abnormality, 206
Animal models, 210
Anomic-repetition disorder, 117
Aphasia, 8, 120, 153
APIB. *See* Assessment of Preterm Infant's Behavior (APIB)
Arithmetic disorder, developmental, 11
Arithmetic skills, deficit, 7–8
Articulation disorder
  developmental, 11
  graphomotor, 14, 15

Asphyxia, 152–153
Assessment of Preterm Infant's Behavior (APIB), 74–75
  differentiation of infant behavior, 81–82*f*
  exploratory group comparisons, 75–81*f*
  newborn vs. 9-month status, 86, 87*f*
Association for Children and Adults with Learning Disabilities, 9
Asynchrony, sound, 140–141
  brain symmetry and, 151–154*f*
  multiple entrainment, 141–151*f*
Attention and interaction system, 68–71
Attention deficit disorder (hyperkinesis), 6–7, 20, 120. *See also* Hyperactivity
  diagnosis, 11
  drug treatment, 21
  educational environment and, 10
  minimal brain damage and, 6–7
Atypical specific developmental disorder, 11
Audiophonic confusion vs. visuospatial confusion, 56
Auditory deficits
  in processing, 17
  reading disability and, 96–97
Auditory learning style, 93–94, 100
Auditory-linguistic subtype, 16
Autism, 201
  entrainment, 154
  left brainstem auditory evoked potential, 153
  multiple entrainment, 145
  orienting responses, 148–151*t*
  process-unit boundaries, 141, 146–147*t*
  post–sound-stimulus behavior, 141–142*t*, 143
  reversed asymmetry, 18
Automatic artifact rejection method, 172
Autonomic system, 68–69

Backward readers, 4

Basal ganglia, 19
Bayley Mental Development Index, 86, 87*t*
BEAM. *See* Brain electrical activity mapping (BEAM)
Beery-Buktenica visual-motor integration test (VMI), 188–189
Behavior, 155. *See also specific behavioral symptoms*
　environmental causation, 1
　investigation by sound-film, 124
　listener, 134–135*f*
　microlevel, 124–125
　neurological causation, 1
　overt, as wave phenomena, 131–133
　post–sound-stimulus, 141–142*t*
　synactive organization model, 72–73*f*
　wave periodicities, 132–133*f*, 154
Behavioral organization. *See* Organization, behavioral
Bender-Gestalt, 188
Blender, phonological, 58*f*, 59
Body language, infant, 75, 76*f*, 77
Body motion
　of listener, 133–140*f*
　of speaker, 126–133*f*
Brain
　abnormalities, EEG topographical distribution, 111
　based mechanisms in reading underachievement, 25
　chemical studies, 20–22
　damage, and classification of dyslexia subtype, 14
　dysfunction
　　differential diagnosis, 158
　　incidence of learning handicaps, 157
　　minimal, 6–7, 8, 20, 159
　　neurometric evaluation, 178–183*f*
　　quantitative electrophysiological evaluation, 159–160
　EEG assessment, 107
　electrical activity, neurometric evaluation, 157–183*f*
　hemispheric asymmetries, 15, 23, 190–191
　　neuroanatomical studies, 17–20
　　sound-induced behavioral asynchrony and, 151–154*f*
　lesions
　　and acquired dyslexia classification, 56
　　brain flow processing and, 152, 153
　　in dyslexia, 209
　　effect on written language competence, 23–24
　　possible abnormalities in dyslexia, 205–206
　　relationships to behavior, 13
　　structural asymmetry, 206–207
　　wave periodicities, 132–133*f*
Brain electrical activity mapping (BEAM), 22, 26
　brain flow process and, 152
　dyslexia study, 114–117
　foot coordination and, 48–49
　implications, 119–120
　methodology, 108–113*f*
　neuropsychological data and CT scan complement, 111–113*f*
Brazelton Neonatal Behavioral Assessment Scale (BNBAS), 69, 74–75
Broca's aphasia, 56, 205
Broca's area, 119

Callosal system, 194
Cataplexy, 24
Central nervous system, 10, 18–19
Cerebellar dysfunction, 187–188
Cerebellovestibular dysfunction, 19–20
Cerebral palsy
　entrainment, 154
　neurometric evaluation, 178–179*f*
　sound-induced motor asynchrony, 143
Child find program, 10
Children, *See also* Infant(s); Newborn(s); *specific aspects of dyslexia*
　unilateral brain lesions, 206
　use of word, 10
Choline acetyltransferase, 20
Classification
　of developmental disorders, 11
　of dyslexia
　　by associated symptoms, 55–57
　　by reading tests, 37–40*t*
　　by subtype, 13–16
Clinical judgment, 23

Coherence, 163
Communication, motivation, 199–201
Computed tomography (CT), 21, 24, 26
  of brain, 18
  complementation of BEAM and neuropsychological data, 111–113*f*
  positron (PCT), 21, 26, 27
Congenital dysorthographia. *See* Developmental dyslexia
Congenital symbol amblyopia. *See* Developmental dyslexia
Congenital word blindness, 3
Coordination. *See* Motor system, coordination
Corpus callosum, 19, 202
Correlational approach, 55
Corsi blocks, 95
Cortical asymmetry, 207
Council for Exceptional Children, 9
Council for Learning Disabilities, 9
Critchley, MacDonald, 4
Cultural background, neurometric EEG features, 174–176*f*

Deafness, 96, 199, 200
Deep dyslexia, developmental analogue, 62–64
Development, human, 68–70
Developmental deviation, 168–169*f*, 181
Developmental disorders. *See specific disorder*
Developmental dyslexia, 4
  correlational classification, 56
  definition, 4
  relationship with acquired dyslexia classification by association, 55–57
    routes to reading, 57–64
  specific, 6
Dextroamphetamine, 21
Diabetes, 23
Diagnosis, 9, 26
Diagnostic and Statistical Manual of Mental Disorders (DSM-III), 11, 35, 50
Dichotic listening tests, 17, 23
Direct route reading, 60–61
Discrepancy scores, 34, 46–47, 50–51
Disparate reduction, 12

Dominance, mixed. *See* Mixed dominance
Dopamine, 20
Dyscalculia, 8
Dyseidetic dyslexia, 16, 17, 24
Dysgraphia, 120
Dyslexia, 8. *See also* Reading *and specific dyslexic subtypes*
  accompaniments of, 207–208
  animal models, 210
  brain abnormalities, 205–206
  brain lesions of, 208
  definition, 12–13, 50–51, 187
    difficulties, 46–47
    by discrepancy score, 34
    exclusionary consensus, 33
    lateral preference and motor skill tests, 43–46
    methods of present study, 35–37*t*
    motor deficit correlates, 48–50
    naming impairment, 47–48
    by reading quotient, 37–40
  developmental. *See* Developmental dyslexia
  descriptive characteristics, 11
  electrophysiological data, 114
  entrainment, 154
  implications for future research, 209–210
  implications for physiological signature, 119–120
  neurological perspective, 1–2
  process-unit boundaries, 146–147*t*
  retrospective analysis, 26–27
  sound-induced motor asynchrony, 142–143
Dyslexia-plus, 14, 15, 17, 26, 187
  association with narcolepsy, 24
  DSM-III classification, 11
Dyslexia-pure, 14, 15, 26
  DSM-III classification, 11
  EEG differences, 114–115, 117–119
  motor behavior, 191–192
  regional differences by BEAM, 120
Dysphasic error, 40–41*t*, 47, 50
Dysphonemic-sequencing disorder, 117
Dysphonetic dyslexia, 16, 17
Dyspraxia, 187

Early visual analysis (EVA), 57, 58*f*

Education of the Handicapped Act of 1970, 7
Electroencephalography (EEG), 18, 22–23, 26
  abnormalities, 161, 176–183f
  abnormality matrix, 169–172f
  adult dyslexia and, 183
  assessment of brain function, 107
  computer analysis, 158
  electrode placement, 162f
  history, 105
  interpretation, 105–107f
  mixed dominance study, 194
  neurometric analysis, 158–159, 178–179f
  relevance to learning disabilities, 160
  test-retest reliability, 173
  topographical mapping method, 108–113f
  typical clinical, 106f
  validation of sample length, 172–173
Elementary and Secondary Education Act of 1969, 7
Emotional problems, 35, 178, 189
Entrainment, interactional, 133–140f
  delayed, 141–142t, 144f
  multiple, 140–141
    and brain processing asymmetries, 152
    in dyslexia, 143, 144f, 145
    out-of-phase pattern, 143, 144f
    and sound, 141–151f
Environmental factors, 8, 199
Epilepsy, 105, 159
Epiphenomena, 4
ERGL (expected reading grade level), 34
Errors, 56
  language (dysphasic), 40–41t, 47, 50
  reading
    in acquired deep dyslexia, 63
    in acquired phonological dyslexia, 63
    in developmental dyslexia, 63
  reversal, 94
  transpositional, 94
  visual-type, 94–95
Ethnic background, neurometric EEG features, 174–176f
Event-related potentials, 158

Evoked potentials (EP), 107–108, 110f, 111
  auditory, 152–153
  dyslexia vs. normal readers, 115
  sensory, 158
  topographical mapping method, 108–113f
  visual (VEP), 108f
Exlusionary clause, 8, 10
Expected reading grade level (ERGL), 34
Eye preference, 3. See also Mixed dominance

Fetus, brain damage, 206
Fine motor coordination, 33, 48–49
Finger agnosia, 11
Finger movement, and verbal fluency, 33
Foot
  movement, 33, 48
  preference, 3
Foundation for Children With Learning Disabilities, 27
Frontal lobe, involvement in linguistic tasks, 120

Gaussianity
  tests of univariate and multivariate features, 173–174
  transformations, 163–164
Genetics, 13, 26
Geographical factors, and reading retardation, 5
Gerstmann syndrome, 207
Gifted children, with written language underachievement, 12
Global language disorder, 117
Glucose metabolism, cerebral, 21
GORT (Gray Oral Reading Test), 35, 37–40t
Government funding patterns, 27
Grapheme, 59
Graphemic parser (P), 57, 58
Graphemic phoneme correspondence, 58–59
Graphomotor discoordination, 14
Gray Oral Reading Test (GORT), 35, 37–40t

Hallucinations, 24

Hand. *See also* Mixed dominance
  lateral preference tests, 43–46t
  preference, 2, 3
Hand-eye coordination, 33
Head, mild injury to, 183
Hearing deficits. *See* Auditory deficits
Heel-toe alteration, 22
Hemialexia, 202–203, 205
Hemispheric specialization. *See* Brain, hemispheric asymmetries
History of dyslexia concept, 1–2, 3
Homophones, 61
Human species, survival, 70–71
Huntington's disease
  entrainment, 154
  multiple entrainment pattern, 146–147t, 151
  process-unit boundaries, 146–147t
  sound-induced motor asynchrony, 143
Hyperactivity, 50, 120, 191. *See also* Attention deficit disorder (hyperkinesis)
  abnormal EEG, 160
  entrainment, 154
  motor coordination, 49
  sound-related self-asynchrony and multiple entrainment, 151
Hyperkinesis. *See* Attention deficit disorder (hyperkinesis)
Hyperlexia, 62, 209

Identification, early, 24–25
Infant(s). *See also* Newborn(s)
  assessment of functioning synactive perspective, 71–73
  body language, 75, 76f, 77
  competence, 68
  developmental assessment, 88
  early, studies, 26
  entrainment to adult speech, 135–140f
  individual patterns of organization, 81–82
  kangaroo-box paradigm, 82–86f, 87f
  preterm, 88
    organizational problems, 75
    school problems, 67
    synactive developmental perspective, 73–75
  synactive development theory, 68–69, 88–89
    assessment, 71–73
    exploratory group comparisons, 75–81t
    prematurity and, 73–75
Institute for Child Development Research, 27
Intelligence, general factor, 2
Intelligence quotient (IQ)
  reading regression and, 34
  verbal, and hemispheric asymmetry, 18
  verbal performance discrepancies, 34
  WISC-R scores, 36–37t
Interaction and attention system, 68–70
International electrode placement system, 10–20, 162f
International Reading Association, 9
Intrauterine damage, 206
IQ. *See* Intelligence quotient (IQ)
Isle of Wight studies, 12, 25
  achievement prediction, 4–5
  incidence of specific reading retardation, 7

Kangaroo-box paradigm (K-box), 82–86f, 87f
Kidney disease, 178
Kimura nonsense figures, 95

Language. *See also* Written language underachievement
  basis of reading, 97–98
  constructs for dyslexia, 12
  correlate, dyslexic, 15
  deficits, 50
  development, relationship to motor proficiency, 33
  difficulties, 2
  disorders, 15
    developmental types, 11
    mixed, 117
    primary, 14
  errors, 40–41t
  expectancy, 47
  faulty lateralization, 3
  foreign, acquisition of, 199–200
  impairment, 33, 47
  oral underachievement, 25

Language—*Continued*
  processing, 97–98, 99, 100
  right-hemispheric, characteristics of, 16
  second, difficulty in mastery, 12
  and selective reading disability, 6
  sign, 199, 200
  tests, 35
  undetected problems, 48
  written
    definition, 12
    origins, 197–198
    specific disability, 3
Language learning handicap, 4
Linguistic deficit patterns for dyslexic subtypes, 117–119
Lateral preference tests, 43–46*t*
Learning difficulties. *See also* Learning disabilities; Learning disorders, differential diagnosis
  differential diagnosis, 157–159
  quantitative electrophysiological evaluation, 159–160
Learning disability specialists, 8
Learning disabilities
  brain flow processing, 152
  classification, 180–181*t*
  definition, 7, 10
  etiology, 10
  motor characteristics, 188–190
  neurometric evaluation, 177–179*f*, 157–183*f*
  relevant EEG studies, 160
  specific, 7–9
  terminology, 7, 9–10
Learning disorders, differential diagnosis, 157–158, 159
Learning styles, 93–94, 100
Left-handedness, 2, 194
Left hemisphere, 190–191, 194, 203
  and dyslexic subtypes, 16–17
  language area lesions, 205
  specialization, 18
Lexical route reading, 59–60, 62–64
Linear prediction models, disillusionment, 67
Listener entrainment, 133–140*f*
Logographies, 101
Lorge-Thorndike word-frequency groups, 40

Mahalanobis distance, 166, 167, 181
Manic-depression, 183
Maturational lag, 50, 160, 181
  neurometric evaluation, 167–169*f*
  statistical analysis, 166–169*f*
Memorized graphic patterns, 101
Memory tasks, by poor readers, 95
Mental retardation, 178–179*f*
Merke's cell mechanoreception, 152
Methyphenidate, 21, 24
Microbehavioral asynchronies
  of body motion, 126–131*f*
  of speech, 124–126*f*
Minimal brain damage, 6–7
Minimal brain dysfunction (MBD), 6–7, 8
  concept, 159
  neurochemical correlates, 20
Mixed dominance, 33, 36, 187, 192–194
Mixed specific developmental disorder, 11
Modality preference, 93–94
  implications for instruction and remediation, 99–101
  reading as language-based skill and, 97–99
  reading disability
    auditory deficit and, 96–97
    visual deficit and, 94–95
Morphological decomposition (MD), 59–60
Mother-infant interaction, 70–71
  K-Box paradigm, 84–85
  synchrony and/or entrainment, 137, 139
Motion pictures, 123. *See also* Sound-film microanalysis
Motor system
  coordination, 187–188, 194–195
    characteristics of learning-disabled children, 188–190
    fine, 33, 48–49
    interpretation of studies, 190–191
    mixed dominance and, 192–194
    proficiency, and language development levels, 33
    tests, 43–46*t*, 50
  deficit correlates, 48–50

development, recent investigations, 191–192
observations, 69

Naming. *See also* Rapid Automatized Naming Test (RAN)
impairment, as deficit correlate, 47–48
of pictured objects, 40–41
plateau in speed and accuracy, 49
tests, 48
Narcolepsy, 24
National Institute of Neurologic and Communicative Disorders and Stroke (NINCDS), 25
National Joint Committee on Learning Disabilities, 9–11
Neuroanatomical studies, 17–20
Neurochemical studies, 20–22
Neurological examinations, 157–158
Neurology
abnormalities, 209–210
disorders
impairing reading, 202–205
neurometric evaluation, 178–183*t*
dyslexia explanation and, 1–2
of language acquisition, 199–200
Neurometric evaluation, 158–159
abnormality or Z-matrix, 169–172*f*
background, 159
procedures
age-regression equations, 164
data acquisition, 162–163
diagnostic utility, 176–183*f*
extraction of univariate features, 163
Gaussian distribution transforms, 163–164
multivariate features, 165–169*f*
objective extraction of univariate features, 163
validation, 172–176
z-transformation, 164–165
requirements, 161–162
sensitivity to brain dysfunction
multivariate features, 181–183*f*
univariate features, 178–179*f*
Neuropharmacology, 21
Neurophysiological concomitants, and EEG, 22–23

Neuropsychological data, complementation by BEAM and CT scan, 111–113*f*
Neuropsychological evaluation, 157–158
Neurotransmitters, asymmetry, 20
Newborn(s). *See also* Infant(s)
APIB classification stability, 86, 87*f*
developmental tasks, 69–70
social environment, 70–71
subsystem differentiation, 71
NINCDS (National Institute of Neurologic and Communicative Disorders and Stroke), 25
Nonsense syllables, 17, 50
Norepinephrine, 20
Norms, developmental, construction of, 176–177
Nuclear magnetic resonance (NMR), 21, 26, 27
Nystagmus, 95

Oldfield-Wingfield picture naming test, 35, 40
Oral word representations (OWR), 58*f*, 59
Organization, behavioral, 123
of body motion, 126–130*f*
individual patterns, 81–82*f*
investigation by sound film, 124
kangaroo-box paradigm, 82–86*f*
microforms, 154
problems, 67–69
speech/body motion hierarchy, 131–133*f*
Orthography, 97
Orton, Samuel Torrey, 1–4, 187
Orton Society (Orton Dyslexia Society), 9, 19, 27
dyslexia neuroanatomy study, 20
NINCDS, 25

Paralexias, 56, 63–64
Parent
K-Box paradigm, 85
screening, 26
Parietal lobe, 119
Parkinson's disease
entrainment, 153–154

Parkinson's disease—*Continued*
  sound-induced motor asynchrony, 143
  sound-related self-asynchrony and multiple entrainment, 151
PCT (positron computed tomography), 21, 26, 27
Peabody Picture Vocabulary Test (PPVT), 35, 163, 176
Perception
  difficulties and out-of-phase processing, 153
  error in, 40–41*t*, 47
  handicap, 8
  motor training and, 6
  separation from motor function, 188
Phenomenological characteristics, 64
Phenylketonuria, 178–179*f*
Phone types, 124, 125
Phoneme, 57–59
Phonetic decoding ability, 50
Phonics reading route, 57–61
Phonological units, apprehension, 98–99
Physicians, and dyslexia, 3–5
Piracetam, 21–22
Planum temporale, 17–18, 19, 207
Polymicrogyria, 19
Positron computed tomography (PCT), 21
Posterior temporal lobe, 119
Postmortem investigations, 27, 55
Power asymmetry, 163
PPVT (Peabody Picture Vocabulary Test), 35, 163, 176
Prematurity, 67, 74, 88
Preschool children, identification program, 10
Process-unit boundaries
  Huntington's disease, 146–147*t*, 151
  prediction, 141
Process units, 126–127, 129, 154
  of listener, 134–135*f*
  reliability of detection, 130–131
  of speaker, 126–133*f*
Psychological tests, 157
Psychometric tests, 157–158
Public Law 91-230, 7
Public Law 94-142, 7, 10
Pulvinar, 20

Rapid Automatized Naming (RAN), test, 35, 49
  latencies, 41–43*t*
  speed of naming and, 47–48
Readers
  backward, 4
  normal, 17, 115–117
  poor, 94–97
Reading
  achievement prediction, 4–5
  acquisition, 198–202
  apprehension of phonological units and, 98–99
  biological foundations, 197–210
  deficit, 33
  definition, 199
  by direct route, 61–62
  disabilities, 8
    auditory deficits and, 96–97
    central auditory dysfunction and, 17
    developmental, 11
    specific, 3
    visual deficits and, 94–95
  disorders
    acquired vs. developmental, 60–64
    correlational classification, 56
  errors, 39, 63
  failure, unexpected, 12
  impairment
    definition, 34
    with language impairment, 33
    relationship to language and motor proficiency, 35
    relationship to test variables, 35
    and RQ, 48
    WRAT and GORT scoring, 39*t*
  instruction
    implications of sensory modalities, 99–101
    visual vs. auditory approach, 93
  neurological substrate, 202–205
  normal mechanisms, 57, 58*f*
  problems, correlation with motor coordination, 44, 45*t*
  process, language basis of, 97–98
  relationship to speed of word retrieval, 47–48
  routes, 57–60
  single word vs. prose, 40

tests, discrepancy scores, 34–35
underachievement, 15, 157
Reading grade level (RGL), 34, 37–40t
Reading quotient (RQ), 48
　calculation, 38
　definition of dyslexia and, 46
　motor coordination and, 44, 46
　relationship to pure reading disability, 49
Reading retardation, 3–5, 25
Relative power, 163
Relative probability, 161
Remediation
　development of methods, 1
　and differential diagnosis, 157–158
　effects on RGL, 46
　implications of sensory modalities, 99–101
　language-pertinent, 6
　perceptual-motor–pertinent, 6
　prerequisites, 157
　selection, 194–195
　services, 8
Research, future implications, 209–210
Response buffer (RB), 59
Reversals, 2, 94
Rey-Osterreith Complex Figure, 189
Right hemispheric specialization, 23
　and dyslexic subtypes, 16–17
　with mixed language disorder, 15
Right-left disorientation, 4
Risk factors, 24

Schizophrenia, 143, 154, 201
Second language, difficulty with mastery, 12
Seizure disorders, 18, 22–23
Self-synchrony, 135, 154
Semantic representations (SR), 58f, 59
Semantics
　errors, 63–64
　interpretation, 61
　reading without, 62
Senile dementia, 183
Sensory deficits, interference with learning, 93
Sensory modalities
　determination of reading instruction, 93
　implications for instruction and remediation, 99–101

Septal cohesion effect, 201
Sex
　correlation with motor coordination in problem readers, 44, 45t
　relationship to dyslexia, 13, 24
Sight vocabulary, 60–61
Significance probability mapping (SPM), 111
　differences between normal readers and dyslexics, 115–117
　technique, 119
Sleep paralysis, 24
Slow learners, and brain damage, 5–6
Social factors
　in newborn environment, 70–71
　of reading retardation, 5
Soft neurological signs, 11
Sound discrimination, impaired, 11
Sound-film microanalysis
　background, 123–124
　of behavioral disorders, 140–141
　　brain asymmetry vs. behavioral asymmetry, 151–154f
　　multiple entrainment vs. sound, 141–151f
　of body motion, 126–131f
　importance, 154–155
　listener entrainment to speaker speech, 133–140f
　overt behavior as wave phenomena, 131–133
　reliability in detection of body motion process units, 130–131
　of speech, 124–126f
Special education, 5–8
Specific learning disability, 7–9, 178–179f
Speech
　delay, and reversed asymmetry, 18
　dyslexic correlate, dyslexic, 15
　listener entrainment to, 133–140f
　microanalysis, 124–125, 126f
　oscilloscope display of, 125, 126f
　perception, 98
　problems, abnormal EEG and, 160
　relationship to body motion, 126–133f
　synchronization and periodicities, 131–133f
　volume, listener response to, 135

Speech/body motion behavior, 131–133f, 154
Spelling underachievement, 12
SPM. *See* Significance Probability Mapping (SPM)
Stanford-Binet Vocabulary Test, 41
Strephosymbolia, 3
Stuttering
  entrainment, 152, 154
  sound-induced motor asynchrony, 143
  sound-related self-asynchrony and multiple entrainment, 151
Subtypes, dyslexic, 13–17
Surface dyslexia, 61
Sylvian fissure, asymmetry, 207
Symbol-word association, memorized, 101
Synactive theory of development, 68–69, 88–89
  assessment of infant functioning, 71–73
  model, 72–73f
  preterm infant, perspective, 73–74
Synchrony, 135
Syncresis, 71
Syntax, 39

Taxonomic Intracellular Analytic System (TICAS), 81
Thalamus, 20
Thinking, 7
Title VI, 7
Topographic mapping procedures, 119
Total absolute power, 163
Transactional model, 67–68
Transformational model, 67, 68
Transformations
  to achieve Gaussian distribution, 163–164
  Z, 164–165

Verbal memorization, deficient, 15
Visual deficits, reading disability and, 94–95
Visual evoked potential (VEP), 108f
Visual learning style, 93–94, 100
Visuospatial confusion vs. audiophonic confusion, 56
Visuospatial disorder, 14–16

VMI (Beery-Buktenica visual-motor integration test), 188–189
Vocabulary. *See also* Peabody Picture Vocabulary Test (PPVT)
  correlation to speed of foot movements, 33, 48
  sight, 59

Wechsler's Intelligence Scale for Children (WISC), 14
Wechsler's Intelligence Scale for Children–Revised (WISC-R), 34–36t, 163, 177, 178
Wepman Test of Auditory Discrimination, 96
Wernicke's aphasia, 56, 205
Wernicke's area, 119, 207, 208
Whole word representations (WWR), 59
Whole-word strategy, 101
Wide Range Achievement Test (WRAT), 35, 37–40t, 163, 176, 178
WISC (Wechsler's Intelligence Scale for Children), 14
WISC-R (Wechsler's Intelligence Scale for Children–Revised), 34–36t, 163, 177, 178
Word blindness, congenital, 55. *See also* Developmental dyslexia
Word retrieval speed, 47–48
Word sequencing, difficulties, 11
World Federation of Neurology, definition of dyslexia, 4, 8, 187
WRAT (Wide Range Achievement Test), 35, 37–40t, 163, 176, 178
Writing disability, specific, 3
Writing systems
  Chinese, 95, 100–101
  history of, 55
Written expression, 7
Written language underachievement. *See also* Language, written
  definition, 12–17
  EEG, 22–23
  future studies, 23–24
  minimal brain damage and, 6–7
  neuroanatomical studies, 17–20
  neurochemical studies, 20–22

physicians and dyslexia, 3–5
specific learning disability, 7–11

Xenon mapping, 119

Z-matrix, 161, 169–172f

Z-statistic, 111, 116, 117
Z transformations, 164–165
   age-regression and, 173–174
   multivariate features and, 165–167f
   relative probability assessment, 161